CELL LINEAGE, STEM CELLS AND CELL DETERMINATION

INSERM Symposia

CELL LINEAGE, STEM CELLS AND CELL DETERMINATION

Proceedings of the International Workshop on Cell Lineage, Stem Cells and Cell Determination held in Seillac, (France), 20-24 May, 1979.
Sponsored by the Institut National de la Santé et de la Recherche Médicale, the European Molecular Biology Organization and the International Society of Developmental Biologists.

Editor: N. LE DOUARIN

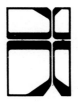

INSERM SYMPOSIUM No. 10

INSTITUT NATIONAL DE LA SANTÉ
ET DE LA RECHERCHE MÉDICALE

1979

NORTH-HOLLAND PUBLISHING COMPANY
AMSTERDAM · NEW YORK · OXFORD

ISBN Series: 0 7204 0653 6
ISBN Volume: 0 7204 0673 0

Publishers:
ELSEVIER/NORTH-HOLLAND BIOMEDICAL PRESS
335 JAN VAN GALENSTRAAT, P.O. BOX 211
AMSTERDAM, THE NETHERLANDS

Sole distributors for the USA and Canada:
ELSEVIER NORTH HOLLAND INC.
52 VANDERBILT AVENUE
NEW YORK, N.Y. 10017

PRINTED IN THE NETHERLANDS

PREFACE

This book contains the proceedings of an International Workshop, held in May 20-24, 1979 in Seillac - France, the aim of which was to assemble scientists from different fields such as Embryology, Hematology and Neurobiology, who shared a common interest in problems related to cell commitment, stem cell properties and cell line segregation. Such subjects, which have always been at the centre of the preoccupations of Embryologists, are of added topicality in view of recent advances in the field of hematology, since the blood-forming system offers particularly suitable models for the study of stem cells functions as well as cell line commitment and differentiation. The methods used to analyze hemopoietic differentiation and the results obtained in this area appeared of considerable relevance for scientists dealing with the more complex problems raised by cell diversification in the embryo itself.

In addition to articles concerned with hemopoiesis, the segregation of cell lines and the stability of the determined state are discussed with reference to various embryonic systems and to the model provided by the mouse teratocarcinoma. In the development of the nervous system, the subjects selected deal with the modulation of both architectural and biochemical differentiation of nervous tissue by environmental factors.

The Scientific Committee of the Workshop, Nicole Le Douarin, Alberto Monroy, Walter Gehring and Fritz Melchers, wish to thank l'Institut National de la Santé et de la Recherche Médicale, the European Molecular Biology Organization and the International Society of Developmental Biologists for their help and support which made this workshop possible.

The Editor

LIST OF PARTICIPANTS

Dr. Cristina ARRUTI
INSERM - U. 18
Unité de Recherches Gérontologiques
29, Rue Wilhem
75016 PARIS

Dr. Philippe AVNER
INSERM U. 152
Lab. d'Immunologie et
Virologie des Tumeurs
Hôpital Cochin
27, Rue du Faubourg St Jacques
75674 PARIS CEDEX 14

Dr. Charles BABINET
Laboratoire de Génétique
Cellulaire
Institut Pasteur
25, Rue du Dr. Roux
75015 PARIS

Prof. Jean-François BACH
Laboratoire d'Immunologie Clinique
INSERM U 25
Hôpital Necker
161, Rue de Sèvres
75730 PARIS CEDEX 15

Dr. Denise BEAUPAIN
Institut d'Embryologie du CNRS
et du Collège de France
49bis, Avenue de la Belle-Gabrielle
94130 NOGENT-sur-MARNE

Dr. Yvonne BERWALD-NETTER
Dept. de Biochimie Cellulaire
Collège de France
11, Place Marcelin Berthelot
75231 PARIS CEDEX 05

Dr. Jeannine BRETON-GORIUS
INSERM U. 91
CHU Henri Mondor
51, Avenue de Lattre de Tassigny
94010 CRETEIL

Dr. Elisabeth CHALMEAU
Laboratoire d'Embryologie
Faculté des Sciences de Nantes
2, Rue de la Houssinière
44072 NANTES CEDEX

Prof. Jean-Pierre CHANGEUX
Laboratoire de Neurobiologie Moléculaire
Institut de Biologie Moléculaire
Institut Pasteur
25, Rue du Dr. Roux
75015 PARIS

M. Pierre COLTEY
Institut d'Embryologie du CNRS
et du Collège de France
49bis, Avenue de la Belle-Gabrielle
94130 NOGENT-sur-MARNE

Dr. Claude CUDENNEC
Institut d'Embryologie du CNRS
et du Collège de France
49bis, Avenue de la Belle-Gabrielle
94130 NOGENT-sur-MARNE

Dr. Françoise DIETERLEN-LIEVRE
Insitut d'Embryologie du CNRS
et du Collège de France
49bis, Avenue de la Belle-Gabrielle
94130 NOGENT-sur-MARNE

Dr. Catherine DRESCH
INSERM ERA N° 4
Hôpital Saint-Louis
2, Place du Dr. Fournier
75475 PARIS

Dr. A.J. DURSTON
Hubrecht Laboratory
Uppsalalaan 8
Universiteitscentrum "De Uithof"
UTRECHT
Pays-Bas

Prof. Günter Von EHRENSTEIN
Abt. Molekulare Biology
Max Planck Institut für experimentelle
Medizin
3400-GOTTINGEN
Allemagne Fédérale

Dr. Harvey EISEN
Laboratoire de Génétique Cellulaire
Institut Pasteur
25, Rue du Dr. Roux
75015 PARIS

Dr. H.H. EPPERLEIN
Max Planck Institute für Virusforschung
Spemanstrasse 35
74 TUBINGEN
Allemagne Fédérale

Dr. Martin EVANS
Dept. of Genetics
Downing Street
CAMBRIDGE CB2 - 3EH
Great-Britain

Dr. Marc FELLOUS
Laboratoire d'Immuno-Hématologie
Institut de Recherches sur les
Maladies du Sang
Hôpital Saint-Louis
75745 PARIS

Dr. Josiane FONTAINE-PERUS
Institut d'Embryologie du CNRS
et du Collège de France
49bis, Avenue de la Belle-Gabrielle
94130 NOGENT-sur-MARNE

Dr. E. FRINDEL
INSERM U 66
Groupe Hospitalier Paul Brousse
94800 VILLEJUIF

Dr. Mark FURTH
MRC Lab. of Molecular Biology
Postgraduate Medical School
Hills Road
CAMBRIDGE CB2 2QH
Great-Britain

Dr. Louis GAZZOLO
Unité de Virologie
Fondamentale et Appliquée
1, Place du Professeur Joseph Renaut
69371 LYON CEDEX

Dr. Walter GEHRING
Biozentrum der Universität
Klingelbergstrasse 70
4056 BASEL
Suisse

Prof. Jacques GLOWINSKY
Groupe NB - Inserm U 114
Collège de France
11, Place Marcelin Berthelot
75231 PARIS CEDEX 5

Dr. Chris GRAHAM
Dept.of Zoology
Oxford University
South Park Road
OXFORD OX1 3PS
Great-Britain

Dr.Pierre GUERRIER
Station Biologique de Roscoff
Place Georges Teissier
29211 ROSCOFF

Dr. Jacques HATZFELD
The Rockefeller University
1230, York Avenue
NEW-YORK N.Y. 10021
USA

Dr. Rolf HEUMANN
Max Planck Institut für Biochemie
8033 MARTINSRIED bei München
Allemagne Fédérale

Dr. Michel HAMON
Groupe NB - Inserm U 114
Collège de France
11, Place Marcelin Berthelot
75231 PARIS CEDEX 05

Melle HOMO
U.7 INSERM
Physiologie et Pharmacologie
vasculaire et rénale
Hôpital Necker
161, Rue de sèvres
75730 PARIS CEDEX 15

Dr. HOPPE
Dept. Biologie
Université de Genève
154, Route de Malagnou
1224-CHENE-BOUGERIE/GENEVE
Suisse

Dr. Michael HORTON
Dept. of Zoology
University College of London
Gower Street
LONDON WCIE 6BT
Great-Britain

Dr. Karl ILLMENSEE
Dept. Biologie
154, Route de Malagnou
1224-CHENE-BOUGERIE/GENEVE
Suisse

Dr. Norman ISCOVE
Basel Institute of Immunology
487, Grenzacherstrasse
4005 BASEL
Suisse

Prof. François JACOB
Lab. de Génétique Cellulaire
Institut Pasteur
25, Rue du Dr. Roux
75015 PARIS

Dr. Robert JACQUOT
Faculté des Sciences
Lab. de Physiologie Animale
Moulin de la Housse
B.P. 347
51062 REIMS CEDEX

Dr. Wilfried JANNING
Zoologisches Institut der
Wilhelms-Universität
Badestrasse 9
D-4400 MUNSTER
Allemagne Fédérale

Dr. Gregory JOHNSON
Cancer Research Unit
Walter and Eliza Hall Institute
of Medical Research
P.O. Royal Melbourne Hospital
3050 VICTORIA
Australie

Dr. Francine JOTEREAU
Laboratoire d'Embryologie
Faculté des Sciences de Nantes
2, Rue de la Houssinière
44072 NANTES CEDEX

Dr. Judith KIMBLE
MRC Laboratory of Molecular
Biology
University Medical School
Hills Road
CAMBRIDGE CB2 - 2QH
Great-Britain

Prof. Jan KLEIN
Max Planck Institute
Dept. of Immunogenetics
42, Correnstrasse
7400 TUBINGEN
Allemagne Fédérale

Dr. Hisato KONDOH
Dept. of Biophysics
Kyoto University
KYOTO
Japan

Dr. Klaus KRATOCHWIL
Institut für Molekularbiologie
Billrothstrasse 11
A-5020 SALZBURG
Autriche

Dr. Claudine LAZARD
Institut d'Embryologie du CNRS
et du Collège de France
49bis, Avenue de la Belle-Gabrielle
94130 NOGENT-sur-MARNE

Prof. Charles LEBLOND
Dept. of Anatomy
Mac Gill University
MONTREAL Québec
Canada

Prof. Nicole LE DOUARIN
Institut d'Embryologie du CNRS
et du Collège de France
49bis, Avenue de la Belle-Gabrielle
94130 NOGENT-sur-MARNE

Dr. Christiane LE LIEVRE
Institut d'Embryologie du CNRS
et du Collège de France
49bis, Avenue de la Belle-Gabrielle
94130 NOGENT-sur-MARNE

Dr. Waldemar LERNHARDT
Basel Institute for Immunology
487, Grenzacherstrasse
4005 BASEL
Suisse

Dr. Marie-Hélène LEVI
Groupe NB - Inserm U 114
Collège de France
11, Place Marcelin Berthelot
75231 PARIS CEDEX 05

Prof. Cyrus LEVINTHAL
Dept. of Biological Sciences
Columbia University
NEW-YORK N.Y. 10027
U.S.A.

Dr. Hilary Ann Mc QUEEN
Imperial Cancer Research Fund
Mill Hill Laboratories
Burtonhole Lane
LONDON NW7-1AD
Great-Britain

Prof. Alfred MAELICKE
Max Planck Institute
Rheinlandamm 201
D-4600 DORTMUND 1
Allemagne Fédérale

Prof. Paul MANDEL
Centre de Neurochimie du CNRS
11, Rue Human
67085 STRASBOURG

Dr. Fritz MELCHERS
Basel Institute for Immunology
487, Grenzacherstrasse
4005 BASEL 5
Suisse

Dr. T. METS
Dept. Internal Medicine and
Geriatrics
Akademisch Ziekenhuis
De Pintelaan 135
9000-GENT
Belgique

Melle MILON
Institut Pasteur
25, Rue du Dr. Roux
75015 PARIS

Prof. Alberto MONROY
Stazione Zoologica
80121 NAPLES
Italie

Dr. Ginès MORATA
Centro de Biologia Molecular
Universidad Autonoma de Madrid
Facultad de Ciencias
Canto Blanco
MADRID 34
Espagne

Dr. Kurt NAUJOKS
Abteilung Neurochemie
Max-Planck Institut für
Psychiatrie
8033 MARTINSRIED bei München
Allemagne Fédérale

Dr. Robert NEGREL
Service de Biochimie
Université de Nice
Parc Valrose
06034 NICE

Dr. Jean-François NICOLAS
Lab. de Génétique Cellulaire
Institut Pasteur
25, Rue du Dr. Roux
75015 PARIS

Dr. Maryvonne NINIO
Centre de Génétique Moléculaire du CNRS
91190 GIF-sur-YVETTE

Dr. Christiane NUSSLEIN-VOLHARD
E.M.B.L.
Postfach 10.2209
D-69 HEIDELBERG
Allemagne Fédérale

Prof. Tokindo OKADA
Institute of Biophysics
Faculty of Science
University of Kyoto
KYOTO 606
Japon

Dr. V.E. PAPAIOANNOU
Dept. of Zoology
Oxford University
South Parks Road
OXFORD OX1 - 3PS
Great-Britain

Dr. Paul PATTERSON
Dept. of Neurobiology
Harvard Medical School
25, Shattuck Street
BOSTON Mass. 02115
U.S.A.

Dr. Elio PARISI
Stazione Zoologica
80121 NAPLES
Italie

Dr. Jean-Michel PAULUS
INSERM U 48
Hôpital de Bicêtre
Institut de Pathologie Cellulaire
94270 LE KREMLIN-BICETRE

Dr. Claude PENIT
IRBM Tour 43
Faculté des Sciences
2, Place Jussieu
75005 PARIS

Dr. R.A. PHILLIPS
The Ontario Cancer Institute
500 Sherbourne Street
TORONTO Canada M4X-1K9

Prof. Edward REICH
The Rockefeller University
1230, York Avenue
NEW-YORK N.Y. 10021
U.S.A.

Dr. Marie-Thérèse de REVIERS
Station de Physiologie de la
Reproduction
Centre de Recherche de Tours
INRA
37380 NOUZILLY

Dr. Roberto REVOLTELLA
Lab. di Biologia Cellulare
Consiglio Nazionale delle Ricerche
Via G. Romagnosi 18/A
00196 ROMA
Italie

Dr. Mary RITTER
Membrane Immunology Lab.
Imperial Cancer Research
Fund Laboratories
P.O. Box n°123
LONDON WC2A 3PX
Great-Britain

Dr. Claude ROSENFELD
INSERM U 50
Institut de Cancérologie
et d'Immunologie Gustave Roussy
14, Avenue Paul-Vaillant Couturier
94800 VILLEJUIF

Dr. Elisabeth ROSS
MRC Cellular Immunology Unit
Sir William Dunn School of Pathology
University of Oxford
OXFORD - OX1 3RE
Great-Britain

Dr. Chica SCHALLER
Lab. Europ. de Biologie Moléculaire
Postfach 102209
69-HEIDELBERG
Allemagne Fédérale

Dr. Trudi SCHUPBACH
Zoologisch-Vergl. Anatomisches
Institut der Universität Zürich
Künstlergasse 16
8006 ZURICH
Suisse

Dr. Martine MENAHEM-SCRIVE
Institut de Microbiologie
Bât. 109 Faculté des Sciences d'Orsay
91405 ORSAY

Dr. Atuhiro SIBATANI
CSIRO - Molecular and Cellular Biology Unit
P.O. Box 184
NORTH RYDE NSW 2113
Australie

Dr. Peter STERN
Dept. of Immunology
Biomedical Center
University of Uppsala
S-751 23 UPPSALA
Suède

Dr. Siegward STRUB
State University of New-York
at Stony-Brook
Dept. of Biology
STONY-BROOK N.Y. 11794
U.S.A.

Prof. Mario TERZI
Lab. di Mutagenesi
10, Via Svezia
56100 PISA
Italie

Dr. Ugo TESTA
INSERM U 91
Unité de Recherche sur les Anémies
CHU Henri Mondor
51, Avenue du Maréchal de Lattre de Tassigny
94010 CRETEIL

Dr. Jean-Paul THIERY
Institut d'Embryologie du CNRS
et du Collège de France
49bis, Avenue de la Belle-Gabrielle
94130 NOGENT-sur-MARNE

Dr. David TURNER
Eidgenossiche Technische Hochschule
Institut für Zellbiologie
Hönggerberg
8093 ZURICH
Suisse

Dr. William VAINCHENKER
INSERM U 91
CHU Henri Mondor
51, Avenue Henri Mondor
94010 CRETEIL

Dr. Jay VALINSKY
The Rockefeller University
1230, York Avenue
NEW-YORK N.Y. 10021
U.S.A.

Dr. Françoise de VITRY
Groupe de Neuroendocrinologie
du Collège de France
11, Place Marcelin Berthelot
75213 PARIS CEDEX 05

Dr. Barbara WALLENFELS
Max Planck Institut
für Virusforschung
Spemannstrasse, 35/II
D-TUBINGEN
Allemagne Fédérale

Dr. Jorma WARTIOVAARA
III Dept. of Pathology
University of Helsinki
SF-00290 HELSINKI
Finlande

Dr. Marie WEISS
Centre de Génétique Moléculaire
du CNRS
91190 GIF-sur-YVETTE

Dr. André WEYDERT
Dept. de Biologie Moléculaire
Institut Pasteur
25, Rue du Dr. Roux
75015 PARIS

Dr. Robert WHALEN
Institut Pasteur
25, Rue du Dr. Roux
75724 PARIS CEDEX 15

Dr. Eric WIESCHAUS
E.M.B.L.
Postfach 10.2209
D-69-HEIDELBERG
Allemagne Fédérale

Dr. Marcia YAROSS
Dept. of Biology
University of Virginia
Gilmer Hall
CHARLOTTESVILLE Virginia 22901
U.S.A.

Dr. Rolf ZINKERNAGEL
Dept. of Immunopathology
Scripps Clinic and Research Foundation
10666 North Torrey Pisses Road
LA JOLLA California 92037
U.S.A.

CONTENTS

xiv

BLOOD FORMING CELL SYSTEM

STABILITY OF THE DETERMINED STATE

SEGREGATION OF CELL LINES, AN EARLY DEVELOPMENTAL EVENT

Cell Lineage, Stem Cells and Cell Determination
INSERM Symposium No. 10
Editor: N. Le Douarin
© 1979 Elsevier/North-Holland Biomedical Press

INTRODUCTORY REMARKS ON THE SEGREGATION OF CELL LINES IN THE EMBRYO

ALBERTO MONROY

Zoological Station, Naples, Italy

In all multicellular organisms, the cleavage of the egg gives rise to cells which differ from one another and which, through successive cell divisions, will eventually give rise to homogeneous cell populations (cell lines) each endowed with its own specific developmental program. This not only implies a process of sorting out of molecules (either pre-existing in the egg before fertilization or being synthetized in the course of development) into the various blastomeres; but also of cells recognizing one another and coordinating their movements, their rate of cleavage, their metabolic activities, and the like.

In this Introduction I shall discuss some examples drawn from our work and from the work of other Laboratories to direct attention to some of the events which I consider as among the most important not only in connection with the segregation of cell lines but indeed with embryonic development as a whole.

Before entering into the subject, I would like briefly to present some speculations on the phylogenetic history of the segregation of cell lines in multicellular organisms.

We have recently suggested (Monroy and Rosati[1]) that one of the major events, if not *the* major event, connected with the appearance of multicellular organisms is the segregation of the somatic from the germ cell line. We have postulated that the dichotomy between the two cell lines involves:

(a) That in the somatic cell line, the genes which in the unicellular organisms code for the surface structures responsible for the recognition of and interaction between cells of the two gametic types, are silenced. The evidence for this is indirect. Although to our knowledge the matter has never been investigated with this question in mind, the formation of mouse chimaeras (Tarkowski[2]; Mintz[3]; see also review by Herbert and Graham[4]) shows that genetically male and female embryonic cells do not discriminate one another as different. Also, hybrid hystotypic aggregates can be formed in culture from such species as far apart as chick and mouse (Moscona[5]; Moscona and Moscona[6]). (However, the possibility should be taken into consideration that *in vitro* conditions may alter the organization of the cell surface in such a way that some of its properties such as the species-specificity are lost while the tissue-specificity is retained). These observations are compatible with the view that the structures discriminating between male and female are not expressed at the surface of these cells.

(b) The retention of a largely derepressed genome by the cells of the germ line. This is inferred from the fact that in the oocyte, the complexity of the transcripts is several-fold greater than in the somatic cells (see e.g. Galau et al.[7]). Although to our knowledge there is no such direct evidence in the case of the male germ cells, it has been shown that at least in *Drosophila*, spermatocytes exhibit lampbrush chromosomes comparable to those of the oocyte (Hess[8]).

In addition, we would like also to argue that the emergence of multicellular organisms has required the establishment of cell junctions; not only as a means of holding the cells together, but as a vehicle of functional coordination between cells (Monroy et al., unpublished).

A classical example of a very precocious segregation of the somatic from the germ line is that of *Ascaris* first described by Boveri[9] (Fig.1). In this nematode while the lineage cells of the germ line retain their full chromosome complement, in the cells of the somatic line pieces of chromosomes are lost; the loss amounts to about 27% of the total DNA of the cell. Interestingly, about one-half of the eliminated DNA consists of repetitive sequences and the other half of unique sequences (Tobler et al.[11])

Chromosome elimination is a frequent occurrence in Hemiptera; one of the most interesting cases is that of *Sciara*, first described by C.W.Metz (see review[12]). In *Sciara coprophila* the zygote carries three X chromosomes, one contributed by the egg and two by the spermatozoon (this results from an equational non disjunction of the maternally derived X chromosome at the second meiotic division in the male following the selective elimination of paternal homologues at the first spermatocyte division). During early cleavage *both* paternal X chromosomes are eliminated from the somatic cell line of the males while only one is eliminated in the female. In the germ line one paternal X chromosome is eliminated both in the female and in the male, but not until the germ cells have reached their final destination in the gonad (Du Bois[12]; Crouse[14]). Chromosome elimination may be thought of as a primitive, and in fact crude mechanism of "gene silencing" (see Sager and Kitchin[15]) to be replaced by more subtle de-

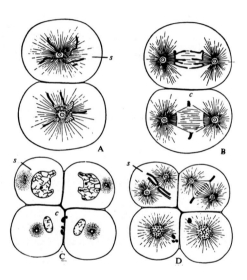

Fig.1. Segregation of the germ and somatic cell lines in *Ascaris*. At the first cleavage (A and B) in the upper blastomere, that is the precursor of the germ cell line (s), the chromosomes remain unchanged, while in the lower blastomere, that is the precursor of the somatic cell line, the heterochromatic ends of the chromosomes (c) are cast off in the cytoplasm and the chromosomes break up in a number of smaller units (side view in B). Two of the resulting 4 blastomeres (C) thus have undiminished chromatin (upper blastomeres) and two have diminished chromatin and hence smaller nuclei (cast off chromatin still visible in the cytoplasm (c)). At the third cleavage (D) one of the two upper blastomeres (upper right) undergoes chromatin diminution thus entering the somatic line, while the other one (s) retains its chromosomes unchanged. (From E.B.Wilson[10]).

vices in the course of evolution. I should like to venture the suggestion that
the eliminated chromosomes, or parts of chromosomes, contain the sexuality
genes.

Next I should like to argue that each cell line is committed to a certain
number of DNA replication cycles before expressing its specific phenotype: in
other words "the program for cell division is a part of the differentiative
program of each cell line" (Rossi et al.[16]). In support of this statement I
shall quote a few examples derived from the study of development of marine
invertebrates. The Ascidian embryo offers unique opportunities to study cell
lineage. Indeed, as the classical work of Conklin[17] has shown the segregation
of the major organ-forming territories occurs before the first cleavage (Fig.2).

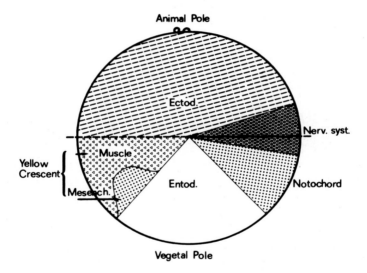

Fig.2. The presumptive organ-forming territories in the fertilized uncleaved
Ascidian egg. Note the two polar bodies which mark the animal pole of the egg.
The dotted horizontal line indicates the approximate position of the equato-
rial line separating the animal and vegetal territories.

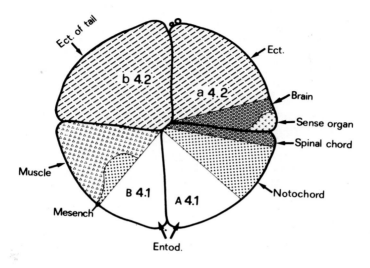

Fig.3.   Segregation of the organ-forming territories in the 8-cell stage of an Ascidian embryo.

Figure 3 shows the situation in the 8-cell embryo; in the 64-cell embryo the individual cell lines are already completely segregated (Table I). The results of a mathematical analysis and its implications of the segregation of the organ-forming territories in the uncleaved Ascidian egg will be discussed by E.Parisi. Table I also gives the total number of cells in each organ in the newly hatched tadpole. As can be seen, the number of cells increases differentially in each organ. In particular, attention is drawn to the nervous system, notochord and muscle. Between the 64-cell stage and the tadpole stage the number of cells in the nervous system increases by 31.2, that of the notochord by 6.7 and that of the musculature by 5. Hence, at the 64-cell stage the lineage cells of the above organs are programmed to undergo on the average 5, 4.5 and 2.3 cell divisions respectively.

TABLE 1

SEGREGATION OF THE MAJOR CELL LINES IN THE ASCIDIAN EMBRYO FROM THE 8-CELL
STAGE TO THE 64-CELL STAGE AND IN THE NEWLY HATCHED TADPOLE.

Blastomeres (in the 8-cell stage)	Derivatives (in the 64-cell embryo)	Number of cells in each cell line in the 64-cell embryo		Number of cells in the newly hatched tadpole
a 4.2	2 nerve cells	Nerve cells	8	250
	5 ectoderm cells	Sense organ	2	
	1 sense organ cell	Ectoderm	26	800
		Entoderm	10	500
A 4.1	3 entoderm cells	Notochord	6	40
	2 nerve cells	Mesenchyme	4	900
	3 notochordal cells	Muscle (tail)	8	40
B 4.1	2 entoderm cells			
	2 mesenchymal cells			
	4 muscle cells			
b 4.2	8 ectoderm cells			

Another interesting example is that of the micromeres of the sea urchin embryo. The micromeres are four small blastomeres which at the fourth cleavage
are segregated at the vegetal pole of the embryo due to the fact that in the
macromeres the spindle is strongly shifted towards the vegetal pole. The micromeres are committed to the formation of the primary mesenchyme and exert two important roles in morphogenesis: 1) they are responsible for the control of gastrulation (Hörstadius[18]); 2) they act as pacemakers of cell divisions during
cleavage (Parisi et al[19]). It was discovered by Driesch[20] that the micromeres
are also programmed for 3 to 4 cell divisions. For example, in the mesenchyme
blastula of *Sphaerechinus* there are about 30 primary mesenchyme cells and about
55 in *Echinus*. Embryos which develop from one of the first two blastomeres isolated after the first cleavage contain half the number of the primary mesenchyme cells: about 14 in *Sphaerechinus* and about 27 in *Echinus*.

It is interesting to note that the micromeres cleave at a lower rate and
their division is out of phase with respect to the other cells of the embryo
(Zeuthen[21]). We have discovered (Parisi et al.[19]) that the cleavage of the first
four micromeres gives rise to eight cells only four of which, namely the outer

ones, continue to divide while the four inner ones appear to have lost the ability to divide any further (at least through the next two division cycles; later the micromeres become undistinguishable from the other cells of the embryo). Thus within the micromere cell population two sub-populations are soon segregated, each of which again appear to be programmed for a different number of cell divisions. Thus far we have no information as to whether or not the inner micromeres are the precursors of a cell line different from that of the other micromeres.

Another example that I would like to mention is that of the mollusc embryo in which in the 16-cell stage, four of the descendants of the first quartet of micromeres, the micromeres $1a^2 - 1d^2$, undergo only two cell divisions and then differentiate into a band of ciliated cells, the larval prototroch (van Dongen and Geilenkirchen[22]).

These observations thus strongly suggest that in the embryo each cell line is programmed for a fixed number of cell divisions. In this context I would like to mention some recent interesting experiments of Dan-Sohkawa and Satoh[23]. These investigators have found that the number of cells of gastrulae obtained from each one of the blastomeres isolated from 2-, 4- and 8-cell starfish (*Asterina pectinifera*) embryos is roughly 1/2, 1/4 and 1/8 the number of cells of the normal gastrulae:

normal gastrulae	4207 cells
1/2 gastrulae	2168
1/4 gastrulae	980
1/8 gastrulae	550

The question is now to what extent the program of cell division - or more precisely the program of the DNA replication cycles - is an absolute requirement of differentiation. To my knowledge there is no clear-cut answer so far. Whittaker[24] has tried to answer this question by studying the effect of arresting the cleavage of the Ascidian embryo on the appearance of acetylcholinesterase in the presumptive muscular cells of the tail. In the normal embryos the enzyme can be detected in the neurula. When cleavage was arrested with Cytochalasin B (the treated embryos remain alive for many hours) the histochemical reaction for the enzyme appeared at the same time as in the normal embryos and

was strictly localized to the lineage cells of the musculature of the tail.How-
ever, since it is not known to what extent DNA replication was affected in these
experiments, it is possible that DNA could have undergone the number of replication cycles that is required for the expression of the acetylcholinesterase
activity.

The next point I would like to discuss concerns the coordination of cell divisions in the cell lines. In the sea urchin embryo such a coordination is quite
clear. I have already mentioned that the cleavage of the micromeres is out of
phase with respect to the other blastomeres; however, they divide synchronously
(with the exception of the four inner ones which divide only once). On the
other hand, the blastomeres divide synchronously only through the fourth cleavage (Fig.4); after the segregation of the micromeres a gradient of cell division sets in whereby the closer the blastomeres are to the micromeres the earlier they enter mitosis (Fig.5) (Parisi et al.[19]). We have postulated the existence within the cells of the sea urchin embryo of a mitotic oscillator from
which chemical signals periodically originate and diffuse from cell to cell.
According to our hypothesis, the blastomeres would behave like oscillators en-
trained on the rhythm of the micromeres acting as a pacemaker. We have also
shown that the pacemaker activity of the micromeres is interfered with by Acti-
nomycin D provided the drug is administered to the embryos prior to the segregation of the micromeres. This suggests that the onset of the pacemaker activity of the micromeres depends on transcriptional event(s) restricted to the time
of their segregation (Parisi et al.[25]).

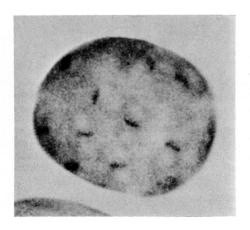

Fig.4. A 16-cell embryo of
Paracentrotus lividus; the
nuclei of all blastomeres are
in metaphase. (From Parisi
et al.[19]).

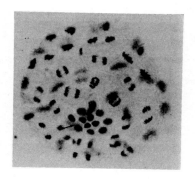

Fig.5. An embryo of *Paracentrotus lividus*
at the 64-cell stage. The micromeres (arrow)
are in interphase. The two rows of cells closer
to the micromeres are in anaphase while those
closer to the animal pole are in metaphase.
(From Parisi et al.[19]

The pattern of cell division in the mollusc embryo is considerably more complex than in the sea urchin. A division asynchrony already becomes apparent at
the 16-cell stage and this seems to be related to the fate of the blastomeres
and to the establishment of the bilateral symmetry (van Dongen and Geilenkirchen[22]). Interestingly, in molluscs the control of the cleavage pattern appears
to depend on the polar lobe. Removal of the polar lobe (in *Dentalium dentale*) at
the first cleavage causes the loss of the division asynchronies between blastomeres in the different quadrants and of the differences in the division patterns whereby the embryo becomes completely radialized (van Dongen and Geilenkirchen[26]).

In this presentation I have confined myself to a few examples drawn from the
study of some,mostly marine,invertebrates in which the analysis of the segregation of cell lines has been investigated in greater detail. These investigations
have been possible due to the fact that the cell lines are segregated very early
during cleavage and that each line is made up of a small number of cells, thus
making it possible to trace the fate of each cell to its final destination.

Two important notions have emerged from this analysis. The first is that the
cells of each line are committed to a definite number of cell divisions. The second concerns the coordination of cell division at least among the stem cells of
each line. How far these findings can be generalized is not at the present
known. It is probable that from the work underway in Dr.Graham's Laboratory
(Kelly et al.[27]; Graham and Deussen[28]; Graham and Lehtonen[29]) detailed informa-

tion will soon be available on the mouse embryo.

It is also extremely important to learn about coupling between cells of the individual cell lines. Indeed, coupling may be a key factor to coordinate both the synchrony and the number of cell divisions (see Parisi et al.[19]; Loewenstein[30]).

REFERENCES

1. Monroy, A. and Rosati, F. (1979) Nature, 278, 165-166

2. Tarkowski, A.K. (1961) Nature, 190, 857-860.

3. Mintz,B. (1962) Am.Zool., 2, 541.

4. Herbert, M.C. and Graham, C.F. (1974) Curr. Topics in Dev.Biol., Acad Press, New York, 8, 151-178.

5. Moscona, A.A. (1957) Proc. Natl. Acad. Sci. USA, 43, 184-194.

6. Moscona, A.A. and Moscona, M. (1965) Dev. Biol., 11, 402-423.

7. Galau, G.A., Klein, W.K., Davis, M.M., Wold, B.J. and Davidson, E.H. (1976) Cell, 7, 487-505.

8. Hess, O. (1968) Molec. Gen. Genet., 103, 58-71.

9. Boveri, Th. (1899) Fetstsch. F.C. von Kapper, pp. 383-430.

10. Wilson, E.B. (1906) The Cell in Development and Inheritance - 2nd Ed. The Macmillan Co., New York, 1906.

11. Tobler, H., Smith, K.D. and Ursprung, H. (1972) Dev. Biol. 27, 190-203.

12. Metz, Ch. W. (1938) Amer. Natur., 72, 485-520.

13. Du Bois, A.M. (1933) Z.Zellforsch. mikr. Anat., 19, 595-614.

14. Crouse, H.V. (1960) Genetics, 45, 1429-1443.

15. Sager, R. and Kitchin, R. (1975) Science, 189, 426-433.

16. Rossi, M., Augusti-Tocco, G. and Monroy, A. (1975) Quart. Rev. Biophys. 8, 43-119.

17. Conklin, E.G. (1905) J. Acad. Nat.Sci. Philadelphia, 13, 1-119.

18. Hörstadius, S. (1939) Biol. Rev., 14, 132-179.

19. Parisi, E., Filosa, S., De Petrocellis, B. and Monroy, A. (1978) Dev. Biol., 65. 38-49.

20. Driesch, H. (1898) Arch. Entw. mech. Org., 6, 198-227.

21. Zeuthen,E. (1951) Pubbl. Staz. Zool. Napoli, 23, 47-69.

22. van Dongen, C.A.M. and Geilenkirchen, W.L.M. (1974) Kon. Nederl. Akad. Wetensch. Amsterdam,)), 57-70.

23. Dan-Sohkawa, M. andSatoh, N. (1978) J. Embryol. exp. Morphol., 46, 171-185.

24. Whittaker, J.r. (1973) Proc. Natl. Acad. Sci. USA, 70, 2096-2100.

25. Parisi, E., Filosa, S. and Monroy, A. (1979) Dev. Biol., in press.

26. van Dongen, C.A.M. and Geilenkirchen, W.L.M. (1975) Kon. Nederl. Akad. Wetensch. Amsterdam, 78, 358-375.

27. Kelly, S.J., Mulnard, J.G. and Graham, C.F. (1978) J. Embryol. exp.Morphol., 48, 37-51.

28. Graham, C.F. and Deussen, Z.A. (1978) J. embryol. exp. Morphol., 48, 53-72.

29. Graham, C.F. and Lehtonen, E. (1979) J. Embryol. exp. Morphol., 49, 277-294.

30. Loewenstein, W.R. (1979) Bioch. Bioph. Acta, 560, 1-65.

Cell Lineage, Stem Cells and Cell Determination
INSERM Symposium No. 10
Editor: N. Le Douarin
© *1979 Elsevier/North-Holland Biomedical Press*

A MODEL FOR EARLY SEGREGATION OF TERRITORIES IN THE ASCIDIAN EGG

G. CATALANO, C.EILBECK[+], A. MONROY[++] and E.PARISI°

Istituto Matematico "G.Castelnuovo", University of Rome, Italy.
[+]Department of Mathematics, Heriot-Watt University, Edinburgh, Scotland.
[++]Stazione Zoologica, Naples, Italy. °Laboratory of Molecular Embryology,
Arco Felice, Naples, Italy.

1. INTRODUCTION

Cleavage of the egg results in the formation of groups of cells from which
the different tissues and organs of the embryo arise (cell lines). The segregation of cell lines is a stepwise process starting from the spatially ordered
territories in the egg and/or in the blastomeres during early cleavage. It is
assumed that this involves the segregation of specific cytoplasmic components
(morphogens) in the different blastomeres. The word "morphogens" as it is used
in this context is not meant as a synonym of *organ-forming substances*; but
rather of factors responsible for the activation or repression of specific sets
of genes in the different blastomeres. Their immediate involvement in the differentiation of certain structures, however, cannot be completely ruled out.
The segregation of the major cell lines is usually completed in the blastula.
However, in most animals by this time the embryo is made up of a very large
number of cells; and this makes the analysis of the "cell lineage" difficult to
follow. A notable exception among chordates is that of the Ascidians in which
the segregation of the major cell lines is completed at the 64-cell stage. Thus,
it is possible to accurately follow the destiny of each presumptive territory
starting from the uncleaved egg (see the accompanying paper by A.Monroy). Thus,
the Ascidian egg provides an example of early segregation of morphogenetic territories. Indeed, following fertilization the egg undergoes a rapid reorganization of its cytoplasm such that before the first cleavage, it is already subdivided into different regions, each having distinct commitments.

Here we shall describe a simple model that is able to explain how regional
patterns are generated in the Ascidian egg. In particular, we propose that the

segregation of the presumptive territories in the egg is the result of the combined action of three factors which are preformed but not prelocalized in the unfertilized egg. A localized distribution of the morphogens is brought about by non-linear reaction-diffusion mechanisms.

For the sake of clarity, we shall first review the main observations of Conklin[1] and of other authors on the cell lineage of the Ascidian egg and the response of the system when parts of it are removed, isolated or grafted together. In the second part we shall briefly discuss a biochemical mechanism capable of forming spatial patterns of chemical substances. A detailed description of the model will follow together with the results of some experiments that appear to be compatible with the proposed model.

2. THE ASCIDIAN EGG AS A MODEL FOR THE SEGREGATION OF MORPHOGENETIC TERRITORIES

Ever since the classical studies of Conklin[1] it has been known that in the Ascidian egg, fertilization is followed by displacement of some of its cytoplasmic components which move towards the vegetal hemisphere where they give rise to four regions. In *Styela partita*, the unfertilized egg is evenly spotted with a yellow pigment but following fertilization the pigment moves towards the vegetal pole, leaving the animal pole filled with yolk except for a small apical cap of clear cytoplasm. Immediately afterwards, the male pronucleus, which originally is located in the vegetal territory, moves towards the centre of the egg following a rather reproducible path. The male pronucleus appears to pull the yellow material inwards as it moves so that a yellow crescent of material arises which extends into the subequatorial half of the egg. Concomitantly with the fusion of the two pronuclei and immediately before the beginning of the first cleavage, new cytoplasmic movements take place resulting in the formation of: the grey yolk, the yellow crescent, the grey crescent (at the opposite side of the yellow crescent), and finally the vegetal pole region rich in yolk (fig.1). These plasm segregations can be observed in other species such as *Halocynthia* (fig.2).

The developmental role of the reorganization that the Ascidian egg undergoes following fertilization is better understood by comparing the development of the egg fragments obtained from the unfertilized egg with those obtained from

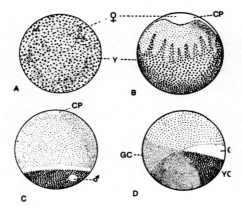

Fig. 1. Plasm reorganization in the egg of *Styela partita*. A. Unfertilized egg; B, C and D time-course plasm reorganization following fertilization. Y=yolk; CP=clear protoplasm; GC=grey crescent; YC=yellow crescent. Black dots represent mitochondria. From Conklin[1].

the fertilized egg[2].Two halves from an unfertilized egg, when fertilized give rise to two essentially complete tadpoles, irrespective of the orientation of the section. The same operation, when performed on a fertilized egg gives an entirely different result. Only egg fragments containing the vegetal territory are able to develop into a normal larva. In particular, as a result of a section of an egg into an animal and vegetal half by an equatorial section, a normal embryo develops only from the vegetal half. On the contrary, the animal half gives rise to a cluster of cells which will never gastrulate (a permanent blastula), even when it contains the zygote nucleus. This result is comparable to that obtained on embryos at the 2-cell stage.The destruction of one blastomere of a 2-cell stage embryo gives a half embryo with entoderm, neuroectoderm and notochord[2].

The most interesting results have been obtained with operations on the 8-cell embryo in which the major organ-forming territories have been precisely mapped (fig.3) (see also fig.3 of the accompanying paper by A.Monroy). The results of these operations show that all the pairs of blastomeres, except for the anterior animal blastomeres, differentiate according to their presumptive fate. The

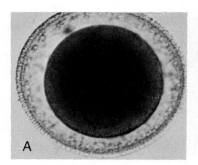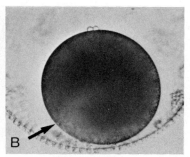

Fig. 2. Plasm segregation in *Halocynthia roretzi*. A. Unfertilized egg; B. Fertilized egg showing the yellow crescent area.

anterior animal blastomeres, when isolated, fail to differentiate into neuroblast unless they are combined with the two anterior vegetal blastomeres (fig. 4)[2]. This situation is similar to that of the Amphibians, where the differentiation of the nervous system is dependent on the chordomesoderm. All the other combinations give rise either to ectodermal vesicles or to structures containing musculature, entoderm and mesenchyme (fig.4)[2].

The results of these observations and experiments thus show that the cytoplasmic reorganization of the Ascidian egg that follows fertilization turns the isotropic structure of the unfertilized egg into a mosaic of territories. The animal hemisphere is entirely ectodermal with its anterior region containing the presumptive territory of the nervous system (which probably extends slightly into the subequatorial hemisphere). In the vegetal hemisphere three territories can be recognized: the chordoblast, corresponding to the grey crescent; the muscle-mesenchyme territory corresponding to the yellow crescent (which is characterized by a high concentration of mitochondria); the entoderm at the vegetal pole, between the notochordal and the muscle territories. However, while the vegetal territories are already committed to differentiation, the nervous system can only differentiate under the influence of the chordoblast.

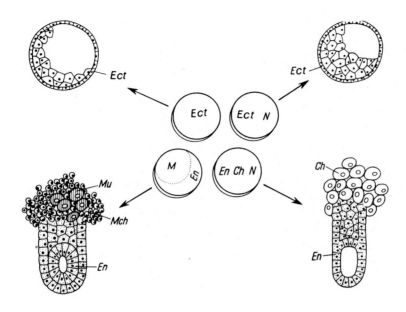

Fig. 3. Developmental fate of the four isolated pairs of blastomeres of an Ascidian embryo at the 8-cell stage. Ect=ectoderm; N=neural territory; En=ento-derm; Ch=notochord; M=Mesodermal territory; Mu=musculature; Mch=mesenchyme. From Reverberi[2].

3. BIOCHEMICAL MECHANISM FOR PATTERN FORMATION

It has been conjectured that formation of differentiated structures during embryogenesis is controlled by concentration gradients of morphogens. Cells in a tissue whould thus respond specifically to morphogens whose concentration is above a certain threshold value.

Several models of morphogen gradient generation have been proposed[3-7]. A way to approach the problem is through the study of open chemical systems exhibit-ing non-linear kinetics and working far from thermodynamic equilibrium. Non-linear kinetics in biological systems can be the expression of feedback, coope-rative and autocatalytic molecular processes involving repressors, activators and allosteric enzymes.When non-linear biochemical reactions occurring in dif-

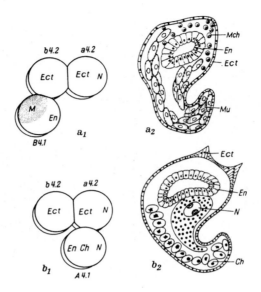

Fig. 4. Combination of blastomeres (a_1, b_1) and their developmental fate (a_2,b_2). Symbols as in figure 3. From Reverberi[2].

ferent regions of space are coupled by diffusion, it may happen that following a perturbation, the system evolves towards a new regime characterized by the spatially inhomogeneous distribution of the chemical substances involved in the process.

In this section we shall discuss a model that is based on a very simple feedback loop in which a certain metabolite U, produced at a constant rate, is converted by an enzymatic reaction into a product V which is destroyed with a rate proportional to its concentration. Moreover, V catalizes its own production by acting as an effector of the allosteric enzyme that transforms U into V. We assume that the allosteric enzyme is a dimer existing under an active and an inactive conformation and that both U and V bind with equal affinities only to the active form. In addition, we assume that transition from one conformation to the other is concerted[8] and that steady-state conditions are valid for the enzymatic forms. This system is a simplified version of the phospho-fructo-kinase model developed by Goldbetter[9-10]. If the metabolites U and V can also diffuse, the evolution equations of the system are given by the boundary value problem:

1)
$$u_t = a - \frac{bu(1+u)(1+v)^2}{c + (1+u)^2(1+v)^2} + D_1 \nabla^2 u$$

$$v_t = \frac{bu(1+u)(1+v)^2}{c + (1+u)^2(1+v)^2} - dv + D_2 \nabla^2 v$$

with appropriate boundary conditions. In (1), u_t and v_t denote time derivatives. ∇^2 is the Laplacian operator, a is production rate for U; b, the V_{MAX} for the allosteric enzyme; c, the allosteric constant; d, the degradation rate constant for V; D_1 and D_2, the diffusion coefficients for U and V respectively. u and v are the concentrations of U and V divided by the dissociation constants (supposed to be equal) of the enzyme complexes.

A detailed analytical and numerical study of (1) has been carried out and will be published elsewhere. Approximate numerical solutions of the boundary value problem (1) with Neuman boundary conditions show that under an appropriate parameter choice the spatially homogeneous stationary state becomes unstable and evolves towards a new non-homogeneous stationary state. Figure 5 shows the solutions in a circular domain of fixed radius after a local perturbation has been applied at one pole. It is possible to see that patterns grow in time until they reach the new non-homogeneous stationary state and that their shape has the form of a monotonic gradient. If a threshold concentration is fixed, an ideal line can be drawn that separates two compartments, one above the threshold and another below it. The orientation of the patterns depends on which point of the domain the initial perturbation is applied. As a direct consequence of this new non-homogeneous stationary state it may happen that two regions separated by the threshold line acquire distinct commitments. Finally, although the above results have been obtained in a two-dimensional domain, they can be assumed to reflect the situation in a three-dimensional case such as that of a spherical egg.

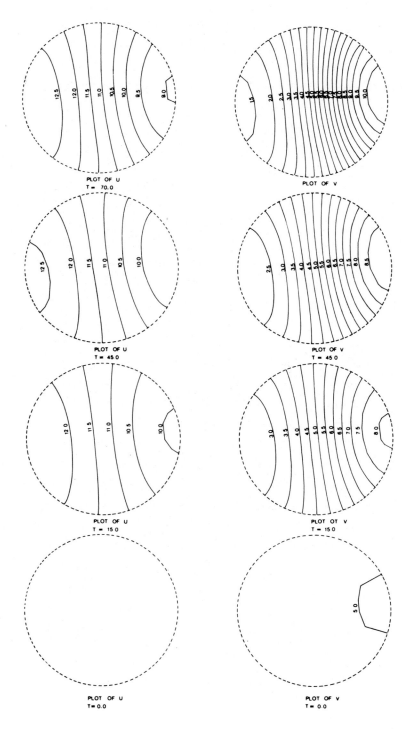

Fig. 5. Time evolution of chemical patterns in a two dimensional domain obtained by numerical integration of (1). Concentrations are constant along the contour lines. The initial perturbation is applied at one point of the domain close to the boundary and on one variable only. The non-homogeneous stationary state is reached after 70 time units. Note that the gradients of U and V go in opposite directions and that pattern orientation depends on where the perturbation was applied. Values of the dimensionless parameters: $a = 5$; $b = 10^4$; $c = 10^7$; $d = 1$; $D_1 = 0.8$; $D_2 = 0.05$.

4. THE MODEL OF THE ASCIDIAN EGG

The results summarized in section 2 may be interpreted as indicating that morphogens which are uniformily distributed in the cytoplasm of the unfertilized Ascidian egg become, after fertilization, organized in a very precise manner. We may assume that spatial distribution of morphogens has the character of gradient systems generated by processes similar to those reported in section 3, i.e. by non-linear reaction diffusion systems.

We postulate that three independent gradients set in consecutively following fertilization along different axes, thus specifying different regions of the egg whose fate is determined by the presence of one or more morphogens. The combined action of three morphogens is sufficient to account for the existence of six distinct compartments in the fertilized Ascidian egg. The sequence of the events leading to the segregation of these compartments is shown in fig.6.

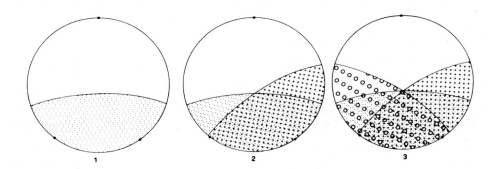

Fig. 6. Sequential formation of compartments in our model of Ascidian egg.
1. Threshold line of the first morphogen gradient dividing the egg into two compartments. 2. The four compartments after the appearance of the second gradient. The yellow crescent would correspond to the left subequatorial section. 3. Final partitioning after the appearance of the third gradient. The various symbols denote the individual morphogens. The symbols indicate those areas where the concentration of the morphogens is above threshold level.

Fertilization triggers the spatial reorganization of the first morphogen along the animal-vegetal axis. Supposing that the threshold line lies in the subequatorial half of the egg, this line would mark the boundary between two regions one above the threshold and one below it. The first gradient therefore subdivides the egg into two unequal parts. Since the first gradient sets in along the animal-vegetal axis, we must assume that the origin of the perturbation is localized at the animal pole of the egg. This is in agreement with Conklin's observations indicating a flow of material from the animal to the vegetal hemisphere.

Soon after this first reorganization a second gradient sets in along an axis forming an angle of approximately 30° with the axis of the first gradient (fig.6). We have at this point, two independent morphogens specifying four compartments. Of these compartments, only the one that contains the first morphogen is clearly recognizable, namely the yellow crescent (see fig.2). The perturbation that triggers the second gradient starts in the vegetal hemisphere in an eccentric position with respect to the animal-vegetal axis. Its point of origin roughly corresponds to the site where the spermatozoon has entered the egg.

It has already been observed by Conklin[1] that in the Ascidians the spermatozoon enters the egg in a narrow area localized at the vegetal pole. This does not depend on the presence of a specialized structure of the chorion that surrounds the egg as the same occurs in dechorionated eggs. Hence we assume (though there is no evidence of this) that this area has a molecular organization different from that of the rest of the egg. There is so far no reliable way to identify the place where, at the vegetal pole, the spermatozoon actually enters the egg. We postulate that the site of sperm penetration causes the perturbation which specifies the direction of the second gradient. This situation is similar to what happens in the Amphibian egg where the dorso-ventral symmetry is specified by the site of entrance of the spermatozoon.

The onset of the second gradient further modifies the constitution of the egg cytoplasm. In particular, we have seen that mitochondria become concentrated in the yellow crescent area. The high density of mitochondria in this region of the egg may cause a variety of metabolic changes including pH change, calcium displacement from a bound to a free form and so on. Any one of these events may function as a trigger for the third gradient which is also tilted with respect to the animal-vegetal axis and which, by interacting with the other two gradients, partitions the egg into six compartments. Each one of these compartments is characterized by having a morphogen concentration that may be either above or below the threshold value. In this context we simply say that a given compartment contains a morphogen when this is present at an above-threshold concentration. Hence, the combined action of the three morphogens specifies the following compartments; 1) a region containing no morphogen, 2) a region containing the second morphogen only, 3) a compartment with the first and the second morphogen, 4) an area characterized by the presence of all three morphogens, 5) a region containing the first and the third morphogen only, 6) a region with the third morphogen only (fig.6). The number of regions specified in this way may, at a first glance, appear redundant since the Ascidian egg seems to contain four territories only i.e. the ectoderm, the notochord, the mesoderm, and the entoderm, the formation of the nervous system being dependent on the induction of the notochordal territory. In particular, the discrepancy seems to concern the animal hemisphere, while for the subequatorial half of the egg the model predicts three regions which correspond to the presumptive territories of the notochord, entoderm and mesoderm. According to our model the ectoderm is not a homogeneous compartment but is subdivided into three regions characterized either by having no morphogens or by having only one morphogen. One should then expect that the animal territories and the blastomeres deriving from them should have different developmental competences. The results of grafting experiments reported in fig.7 show that this is in fact the case. Indeed, if the posterior pair of blastomeres is substituted for the anterior one, in spite of its contact with the anterior vegetal blastomeres containing the notochordal territory, no nervous tissue differentiates[2]. An identical result has been obtained when the whole animal quartet is rotated 180° with respect to the vegetal quartet (Ortolani, personal communication).

Every model of pattern formation based on the concept of morphogen gradients must deal with the problem of the regulatory capacity of the system. Within certain limits, chemical patterns can be re-established after they have been perturbed, for instance by cutting or reducing the size of the system[11]. This is

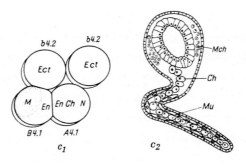

Fig. 7. Substitution of the posterior animal blastomeres for the anterior ones (C_1) resulting in a larva-lacking nervous system (C_2). From Reverberi[2].

exactly what happens in the Ascidian egg before fertilization. The regulatory capacity of the egg is lost after fertilization, as isolated blastomeres have now become unable to give rise to a complete larva. This means that any local change in morphogen concentration within the egg cytoplasm is somehow recorded and maintained under the form of an irreversible change of some structures of the egg such as, for instance, the plasma membrane. A possible interpretation of our model is that following fertilization the plasma membrane of the Ascidian egg undergoes a series of modifications related to those of the underlying cytoplasm. Weight is given to this interpretation by the observation that the receptor-sites of the *Dolichos* anti-A lectin which are evenly distributed at the surface of the unfertilized egg become, after fertilization, concentrated at the vegetal pole of the egg[12]. Displacement of the egg surface from the animal to the vegetal pole following fertilization has also been described[13]. It is likely that the mosaic character of the egg determined by cytoplasmic rearrangements remains, by a modification of the structural architecture of the membrane, in a "frozen" state. We suggest that the distribution of a number of specific factors in the plasma membrane plays a major role in determining the developmental fate of the individual blastomeres.

Evidence that differentiation of the Ascidian egg is, at least in part, controlled by the plasma membrane is provided by experiments carried out on iso-

lated blastomers at the 8-cell stage. The blastomeres of the animal quartet
that when isolated give rise to ectodermal vescicle, are able to develop neural
structures following a short treatment with trypsin[14]. These results further
support the hypothesis that surface specialization may play an important role
in the formation of spatially ordered differentiated structures.

5. CONCLUSIONS

The Ascidian egg provides a clear example of a regulative egg turned into
a mosaic egg by the effect of fertilization. In the model presented here we
have interpreted the sequence of cytoplasmic rearrangements occurring between
fertilization and cleavage as a consequence of the segregation of three distinct morphogens produced by biochemical reactions exhibiting non-linear kinetics. The combined action of these morphogens specifies six presumptive territories of the future embryo. Of these compartments only one, corresponding to
the posterior region of the ectoderm, has never been observed, but it can be
tentatively identified as the presumptive territory of the tail. Whether the
full development of this region depends on the interactions with neighbouring
structures, as in the case of the neural ectoderm, remains to be established
and may constitute a test of the model.

In order to explain the lack of regulatory capacity of the fragments obtained from the fertilized egg or from embryos at early stages, we have postulated that the cytoplasmic information of the mosaic egg is irreversibly converted into a specialization of the plasma membrane. While some experimental
observations seem to support this hypothesis, very little evidence is available
on how patterns of membrane components exert their regulatory role on cell differentiation. It might also be of interest to know whether organ-specific antigens can be identified and localized in the presumptive territories of embryos
at very early stages of development.

Finally, we have to point out that even though in non-linear kinetics systems chemical patterns can in principle arise by means of random fluctuation,
the morphogenetic patterns observed in the Ascidian egg display a predictable
orientation. This means that a limited number of physical asymmetries already

exist in the unfertilized egg that, however, are not sufficient to give the mosaic character typical of the post-fertilization stages. Often these asymmetries have the features of self-regulating prepatterns as demonstrated by the fact that in the egg fragments polarity along the animal-vegetal axis is promptly re-established. It is evident that further investigations on the origin and nature of these prepatterns will contribute towards understanding the formation of the developmental compartments in the egg.

REFERENCES

1. Conklin, E.G. (1905) J. Acad. Natur. Sci. (Philadelphia), 13, 1-119.

2. Reverberi, G. (ed.) (1971) Ascidians in *Experimental Embryology of Marine and Freshwater Invertebrates*. North-Holland, Amsterdam.

3. Wolpert, L. (1969) J. Theoret. Biol. 25, 1-47.

4. Meinhardt, H. (1977) J. Cell Sci. 23, 117-139.

5. Meinhardt, H. (1978) J. Theoret. Biol. 74, 307-321.

6. Crick, F.H. (1971) Symposia Soc. Exptl. Biol. 25, 429-438.

7. Kauffman, S.A., Shymko, R.M. and Trabert, K. (1978) Science, 199, 259-270.

8. Monod, J., Wyman, J. and Changeux, J.P. (1965) J. Mol. Biol. 12, 88-118.

9. Goldbeter, A. and Lefever, R. (1972) Biophys. J. 12, 1302-1315.

10. Goldbeter, A. (1973) Proc. Natl. Acad. Sci. 70, 3255-3259.

11. Lacalli, T.C. and Harrison, L.G. (1978) J. Theoret. Biol. 70, 273-295.

12. Ortolani, G., O'Dell, D.S. and Monroy, A. (1977) Exptl. Cell Res. 106, 402-404.

13. Ortolani, G. (1955) Riv. Biol. 42, 169-178.

14. Ortolani, G., Patricolo, E. and Mansueto, C. Exptl.Cell Res. (in press).

Cell Lineage, Stem Cells and Cell Determination
INSERM Symposium No. 10
Editor: N. Le Douarin
© *1979 Elsevier/North-Holland Biomedical Press*

INTRACELLULAR ACTIVATION AND CELL INTERACTIONS IN SO-CALLED MOSAIC EMBRYOS.

P. GUERRIER and J.A.M. van den BIGGELAAR

Station Biologique, 29211 Roscoff (France) and the Zoological Laboratory, University of Utrecht, Padualaan 8, Utrecht (The Netherlands)

INTRODUCTION

The eggs of Molluscs and Annelids still figure in many textbooks of embryology as clear cut examples of mosaic development in which the fate of each blastomere is determined right from its origin by intrinsic factors inherited from the uncleaved egg. According to this conception, it has been proposed that the environment (follicle cells for example) may regionally organize the oocyte cortical layer which, divided among the blastomeres, will direct their individual evolution[1].

Despite some provocative results which, like those of Clement[2] and Cather[3], pointed to the importance of cell interactions in *Ilyanassa*, the idea remained strong however that, at least, the two foundamental axes which defined the plane of symmetry were definitively settled down into the oocyte structure[4]. Accordingly, it was considered that individual blastomeres, whether isolated or still part of the embryo, evolved irremediably according to their known position in this system (by which possible interactions were restricted to specific cell line), and that they were deprived of extensive regulative capacities.

During the past 10 years, we have reinvestigated this problem, tackling it directly by changing the usual relationships that classical cell lineage studies depicted to occur between such an eventual preformed pattern and the disposition of the cleavage planes (Fig. 1).

Our results concerning the progressive fixation of the polar and dorsoventral axes[5] definitively ruled out the possibility of maintaining such a preformative interpretation. The early differentiation of the mosaic egg actually proceeds epigenetically. It involves intracellular as well as intercellular interactions, depending both on the course and orientation of cell division and on dynamic rather than fixed properties of the plasma membrane. In brief, dorsoventral membrane determination involves intracellular activation and occurs quite early in unequally cleaving eggs. It is postponed and results from the development of determinant intercellular contacts in equally cleaving eggs.

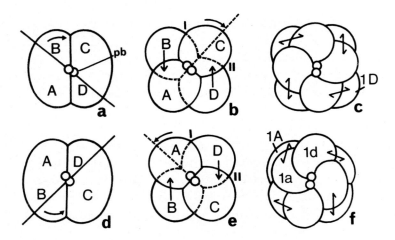

Fig. 1. - Spatial organization in enantiomorphic spiral cleavage, views from the animal pole. The first row of drawings refers to dextral forms (D type), the second row to sinistral forms (L type). p.b., polar bodies.

a - d : Two cell stage. The first furrow is on the right (D type) or on the left (L type) of the presumptive plane of symmetry (S).

b - e : Four cell stage with internal arrows indicating the orientation of second spindles. Dashed line indicates the position of the vegetal cross-furrow which is on the right (D type) or on the left (L type) of the first cleavage plane (I). B and D cells contact each other at this level.

c - f : Formation of the first quartet of micromeres during the third cleavage.

INADEQUACY OF THE MOSAIC CONCEPT IN THOSE EGGS WHICH PRESENT AN UNEQUAL 1st AND 2nd CLEAVAGE. INTRACELLULAR INTERACTIONS VERSUS PREFORMED MORPHOGENETIC MATERIAL.

In those eggs, the 1st cleavage plane is not truely meridian, although it cuts through the polar bodies which mark the animal pole. It isolates a small cell AB from a bigger cell CD. At the end of the 2nd cleavage, one gets three cells of equivalent size A, B and C, while D is the biggest cell which contains most of the vegetal region of the egg· We know, from cell lineage studies, that this D quadrant always represents the dorsal side of the embryo, since it gives rise to the mesoderm mother cell 4 d, at the sixth division.

In bivalves, where D forms opposite to the entrance point of the sperm, we demonstrated that this relation could not result from some kind of preformation, since centrifuging the egg could make this blastomere to appear in a different position[6]. Moreover, when first cleavage was made to be equal, two large cells formed at 2nd cleavage, which contained a part of the vegetal region and were located either side by side (CCDD embryos) or in opposition (CDCD embryos). These cells behaved in every way (including the rather particular pattern of successive spindle orientations) as true dorsal blastomeres, by which double embryos with two shells were produced. In any case, the type of evolution of each individual blastomere, obtained either after normal or equalized cleavage, was found not to depend on its endoplasmic composition but on the fact that it included or not a part of the vegetal cortex. It is thus clear that this structure is able to organize any of the presumptive quadrants one can arbitrarily trace over the oocyte.

Another mechanism to direct the vegetal region of the egg towards the D quadrant involves a transitory bulging out of the vegetal pole (polar lobe) at 1st and 2nd cleavage. By this mechanism, the vegetal region of the egg is shunted to the CD and then to the D blastomere. After removal of the polar lobe, the D quadrant shows the same developmental characteristics as the other quadrants and the embryo becomes completely radialysed : no sign of dorsoventrality is apparent. This holds true for the eggs of the Annelid *Sabellaria*[7,8], the Bivalve *Mytilus*[9], the Gastropod *Ilyanassa*[10] and the Scaphopod *Dentalium*[11-13]. These observations point to the importance of polar lobe material but do not answer the very old and disputed question according to which polar lobe fusion may depend on a preformed dorsoventral organization of the oocyte[14]. We demonstrated however that this was not the case for *Sabellaria*[15], since, changing 1st spindle orientation, either by pressure or centrifugation, allowed us to obtain dorsoventral differentiations from any of the presumptive blastomeres which has accepted the polar lobe. Double embryos were also obtained after equalization of 1st cleavage. In any case, it was found again that dorsoventrality did not depend on the plasmatic composition of the blastomeres but only on the inclusion of the vegetal cortex. These first conclusions have been now extended to the egg of *Dentalium*[16] where the polar lobe has been shown to be able to fuse with either of the prospective AB or CD regions of the egg and where double embryos may be obtained after a transient treatment with cytochalasin B. Even 1/8th of the volume of the polar lobe seems to be able to induce a prospective AB cell to cleave and behave as CD, thus producing a supernumerary mesentoblast. These results strongly suggest that cell activation rather than ooplasmic segregation must play a cardinal role in differentiation.

That the concept of "formative material" which derives from classical experiments involving blastomere isolation or polar lobe removal is inadequate was also illustrated in our experiments on *Sabellaria*. In this material, microsurgical experiments[7,8] have shown that the factors for development of the post-trochal region remained apparently located in the vegetal part of the embryo since they were present in the 1st, 2nd and 3rd polar lobe before they concentrated in the 1D macromere. Despite this, we found repeatedly[15] that "lobeless embryos" (i.e. embryos deprived of posttrochal differentiations), similar to those resulting from 1st polar lobe removal, could be obtained from whole eggs which have been induced to cleave with an aequatorial 1st cleavage plane instead of the usual meridian one. It is worth to stress that this occurred also when such a cleavage was obtained from eggs previously centrifuged perpendicular to the polar axis and, thus, provided with an equivalent set of each type of plasmatic inclusions in the resulting animal and vegetal blastomeres. On the contrary, normal development was preserved if the aequatorial cleavage was only induced during the 2nd division.

Taken together, these results indicate that intracellular activation phenomena depending on cleavage orientation must play a key role in blastomere differentiation. In the present case, these phenomena, which occur during the first cleavage and the following interkinetic period, are likely to involve an interaction between the endoplasm and the cortex of both the animal and vegetal regions of the embryo since they occur only when these are present in the same blastomere.

Other intracellular interactions are also needed to explain the absence of apical cilia development in their mother blastomeres, when these have been made to include part of the polar lobe[12, 15, 17].

THE CASE OF EGGS WITH AN EQUAL 1st AND 2nd CLEAVAGE. INTERCELLULAR INTERACTIONS AS A FACTOR OF DIFFERENTIATION.

In these forms, it is quite unlikely that the cortex of the vegetal hemisphere determines the dorsal blastomere since each first four blastomeres or, at least two of them, which meet at the vegetal cross furrow (B and D), contain an equal amount of that material. Until recently, it was therefore considered that this differentiation depended on a true dorsoventral organization which extended perpendicular to the polar axis[4]. Our experiments on the egg of *Limax maximus* demonstrated however that this assumption was incorrect since (1) normal development always resulted[18] with a new dorsoventral polarity, after we have changed the orientation of the polar axis and of the ooplasmic segregation by shifting the position of extrusion of the 2nd polar body; (2) normal development always followed[19] after a displacement of the 1st spindle in the aequatorial plane such as cleavage planes occupy a new position relative to any eventual preformed dorsoventral pattern; (3) blastomeres isolated at the two-cell stage exhibited equivalent developmental potencies[20].

This last observation has been now confirmed and extended by Morill & al.[21] and by Verdonk[22], who obtained perfect normal embryos from isolated first blastomeres of *Lymnaea* and *Physa*. In these cases, regulation was even more complete than with the sea urchin embryo, since the only blastomeres which developed normally did not cleave as the half of one embryo but as a whole egg (Fig. 2). In these conditions, the 3rd and 4th cleavage reproduce the disposition found during normal 2nd and 3rd cleavage.

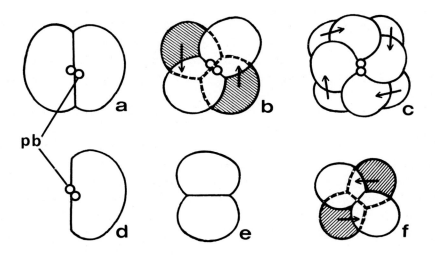

Fig. 2. - Comparison between the cleavage of a normal embryo and that of an isolated blastomere from the 2-cell stage, dividing "as a whole egg".

Second (e) and third (f) cleavage of the isolated blastomere reproduce normal first (a) and second (b) cleavages. Normal third cleavage (c) will be exhibited by the isolated blastomere during the fourth cleavage cycle. Since both 4-cell stages are produced laetropically, it results that the blastomeres which contact each other at the vegetal pole (dashed) are differently oriented relative to the first spindle orientation.

Polar bodies (p.b.) indicate the position of the animal pole, arrows indicate spindle orientation.

It results that normal cell relations are reestablished in these half embryos except that the two blastomeres which contact each other at the vegetal pole are disposed perpendicular to the normal orientation and arise from lateral presumptive parts of the original embryo. These results suggest that the dorsoventral determination of the embryo may depend directly on the form of the cleavage and on the nature of the cell contacts which develop between individual cells. Such a conclusion also emerged from a detailed study of the evolution of external and internal cell contacts as observed during the normal development of *Lymnaea*[23] and *Patella*[24]. In both cases, a dramatic change was noticed to occur during the period of mitotic inactivity which followed the formation of the 3rd quartet of micromeres, i.e. after the 24-cell stage in *Lymnaea* and the 32-cell stage in *Patella*. Briefly, the two vegetal cross-furrow macromeres 3 B and 3 D tended to contact the first quartet cells up to a stage when only one of these vegetal cells maintained this contact. From that moment, it may be thus defined, for the first time, as the true dorsal 3 D cell. It is indeed this internal blastomere which will give rise to the mesentoblast 4 d; i.e. the mother cell for the right and left mesodermic bands. In *Lymnaea*, this internal 3 D macromere is the first macromere to divide next whereas, in *Patella*, it cleaves about 18 minutes after the three other simultaneously dividing macromeres 3 A, 3 B and 3 C.

The experiments we performed on the embryo of *Patella*[25] definitively demonstrated that the determination of that 3 D cell and, thus, that mesoderm differentiation is not included in the original structure of the egg but that it rather results from an essentially arbitrary although unescapable choice effected through contact with the micromeres. This follows from two main types of experiments which included either a deletion of the first quartet cells or the selective destruction of one of the vegetal cross-furrow macromeres 3 B or 3 D. In the first case, the maximal delay observed in the cleavage of the macromeres amounted for less than 5 minutes (versus the 18 minutes usually observed in normal conditions) and no mesentoblast could develop. By deleting a decreasing number of first quartet cells, an increasing percentage of embryos was able to differentiate normally. It is worth to notice, moreover, that the deletion of two adjacent micromeres seems to favour a situation where not only cross-furrow macromeres but also non cross-furrow macromeres (A or C) may function as the pivot cell whose cleavage is retarded.

Results from the second crucial test, which has been performed on 24 embryos, were even more conclusive since they showed that the remaining cross-furrow macromere or one of the two lateral macromere was able to form a normal mesentoblast cell in 92% of the cases. The remaining 8% corresponded to embryos where no macromere could enter the cell mass, which resulted in the absence of mesoderm differentiation.

It is thus clear that any one of the vegetal macromeres has the same developmental potencies and that a differentiation as important as that which will lead to mesoderm differentiation cannot be accounted for on the basis of a mosaic network. In this new model, it appears that the cell membrane structure continues to play a major role in cell differentiation. However, it does not exert its influence by maintaining preformed regional differencies but rather acts as a dynamic relay which may recognize, transfer and amplify various signals. Translated in the competent cells, these signals may be further active either in controlling nuclear functions or in regulating cellular mechanisms at a post-transcriptional or posttranslational level.

REFERENCES

1. Raven, C.P. (1963) Develop. Biol., 7, 130-143.

2. Clement, C.A. (1962) J. Exp. Zool., 149, 193-216.

3. Cather, J.N. (1967) J. Exp. Zool., 166, 205-224.

4. Raven, C.P. (1974) J. Embryol. Exp. Morphol., 31, 37-59.

5. Guerrier, P. (1971) Année Biol., 10, 152-192.

6. Guerrier, P. (1970) J. Embryol. Exp. Morphol., 23, 667-692.

7. Hatt, P.(1932) Arch. Anat. Microsc., 28, 81-98.

8. Novikoff, A.B. (1938) Biol. Bull., 74, 211-234.

9. Rattenbury, J.C. and Berg, W.E. (1954) J. Morphol., 95, 393-414.

10. Clement, C.A. (1952) J. Exp. Zool., 121, 593-626.

11. Dongen, C.A.M. van and GEILENKIRCHEN, W.L.M. (1975) Proc. Kon. Ned. Akad. Wetensch., Ser C 78, 358-375.

12. Dongen, C.A.M. van (1976) Proc. Kon. Ned. Akad. Wetensch., Ser C 79, 245-266.

13. Wilson, E.B. (1904) J. Exp. Zool., 1, 1-74.

14. Verdonk, N.H. (1968) J. Embryol. Exp. Morphol., 20, 101-105.

15. Guerrier, P. (1970) J. Embryol. Exp. Morphol., 23, 639-665.

16. Guerrier, P., Biggelaar, J.A.M. van den, Dongen, C.A.M. van and Verdonk,N.H. (1978) Develop. Biol., 63, 233-242.

17. Cather, J.N. (1973) Malacologia, 13, 213-223.

18. Guerrier, P. (1968) Ann. Embryol. Morphog., 1, 119-139.

19. Guerrier, P. (1970) J. Embryol. Exm. Morphol., 23, 611-637.

20. Guerrier, P. (1970) Ann. Embryol. Morphog., 3, 283-294.

21. Morrill, J.B., Blair, C.A. and Larsen, W.J. (1973) J. Exp. Zool., 183, 47-56.

22. Verdonk, N.H., Unpublished results.

23. Biggelaar, J.A.M. van den (1976) Proc. Kon. Ned. Akad. Wetensch., Ser C 79, 113-126.

24. Biggelaar, J.A.M. van den (1977) J. Morphol., 154, 157-186.

25. Biggelaar, J.A.M. van den and Guerrier, P. (1979) Develop. Biol., 68, 462-471.

Cell Lineage, Stem Cells and Cell Determination
INSERM Symposium No. 10
Editor: N. Le Douarin
© *1979 Elsevier/North-Holland Biomedical Press*

ANALYSIS OF CELL BEHAVIOUR IN THE PREIMPLANTATION MOUSE LINEAGE

C.F. GRAHAM AND E. LEHTONEN*

Zoology Department, South Parks Road, Oxford OX1 3PS, Great Britain.

* Present address, Department of Pathology, University of Helsinki,
  Haartmaninkatu 3, SF-00290 Helsinki 29, Finland.

INTRODUCTION

The aim of this article is to review recent studies on the cell lineage of
the preimplantation mouse embryo and then to assess the cellular and molecular
mechanisms which may control the lineage. There are several reasons for being
interested in this cell lineage. First it appears to depend on cell interactions from the 2-cell stage onwards. Second, the cell lineage is the normal
device by which cells reach different relative positions, and third these
relative positions appear to be important in initiating the formation of the
inner cell mass cells which both express different genes to those synthesized
by the outside cell layer in the blastocyst (the trophectoderm) and which
eventually form all the tissues of the embryo (recently reviewed)[1,2,3]. There
are also several reasons for being disinterested in the cell lineage. First,
it does not matter very much how cells eventually move to different relative
positions for the embryologist can intervene, change their relative positions
and development will still proceed to completion. Second, half the cytoplasm of
the embryo may be removed or two or three embryos added together and the embryology still works (e.g.[4,5,6]); it is clear that parts or combinations of embryos
can self organize into a single complete body and that the "normalcy" of
undisturbed development is irrelevant to the basic processes involved in making
a mouse.

There remains, however, a fascination for studying how a biological system
usually proceeds. Cell lineage must be the consequence of selection and it is
perhaps unfortunate that our work has concentrated on inbred mice which have
lived in laboratory conditions for twenty or more years. In many ways the
lineage of the wild mouse would be more interesting for it would show the
lineage with the greatest selective advantage and this, like the cleavage planes
of planarians, might change with the seasons of the year[7].

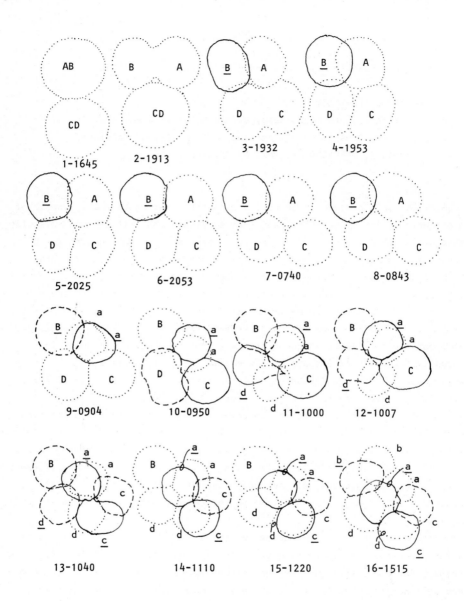

1-1645 2-1913 3-1932 4-1953

5-2025 6-2053 7-0740 8-0843

9-0904 10-0950 11-1000 12-1007

13-1040 14-1110 15-1220 16-1515

ORDERED PREIMPLANTATION DEVELOPMENT

The preimplantation development of the mouse occurs in the first four and a half days after fertilization. During this time about 120 cells are formed and about two thirds of these are in the outside trophectoderm layer while the other third are grouped in a central inner cell mass[8,9,10]. This blastocyst structure is asymmetric and hollow with a blastocoel at the opposite end to the inner cell mass; the blastocoel starts to form when the embryo contains between twenty and thirty cells[11] and when the outside cells are linked by focal tight junctions[12,13].

During preimplantation development, there is little cell migration or intermingling. Direct observation of development from the 2-cell to the 8-cell stage has shown that the daughter cells at both divisions remain beside each other and consequently each clone remains coherent[14] (Figs. 1-16). This coherence has also been shown during development from the 8-cell stage in two types of experiment. First whole embryos have been labelled with tritiated thymidine and each recombined with an unlabelled embryo to form a chimaera[15,16], and second, individual embryos have been disrupted into single cells, one of

---

Cell lineages on the second and third day of development

Tracings from photographs of a single zona free embryo. The drawing conventions are that cells with dotted outlines are away from the reader (on the bottom of the culture dish), those with continuous outlines are towards the reader, and those circumscribed by a broken line are in between. Cells at the 4-cell stage are marked with capitals and those at the 8-cell stage with lower case letters; in either case the cell letter is in or close to the periphery of the cell it nominates. An underlined letter indicates that it marks a cell close to the reader.

Figures 1-4. Division to the 4-cellstage. Note how both cells elongate and narrow as they divide. The cells are arranged as a rhomboid.

Figures 4-8. The 4-cell stage. Note that the maximum extent of cell contact is established soon after division and that there is little relative cell movement until cell A reduces cell contact as it starts to divide.

Figures 8-12. The 5-cell to 6-cell stages. Note that cell A has elongated towards the reader and as it narrows so B and C are drawn together. Cell D divides similarly and has the same effect on relative cell position.

Figures 12-16. The 6-cell to 8-cell stages. Note that the last two cells to divide to the 8-cell stage (B and C) are excluded from the centre of the embryo by the daughters of the early dividing A and D which pack against each other. Consequently the daughters of A and D lie deep in the structure of the 8-cell cell stage; they make many contacts with other cells on the surface of the embryo (5,6 and 4,4 cell contacts respectively). In contrast the daughters of the last two cells to divide to the 8-cell cell stage are more superficial and have fewer cell contacts (B daughters have 4 and 2 contacts while C daughters have 4 and 3 contacts).

the cells labelled, and each embryo rebuilt[17,18]. In both situations the
clones of labelled cells remained together and labelled cells were only
separated from each other when the blastocoel formed between them.

During preimplantation development, there is no major reorganization of the
cytoplasm which can be detected. The experiments which favour this view are
those of Wilson et al.[19] who injected oil droplets beneath that part of the
cell membrane which is away from the centre of the embryo at the 2-cell, 4-cell,
8-cell, and 16-cell stages. In each case the oil droplets segregated into the
outside trophectoderm layer of the blastocyst; this experiment and result has
been repeated[14].

It would then be reasonable to suppose that the ordered division of the
zygote was no more than the expression of some masterplan, however vague
(prepattern), in the egg. Here we will argue the view that the special
properties of this zygote are principally those of being able to form other
cells which have the capacity to interact with each other; this zygote sets
development in motion but it does not appear to anticipate the organization of
the early embryo.

TENDENCIES IN THE CELL LINEAGE

The cell lineage of early preimplantation development does not follow a
fixed pattern and varies from one embryo to another within the same inbred
strain[14]. For this reason, tendencies and regularities common to different
cell lineages are discussed in this section.

The daughter cells of each division do not have equal opportunity

Each parental cell forms two daughter cells whose relationship with other
cells in the embryos usually differs. In most cases only one of these daughters
maintains the cell contact relationships of the parental cell while the other
is formed away from the visual centre of the embryo and is placed superficially.
This process occurs at the 2-cell to 4-cell stage division; see for instance
that the zona free 4-cell stage illustrated in Figs. 1-16 has two superficial
cells, B and C. It occurs again during division to the 8-cell stage, where in
the 80 cases studied, one daughter cell maintained the contacts of the parental
cell in all except eight cases, while the other daughter cell was formed
superficially and rarely maintained the contact relationships of the parental
cells (11/80 cases)[14]. This discrepancy in the relative position of the
daughter cells of each mitosis also occurs again at the 8-cell to 16-cell stage
division (see later)[14]. Clearly the direction of mitosis and the unequal
disposition of the progeny of each division with respect to the main bulk of

the embryo is a regular tendency in the lineage.

The first shall be first and the last shall be last

For a long time it has been known that cells at the 2-cell stage rarely divide synchronously to the 4-cell stage and it seemed likely that those which reached the 4-cell stage first also divided first to the 8-cell stage[20,21]. These impressions have been confirmed with continuous recording techniques and by studying large numbers of embryos. In fact in batches of eggs studied with cinematic[22] or video equipment (personal observations) only one in twenty or so 2-cell stages show division of both cells within one minute of each other to the 4-cell stage; the other embryos clearly show asynchronous division and on average there is a 40-60 mins interval between the division of the first and the last divider[18]. During the subsequent development of the embryo up to the blastocyst stage, the first divider to the 4-cell stage also tends to divide ahead of its slower neighbour at all subsequent rounds of division; this has been shown by observing divisions in the intact embryo up to the 8-cell stage and by dissociating 2-cell embryos and counting the time of division of the descendants of the first and last dividers at the 4- to 8-cell, 8- to 16-cell, 16- to 32-cell, and 32- to 64-cell stages[18].

The first shall be deeper and the last shall be more superficial

After the 2- to 4-cell division in either zona enclosed or zona free embryos it is noticeable that one daughter of the last cell to divide does not push tightly into the structure of the embryo; the impression is difficult to quantify (see Figs. 1-8). However, soon after the start of the 8-cell stage it is apparent that the first cells to reach the 8-cell stage tend to lie deep in its structure. In this case it is possible to put numbers to this arrangement for deep cells touch several other cells (usually five or more) while superficial cells are exposed on the surface of the embryo and usually touch four or less other cells (note that these cell contacts are contacts on the surface of the embryo). Taking the daughters of the first cell to reach the 4-cell stage, then the first of these to divide to the 8-cell stage always has a significantly greater number of cell contacts than the last to reach this stage. Similarly the first daughters to reach the 8-cell stage from the descendants of the last cell to divide from the 2-cell stage, tend to have a greater number of cell contacts than their slower partners[14] (see Figs. 9-16).

This process of internalization of fast dividers continues into the development of the blastocyst. In these next experiments there was some disruption of normal development for embryos were dissociated at the 4-cell stage, the first or last divider to the 8-cell stage labelled with tritiated thymidine, and the embryo rebuilt. These combinations developed to the blastocyst stage and sectioning, reconstruction, and autoradiography showed that the descendants of the fast dividers had contributed significantly more cells to the inner cell mass than had the descendants of the last dividers[18].

The deep shall tend towards inner cell mass and the superficial shall tend towards trophectoderm.

At the 8-cell stage there are rarely any completely enclosed cells in the embryo while in the 16-cell stage embryos there are usually two. Disruption and reassociation experiments suggest that these internal cells will principally contribute to the inner cell mass while the superficial cells will usually form trophectoderm[23,24]. In the intact embryo, there is considerable regularity in contribution of descendants from the 8-cell to the blastocyst. It seems likely that every cell of the 8-cell stage forms at least one trophectoderm cell for nearly every oil droplet placed beneath the exterior membrane of 8-cell stage cells has eventually been found in the trophectoderm layer[14,19]. Contrast this behaviour with the segregation of oil droplets placed beneath that part of the cell membrane which is near the centre of the embryo; when such drops are placed in deep cells with five or more cell contacts then they are usually found in the inner cell mass of the blastocysts which develop, while if they are placed in superficial cells with four or less cell contacts then they most frequently segregate to the trophectoderm. It is clear that deep cells contribute at least one daughter cell to the inner cell mass. Since most embryos have about four deep cells at the 8-cell stage and only two enclosed cells at the 16-cell stage it follows that at least some inner cell mass cells reach the interior of the developing embryo after the 16-cell stage[9,14].

ANALYSIS OF THE LINEAGE

We next analyse the behaviour of isolated single cells and of isolated groups of two and four cells at different stages of development to find out if alterations in simple cellular properties could account for the tendencies and regularities which have been noticed within the cell lineage.

Directional Mitosis depends on cell interactions

Cells elongate as they divide and consequently their shape changes and they can establish new cell contacts at each division. This change in form of cells has been studied with time lapse video equipment and the cells were isolated from 1-cell, 2-cell, 4-cell, and 8-cell stages[25]; after each division the maximum elongation amounted to a 53 to 61% increase in one diameter of the

original parental cell (Figs. 1-16). Mitosis and the subsequent arrangement of
the daughter cells is therefore directional. Notice how cell narrowing at
mitosis can alter cell arrangements (Figs. 8-12).

Studies have been conducted on two stages of development to observe the
mechanisms which might be invloved in controlling the direction of mitosis.
These studies are still incomplete but they do show that the direction of
mitosis is controlled by cell contacts. First the 2- to 4-cell stage division
was observed in zona free embryos and it was found that the contact between
the daughters of the first cell to divide and its undivided slower partner, was
related to the mitotic direction of the slower cell. With this association
established, it could further be shown that when embryos were dissociated at
the 2-cell stage and recombined, then the direction of mitosis of the slower
cell was still related to its contacts with the daughters of the fast divider.
It follows that brief cell contacts established after recombination must
control the direction of mitosis of the slower cell[26].

Second the division from the 8-cell to the 16-cell stages was studied
because it is at the 16-cell stage that enclosed cells are usually formed for
the first time. Unfortunately it was not possible to make these observations
on intact embryos because cell overlap obscures cell outlines, and it was
necessary to partially dissociate the 8-cell stage embryos into two groups of
four cells lying flattened in a microdrop. In these four cell groups, those
cells lying deep in the structure and making a cell contact near its centre
usually formed the one enclosed cell in the eight cell cluster which developed
after all the cells in the original group had divided. In nearly all cases the
first deep cell to divide formed the enclosed cell. Once again it could be
shown that the direction of mitosis was controlled by cell contacts, because
exactly the same relationship occurred when 8-cell stage embryos were completely
dissociated and then recombined into new four cell groups just before
division[26].

These studies on the relationship between the direction of mitosis and cell
contacts demonstrate that the lineage of the preimplantation mouse embryo
depends on a series of cell interactions.

The Change in Cellular Dimensions During Division to the 16-cell Stage

The changes in cellular dimensions during cleavage to the 16-cell stage have
been studied to see if their alteration can account for the development of the
form of the preimplantation embryo. The dimensions of cells have been measured
by isolating cells from the embryo after each division and following their
appearance with time lapse video equipment as they proceed through one cell

division in culture[25].

From the late 2-cell stage to the early 16-cell stage the total cellular volume of the embryo does not change significantly and consequently cellular volume is approximately halved at each cell division and average cell diameter is reduced from 53 μm at the 2-cell stage to 27 μm at the 16-cell stage. The most noticeable change in cellular form is seen in the relationship between the two daughter cells of each division. When isolated cells from the 2-cell stage divide then they usually establish contact with each other, but the extent of this contact never exceeds 35% of the average diameter of the two daughter cells. In contrast, when isolated cells from the 8-cell stage divide, then an extensive cell contact is rapidly established between the two daughter cells; this cell contact is usually 99% of the diameter of the two daughter cells and the form of the pair of daughter cells is nearly spherical. It is probable that these changes in the extent of contact between the daughter cells of each division also occur in the extent of contact between all the cells of the embryo and if this assumption is correct then the change in this dimension can account for the loose packed appearance of 2- and 4-cell stage embryos and the compacted form of the late 8-cell and 16-cell stages. Certainly the relative positions of cells can change as a consequence of a change in this dimension (Figs. 1-16).

It is not a simple matter to discover how the extent of cell contact is controlled. The two daughters of cells isolated from the 2-cell stage establish new maximum contact (average 14.5 μm) soon after division while the contact diameter between the daughters of cells isolated from 4- and 8-cell stage embryos increases progressively during the early part of the cell cycle; the rate of increase in contact slows down respectively at 7 to 8 hours after division and at two to three hours after division and plateaus for the rest of the cell cycle until cells loosen up just before division.

We have considered several possible explanations of this behaviour. First it was possible that the principal organelles involved in drawing the cells together were microvilli. Microvilli in early mouse embryos contain actin-like structures which may be contractile[27] and if the number of microvilli was related to the movement of the two daughter cells together then their density on the cell surface should alter at different stages of cleavage. In scanning electron microscopy it is difficult to obtain accurate counts of the density of microvilli at the junction between the two daughter cells and counts of microvillar density were therefore made on the exposed surface of the interacting cells away from the points of cell contact. These counts show that the density of microvilli are similar at the late 4-cell stage and late 8-cell stage and that although microvillar density drops for about 2 hours after division from the 4- to 8-cell stages it soon returns to a steady level for the rest of the cell cycle (Lehtonen, unpublished). It is clear from these preliminary observations that microvillar density by itself does not account for the extent of contact between the daughter cells of each division for the average maximum contact line between two 4-cell stage cells is 14.5 μm and that between two 8-cell stage cells is 35.9 μm.

Second it was possible that the extent of cell contact was controlled by the number of adhesive molecules on the cell surface. Again this seems an unlikely explanation of our results for we have preliminary evidence that the extent of contact between two daughter cells is not greatly reduced if one of the two daughters is sticking to another cell.

Lastly it is likely that a whole range of cell functions are involved in controlling the extent of cell contact. These may include the deformability of the cell cortex near the contact line where it curves sharply, internal pressure in the cells flattening against each other, and the general organization of the cytoskeleton.

CONSEQUENCES OF DIRECTIONAL MITOSIS AND CYCLE DEPENDENT CELL CONTACT

Although the molecular control of mitotic direction and cell contact extent is not understood, certain features of the cell lineage follow directly from these two phenomena.

Mitotic direction and segregation

At the second, third, and fourth division of the zygote it has been shown that one daughter of each divider tends to maintain the contacts of the parental cell while the other does not and is formed towards the periphery of the embryonic structure. This phenomenon is probably responsible for the segregation of oil drop placed in interior and superficial cytoplasm of 2-cell and 4-cell stage embryos[19]. The control of this unequal allocation of daughter cells has been shown to depend on cell interactions.

Cycle dependent extent of cell contact and internalization

There is a tendency in the lineage for descendants of fast dividers from the 2-cell stage to lie deep in the structure of the embryo and to eventually internalize and contribute disproportionately more cells to the inner cell mass. Now the descendants of fast 2-cell stage dividers tend to be ahead at all

subsequent rounds of division and consequently, at the start of each interphase, these descendants will have extended cell contacts with each other;
these contacts will be longer than those between the descendants of the slower
cell at the 2-cell stage which will tend to be behind in cell cycle. This
difference will tend to curve the form of the embryo around the fast
descendants which start to internalize (Figs. 8-16). However, this curvature
and internalization would not be maintained if all the cells in the embryo
behaved as they do when isolated from each other; for instance, after the first
two-thirds of the 8-cell stage cycle, maximum contact between the daughter
cells of cells isolated from 4-cell stage embryos is achieved and this allows
ample time for any cell cycle differences in the extent of contact to equalize
out towards the end of each cycle. And so we must also assume that in addition
to cycle dependent cell contact there must also be other mechanisms operating
in the intact embryo which "freeze" its form after the descendants of fast
dividers reach maximum contact.

CONCLUSION

This analysis has attempted to identify the cellular properties and interactions which are responsible for the normal preimplantation mouse lineage; they
appear to underlie the processes by which cells start to become different from
each other in normal development.

ACKNOWLEDGEMENTS

We thank the MRC for research grants and EMBO for providing a Research
Fellowship (E.L.)

REFERENCES

1. Gardner, R.L. (1978) Results and Problems in Cell Differentiation,
   Volume 9, Ed. W.J. Gehring, Springer-Verlag, Berlin, Heidelberg, pp. 205-241.

2. Johnson, M.H. (1979) J. Reprod. Fert., 55, 255-265.

3. Papaioannou, V.E., Rossant, J. and Gardner, R.L. (1978) Stem Cells and
   Tissue Homeostasis, Ed. B.I. Lord, C.S. Potten, and R.J. Cole, Cambridge
   University Press, pp. 49-69.

4. Tarkowski, A.K. (1977) J. Embryol. exp. Morph. 38, 187-202.

5. Mintz, B. (1964) J. Exp. Zool. 157, 273-292.

6. Markert, C.L. and Peters, R.M. (1978) Science, N.Y., 202, 56-58.

7. Skaer, R.J. (1971) Experimental Embryology of Marine and Fresh-water
   Invertebrates, Ed. G. Reverberi, North Holland, Amsterdam, pp. 104-125.

8. Bowman, P. and McLaren, A. (1970) J. Embryol. exp. Morph. 24, 203-210.

9. Barlow, P., Owen, D.A.J., and Graham, C.F. (1972) J. Embryol. exp. Morph.
   27, 431-445.

10. Copp, A.J. (1978) J. Embryol. exp. Morph. 48, 109-125.

11. Smith, R. and McLaren, A. (1977) J. Embryol. exp. Morph. 41, 79-92.

12. Ducibella, T., Albertini, D.F., Anderson, E. and Biggers, J.D. (1975) Develop. Biol. 45, 231-250.

13. Magnuson, T., Jacobson, J.B. and Stackpole, C.W. (1978) Develop. Biol. 67, 214-224.

14. Graham, C.F. and Deussen, Z.A. (1978) J. Embryol. exp. Morph. 48, 53-72.

15. Garner, W. and McLaren, A. (1974) J. Embryol. exp. Morph. 32, 495-503.

16. Mintz, B. (1974) Preimplantation Stages of Pregnancy, Eds. G.E.W. Wolstenholme and M. O'Connor, Churchill, London, pp. 194-207.

17. Kelly, S.J. (1979) J. Exp. Zool. 207, 121-130.

18. Kelly, S.J., Mulnard, J.G. and Graham, C.F. (1978) J. Embryol. exp. Morph. 48, 37-51.

19. Wilson, I.B., Bolton, E. and Cuttler, R.H. (1972) J. Embryol. exp. Morph. 27, 467-479.

20. Lewis, W.H. and Wright, E.S. (1972) Contrib. Embryol. Carnegie Instn. 148, 115-143.

21. Borghese, E. and Cassini, A. (1963) Cinemicrography in Cell Biology, Ed. G.G. Rose, Academic Press, New York, pp. 263-277.

22. Mulnard, J.G. (1967) Archs. Biol. (Liège), 78, 107-138.

23. Hillman, N., Sherman, M.I. and Graham, C.F. (1972) J. Embryol. exp. Morph. 28, 263-278.

24. Kelly, S.J. (1977) J. Exp. Zool. 200, 365-376.

25. Lehtonen, E. (1979) Unpublished observations.

26. Graham, C.F. and Lehtonen, E. (1979) J. Embryol. exp. Morph. 49, 277-294.

27. Ducibella, T., Ukena, T., Karnovsky, M. and Anderson, E. (1977) J. Cell Biol. 66, 568-576.

Cell Lineage, Stem Cells and Cell Determination
INSERM Symposium No. 10
Editor: N. Le Douarin
© *1979 Elsevier/North-Holland Biomedical Press*

CELL LINEAGES OF THE WILD TYPE AND OF TEMPERATURE-SENSITIVE EMBRYONIC ARREST
MUTANTS OF <u>CAENORHABDITIS</u> <u>ELEGANS</u>

GUNTER von EHRENSTEIN, EINHARD SCHIERENBERG, and JOHJI MIWA
Department of Molecular Biology, Max-Planck-Institute for Experimental
Medicine, 3400 Göttingen (Federal Republic of Germany)

INTRODUCTION

<u>Caenorhabditis</u> <u>elegans</u>, a free-living nematode, is the subject of intensive
genetic and developmental studies[1,2].

Embryogenesis in <u>C</u>. <u>elegans</u>, like other nematodes, is strictly determinate
and virtually invariant among individuals[3]. The newly hatched juvenile has only
about 550 cells arranged quite predictably[4]. Postembryonic development is also
quite regular and the number of nongonadal cells increases to only about 810
in the adult hermaphrodite[4].

Here we will summarize results of embryonic cell lineage studies in our
laboratory including the wild type and temperature-sensitive embryonic arrest
mutants. We will also compare the developmental mechanisms of <u>C</u>. <u>elegans</u> to
those of higher animals, and speculate about the possible role of histones in
the timing of cell divisions in embryogenesis.

<u>Methodology</u>. Embryonic cell lineages in <u>C</u>. <u>elegans</u> are determined by tra-
cing the times and the directions of the divisions and migrations of individual
cells continuously in living embryos using Nomarski differential interference
contrast microscopy and high resolution video recording[3]. The light microscopic
observations are combined with the detailed analysis of the cellular anatomy of
embryos reconstructed in three dimensions from serial-section electronmicro-
graphs with a computer system[5].

EMBRYONIC CELL LINEAGES OF THE WILD TYPE

<u>Time is measured in developmental events</u>. Embryogenesis in <u>C</u>. <u>elegans</u> can
be described in a general way using easily identifiable developmental events
to stage embryos, thus, counting "developmental time", not by time units, but
directly by developmental events, for example, by cell stages.

<u>Two developmental phases: proliferation and morphogenesis</u>. The first half
of embryogenesis involves cell divisions from one to more than 500 cells with
considerable rearrangement of cells. At the end of the proliferation phase,

the embryo has already reached its final number of about 550 essentially undifferentiated cells.

Organ formation and terminal differentiation of cells occur in the second half of embryogenesis. During the morphogenesis phase, the ball-shaped embryo takes form as an animal with fully differentiated tissues and organs without additional cell division. Morphogenesis begins with a ventral indentation in the posterior third of the embryo: "lima bean" stage, during its gradual elongation, the embryo passes through a "comma", "tadpole", "plum", and "loop" stage, shaping into a worm rolled up in the egg: "pretzel" stage[5,6].

Stem cells and cell lineages. By an invariant pattern of cleavage divisions, six stem cells, AB, MSt, E, C, D, and P_4, are generated. These stem cells are the founders of six cell lines. These give rise to: anterior ectoderm, anterior mesoderm, endoderm, posterior ectoderm, posterior mesoderm, and gonad primordium, respectively[6,7,8].

The stem cells arise by asymmetric divisions from the germ line in a typical stem cell pattern[3]. In these divisions, the smaller daughter is the precursor of the germ line.

In C. elegans embryogenesis, a stem cell is defined as one whose descendants arise by a series of synchronous and symmetrical divisions. This type of division pattern, generating new cells of one type, is different from the stem cell pattern. To date, the lineages of 232 embryonic cells have been determined[3,6,7].

Autonomous cell cycle clocks and rounds of cell division. Each cell line has its own clock, i.e., a specific autonomous rhythm of essentially synchronous cell divisions[3]. The rhythms are maintained in spite of extensive cellular rearrangement. Rounds of cell divisions are initiated periodically, each round starting with the AB cell line.

Preprogramming of the egg involves the cell cycle clocks. The site of origin of the stem cells in the egg relates to the setting of the rhythm of the cell cycle, suggesting intracellular preprogramming of the egg involving at least the rates of the autonomous cell cycle clocks[3].

The final number of cells and their destiny depends on the lineage history. The rates and orientations of the cell divisions are essentially invariant, and each stem cell gives rise to a predetermined number of cells. The state of determination, at least the length and the number of cell division cycles, is inherited by all the offspring of a given stem cell[3]. Thus, the destiny of cells seems to depend primarily on their lineage history.

The sequence of developmental events is rigidly ordered. Gastrulation is defined as the migration of the two E-cell descendants, the precursor cells for the intestine, into the interior of the embryo[3]. The E-cells start their migration invariably at the 26-cell stage, they complete migration at the 44-cell stage, and divide invariably after migration[6,7]. Thus, the timing (relative to cell stage) and, therefore, the order of the events migration and division is rigidly determined. Other divisions and migrations are also strictly ordered.

Decisions about migration and their execution are separated in time. Bilateral symmetry in C. elegans is established in the case of the MSt, C, and D cell lines by equivalent cells migrating to matched left-right positions[6,7,9]. The decision to migrate or not is segregated to the daughter cells in the first division of the three stem cells and executed three (for C and MSt) and two (for D) cell divisions later. Thus, the decision about cell migration and its execution are separated in time, and a binary state of determination is inherited through several divisions by all descendants. The paths and extents of these cell migrations are rigidly determined including reproducible starting and stopping sites.

CELL LINEAGES OF MUTANTS

Temperature-sensitive mutants causing embryonic arrest in C. elegans have been isolated and characterized[10,11,12]. Eleven mutants have recently been characterized in detail in our laboratory including determination of early cell lineages and developmental defects[13,14].

Mapping of embryonic arrest mutants. The eleven mutations define nine genes (emb-1 - emb-9). Eight mutations, tentatively assigned to six separate genes on the basis of complementation tests, map close to one another on chromosome III. The other three genes map on three different chromosomes.

The function of six genes seems to be required exclusively for embryogenesis. Mutants in these genes have no other detectable phenotype at the permissive (16°) or non-permissive (25°) temperature. The function of the other three genes is also required for postembryonic development.

The egg is preprogrammed by the action of maternal genes. Progeny tests for parental effects on embryogenesis define 5 classes of mutants[12]. The eleven mutants belong to three of these classes[13]. For seven genes, maternal gene expression is necessary and sufficient for normal embryogenesis (GM class); for one gene, emb-2, either maternal or zygotic expression is sufficient (GZ class); for one gene, emb-9, zygotic expression is necessary and sufficient (ZZ class). The high proportion of embryonic arrest mutants with maternal gene

expression in C. elegans indicates that much of embryonic development is
preprogrammed in the egg by the action of maternal genes.

Irreversible defects are generated in mutant embryos at the non-permissive
temperature. Temperature-shift experiments indicate the developmental stages
at which mutant embryos are irreversibly affected. Two stages have been
defined[13]: (1) the normal execution stage indicating the irreversible
execution of the normal event at 16°; (2) the defective execution stage
indicating the execution of an irreversible defect at 25°.

The function of the wild-type alleles of the emb genes is required for
specific stages of development, and the strict maternal (GM) class has been
subdivided into genes executing their function before fertilization and into
genes executing after fertilization[13].

Arrested embryos of many mutants are monsters. The mutants are also classified by the stage of arrest at 25°. Mutants in three genes stop at different
stages during the proliferation phase, and the only zygotic mutant stops late
in morphogenesis. Six mutants in five genes complete proliferation and stop at
the beginning of the morphogenesis phase (around the 550 cell lima bean stage:
"lima bean stoppers") with a grossly abnormal terminal phenotype.

Some mutants stop developing close to the defective execution stage,
whereas the lima bean stoppers continue developing after an irreversible early
defect. They apparently exit from the normal sequence of developmental events,
continue cell division, and arrest much later as monstrous lima beans. Thus,
the periodic cell lineage clocks[3] continue to run, in spite of irreversible
defects.

Mutants in maternal genes affect the timing of cell divisions in cleavage.
Cell lineages and development to the 50-cell stage at 16° and 25° have been
determined in the mutants in the emb genes[14]. All but the single zygotic
mutant have visible defects before the 50-cell stage, even if they arrest much
later.

The cleavage pattern and the generation of stem cells are essentially normal
in the mutants studied, but the timing of the cleavage divisions is altered in
many mutants. The overall rate of all cell divisions is faster than in the
wild type in mutants in two genes, (GM class), and slower in mutants in five
genes, (4 GM; 1 GZ). In mutants in four of these genes, the relative rate
of division of specific stem cell lines is altered. Thus, programming of
the egg by maternal genes involves the timing of cell divisions in cleavage.

A timing defect leads to an abnormal cell pattern. The division rhythm of
the E-cell line is too fast relative to that of the other cell lines in both

mutants in gene _emb-5_. The timing defect leads to an abnormal cell pattern in the 4-E cell intestinal primordium, presumably because E-cell division occurs before migration at gastrulation. This reversal closely coincides with the independently determined _defective execution stage_. The temporal coincidence indicates that the observed defect might be responsible for the later death of the embryo. Thus, timing seems to be involved in establishing regional differences in the development of _C. elegans_.

DISCUSSION

Caenorhabditis elegans, a model for animal development

The complete cell by cell description of the development of an animal is possible. Beginning with the egg, the lineage of 232 of the 550 embryonic cells of _Caenorhabditis elegans_ has been determined[3,6,7], and the development of the animal until hatching has been described at the level of cell groups and tissues[5,6,7,8]. Other workers have determined the complete lineages of the 260 postembryonic non-gonadal cells[4] and of the 143 cells of the somatic structures of the gonad[15]. In principle, it is possible to determine the lineages of all embryonic cells, to follow these cells through organ formation, and to provide a complete cell by cell description of the development of an animal from egg to adulthood.

C. elegans has very favorable genetics[1] and the cellular phenotype of embryonic arrest mutants can be analyzed in great detail[14]. Recombinant DNA and related technologies including restriction analysis[16] and gene cloning[17] are being applied to _C. elegans_. Thus, a genetic, biochemical, and cellular approach can be combined in _Caenorhabditis elegans_ to help clarify the molecular basis of cell behavior in development.

C. elegans development compared to higher animals

Many of the fundamental mechanisms of development operating in _C. elegans_ are common to higher animals as well. These include instances of regulation in _C. elegans_, common lineage patterns, and the segregation and maintenance of developmental decisions.

Regulative vs. mosaic development. The embryos of many animals have regulative properties, i.e., they develop normally regardless of absolute cell number or of the removal of part of the cells at an early stage. The developmental fate of a cell depends on its position within the multicellular assembly and the regenerative capacity of cell groups depends on their relative positions within the organism.

But also in mammalian cells, self-renewal appears to be indefinite only following malignant transformation; the capacity for proliferation of normal cells is limited. Diploid cells in culture are capable of only about 50 doublings[18]. In vivo, hemopoietic tissue can be transplanted successfully for only a limited number of transfer generations[19].

Nematodes, including C. elegans, have very limited regulative and regenerative capacity, providing a classic example of mosaic development. Compensatory cell divisions are virtually absent and the capacity of cells to divide is limited and tightly controlled.

On the other hand, in C. elegans, there are instances of positional influences, where the decision of a cell to divide or not depends on external signals. Particularly in the postembryonic development of the accessory sexual structures[4] and in gonad development[15], the developmental fate of some cells depends on their position in one of two alternative cellular configurations, but their subsequent division programs are again rigidly determined. Thus, as in mammalian myogenic and chondrogenic lineages[20], external positional signals (in C. elegans, for example, from the gonad[4]) simply permit a cell to express one of its predetermined, inherited developmental options, but external signals apparently do not determine the options.

Thus, there may not be a fundamental difference between the regulative and the mosaic modes of development. The apparent difference may only be quantitative, depending on the number of cells in an animal.

Two fundamental lineage patterns. Two basic types of lineage pattern have been observed in C. elegans development[3,4,15]. A stem cell pattern of asymmetric divisions generates two different cells, one daughter identical to the mother cell in morphology and developmental fate, and the other daughter of a new type. Alternatively, apparently symmetrical divisions generate daughter cells of equivalent morphology and, often, of equivalent developmental fate. All cell lineages in C. elegans may be viewed as combinations or modifications of the two basic patterns.

Symmetrical cell divisions (also termed amplifying or proliferation divisions) and asymmetrical stem cell divisions have been described in several mammalian tissues including human[20,21]. The two fundamental mechanisms for segregating developmental potential may be common to all animals.

Developmental decisions are binary and the state of determination is inherited in cell division. In C. elegans embryogenesis, developmental decisions (for example, positional decisions involving cell migration[9]) are segregated at particular cell divisions, and a binary state of determination is inherited through several cell generations by all descendants. Thus, the behavior of cells in C. elegans development follows a binary pattern.

Similarly, determination of mammalian cells[20] and transdetermination of imaginal disc cells of Drosophila[22] are strictly dependent on cell division. In both systems, the capacity to differentiate, i.e., to express the state of determination, is inherited over many generations of growth and division. Lineages based on binary decisions have been proposed for the development of myogenic clones in chick embryos[23], and a binary code has been proposed for imaginal disc determination and transdetermination in Drosophila[24].

Cell lineage and chromosome lineage. The developmental decisions may be stored in the structure of the chromosomes. Examples of chromosome imprinting have been described in many animals, including man[25]. Models for generating and distinguishing specific chromosome structures have invoked DNA modification[26], differential arrangement of histones[27,28] or segregation of oldest DNA strands[29].

In any chromosomal model, sets of chromosomes must be segregated specifically at cell divisions. In his classical studies on Parascaris equorum (another nematode), Theodor Boveri followed individual chromosomes through single cell cycles in early cleavage[30]. It might be possible to follow sets of chromosomes in development in C. elegans and to correlate chromosome lineage and cell lineage.

Timing plays a key role in development

The developmental decisions include the timing and the final number of cell divisions in embryogenesis.

Observation of intact embryos allows detection of timing defects in mutants. The direct comparison of the predictable behavior of cells in living wild-type embryos with that in mutant embryos has allowed the identification of defects that would have been impossible to detect otherwise (e.g., in cell culture). Defects are detectable in the directions of cell divisions and cell migrations, and, most importantly, in the timing of the embryonic cell divisions.

The timing of embryonic cell divisions must be closely controlled. With this reproducible and sensitive reference system, defects in timing have been detected in mutants in seven of the nine emb genes studied. In the case of the mutants in emb-5, the timing defect may be the direct cause of

death of the embryo. Clearly, the timing of the embryonic cell divisions
must be closely controlled.

One aspect of this control involves the timing of chromosome replication.
In the cell division cycle mutant in gene lin-5 of C. elegans, the control of
chromosome replication, i.e., the mechanisms for timing, further replication,
or cessation of replication, possibly continues to operate within a single,
polyploid nucleus, independent of cell division[31]. Thus, chromosome replication
might be inherently controlled by the chromosome structure.

Histones may play key roles in the timing of cell divisions in development

Here we speculate that histones may be involved in regulating the timing of
embryonic cell divisions.

The time required to replicate the chromosomal DNA molecules in cleavage is
determined by the number of initiation sites on the DNA, rather than by the
rate of replication fork movement[32,33]. The control mechanism for origin
activation may operate through specific configurations of DNA with chromosomal
proteins[34], perhaps histones.

Histones of higher eukaryotes show very little sequence variation in the
course of evolution. But the amino acid sequence of Tetrahymena histone H4
differs substantially from the H4 sequence of calf or pea[35]. This suggests that
the rate of evolution of this most highly conserved protein known is considerably more rapid in this single-cell eukaryote than in multicellular
eukaryotes. This is consistent with a key role of histones in development,
particularly in the timing of embryonic cell divisions, since even minor
timing defects are amplified due to derangement of the normal sequence of
developmental events.

Histones are synthesized on maternal messenger RNA[36]. In sea urchin embryogenesis, different histone subtypes are synthesized in specific developmental
stages[27,37,38,39]. Separate genes code for these variants. Thus, histones
are highly regulated temporally in development. All subtypes made early are
retained in chromatin long after their synthesis ceases; they are inherited
through several cell divisions[27].

It has been shown in chicken myoblasts that the octameric core of the
nucleosome is assembled and segregated as a conserved unit[40]. Histone octamers
remain stable over at least three to four divisions and adjacent octamers
segregate together. In this way, variegated chromosomes carrying developmental
decisions might be generated and propagated in development[27,28].

The genes for the histones are clustered in the genome, both in sea urchin[41,42] and in _Drosophila_[43]. The histone gene heterogeneity in the sea urchin cluster is consistent with the developmental variants of the histones in this organism[44,45]. Non-allelic histone variants have also been found in mammals[46].

The postulated role of histones in development specifically in timing could be studied in _C. elegans_. We are exploring the possibility that there might be mutants in _emb_ genes, which affect developmental variants of histones.

ACKNOWLEDGEMENT

We thank our colleagues of the Göttingen _C. elegans_ group for cooperation and Randall Cassada, Joseph Culotti and Shahid Siddiqui for stimulating discussions. We also thank Judith Kimble and David Hirsh for sharing unpublished results.

E.S. and J.M. are supported by postdoctoral research fellowships of the Max-Planck-Society.

REFERENCES

1. Brenner, S. (1974) Genetics, 77, 71-94.

2. Edgar, R.S. and Wood, W.B. (1977) Science, 198, 1285-1286.

3. Deppe, U., Schierenberg, E., Cole, T., Krieg, C., Schmitt, D., Yoder, B., and von Ehrenstein, G. (1978) Proc. Nat. Acad. Sci. USA., 75, 376-380.

4. Sulston, J.E. and Horvitz, H.R. (1977) Develop. Biol., 56, 110-156.

5. Krieg, C., Cole, T., Deppe, U., Schierenberg, E., Schmitt, D., Yoder, B., and von Ehrenstein, G. (1978) Develop. Biol., 65, 193-215.

6. Schierenberg, E. (1978) Doctoral Thesis, University of Göttingen, Germany.

7. von Ehrenstein, G. and Schierenberg, E. (1979) In: Nematodes as Model Biological Systems (B.M. Zuckerman, ed.) Academic Press, New York, in press.

8. von Ehrenstein, G., Krieg, C., Cole, T., Schierenberg, E., Schmitt, D., and Yoder, B., unpublished results.

9. von Ehrenstein, G. and Schierenberg, E., unpublished results.

10. Hirsh, D. and Vanderslice, R. (1976) Develop. Biol., 49, 220-235.

11. Vanderslice, R. and Hirsh, D. (1976) Develop. Biol., 49, 236-249.

12. Hirsh, D., Wood, W.B., Hecht, R., Carr, S., and Vanderslice, R. (1977) In: Molecular Approaches to Eucaryotic Genetic Systems (G. Wilcox, J. Abelson, and C.F. Fox, eds.) Academic Press, New York, pp. 347-356.

13. Miwa, J., Schierenberg, E., and von Ehrenstein, G. (1979) Develop. Biol., submitted.

14. Schierenberg, E., Miwa, J., and von Ehrenstein, G. (1979) Develop. Biol., submitted.

15. Kimble, J. and Hirsh, D. (1979) Develop. Biol., in press.

16. Emmons, S.W., Klass, M.R., and Hirsh, D. (1979) Proc. Nat. Acad. Sci. USA. 76, 1333-1337.

17. Cortese, R., Melton, D., Tranquilla, T., and Smith, J.D. (1978) Nucleic Acids Res., 5, 4593-4611.

18. Littlefield, J.W. (1976) Variation, Senescence, and Neoplasia in Cultured Somatic Cells, Harvard University Press, Cambridge, Mass., pp. 1-163.

19. Siminovitch, L., Till, J.E., and McCulloch, E.A. (1964) J. Cell. Comp. Physiol., 64, 23-31.

20. Holtzer, J. (1978) In: Stem Cells and Tissue Homeostasis (B.I. Lord, C.S. Potten, and R.J. Cole, eds.) Cambridge University Press, Cambridge, England, pp. 1-27.

21. Potten, C.S. (1978) In: Stem Cells and Tissue Homeostasis (B.I. Lord, C.S. Potten, and R.J. Cole, eds.) Cambridge University Press, Cambridge, England, pp. 317-334.

22. Hadorn, E. (1966) In: Major Problems in Developmental Biology (M. Locke, ed.) Academic Press, New York, pp. 85-104.

23. Abbott, J., Schiltz, J., Dienstman, S., and Holtzer, H. (1974) Proc. Nat. Acad. Sci. USA., 71, 1506-1510.

24. Kauffman, S.A. (1973) Science, 181, 310-318.

25. Chandra, H.S. and Brown, S.W. (1975) Nature, 253, 165-168.

26. Holliday, R. and Pugh, J.E. (1975) Science, 187, 226-232.

27. Newrock, K.M., Alfageme, C.R., Nardi, R.V., and Cohen, L.H. (1977) Cold Spring Harbor Symp. Quant. Biol., 42, 421-431.

28. Weintraub, H., Flint, S.J., Groudine, M., and Grainger, R.M. (1977) Cold Spring Harbor Symp. Quant. Biol., 42, 401-407.

29. Cairns, J. (1975) Nature, 255, 197-200.

30. Boveri, Th. (1888) Jena. Z. Naturw., 22, 685-882.

31. Albertson, D.G., Sulston, J.E., and White, J.G. (1978) Develop. Biol., 63, 165-178.

32. Callan, H.G. (1973) Cold Spring Harbor Symp. Quant. Biol., 38, 195-203.

33. Blumenthal, A.B., Kriegstein, H.J., and Hogness, D.S. (1973) Cold Spring Harbor Symp. Quant. Biol., 38, 205-223.

34. Hand, R. (1978) Cell, 15, 317-325.

35. Glover, C.V.C. and Gorowsky, M.A. (1979) Proc. Nat. Acad. Sci. USA., 76, 585-589.

36. Davidson, E.H. (1976) Gene Activity in Early Development, 2nd. ed., Academic Press, New York, pp. 1-452.

37. Cohen, L.H., Newrock, K.M., and Zweidler, A. (1975) Science, 190, 994-997.

38. Grunstein, M. (1978) Proc. Nat. Acad. Sci. USA., 75, 4135-4139.

39. Newrock, K.M., Cohen, L.H., Hendricks, M.B., Donelly, R.J., and Weinberg, E.S. (1978) Cell, 14, 327-336.

40. Leffak, I.M., Grainger, R., and Weintraub, H. (1977) Cell, 12, 837-845.

41. Schaffner, W., Kunz, G., Daetwyler, H., Telford, J., Smith, H.O., and Birnstiel, M.L. (1978) Cell, 14, 655-671.

42. Sures, J., Lowry, J., and Kedes, L.H. (1978) Cell, 15, 1033-1044.

43. Lifton, R.P., Goldberg, M.L., Karp, R.W., and Hogness, D.S. (1977) Cold Spring Harbor Symp. Quant. Biol., 42, 1047-1051.

44. Kunkel, N.S., and Weinberg, E.S. (1978) Cell, 14, 313-326.

45. Overton, G.C. and Weinberg, E.S. (1978) Cell, 14, 247-257.

46. Franklin, S.G. and Zweidler, A. (1977) Nature, 266, 273-275.

Cell Lineage, Stem Cells and Cell Determination
INSERM Symposium No. 10
Editor: N. Le Douarin
© *1979 Elsevier/North-Holland Biomedical Press*

REGULATIVE DEVELOPMENT IN THE POST-EMBRYONIC LINEAGES OF CAENORHABDITIS
ELEGANS

J. KIMBLE, J. SULSTON, J. WHITE

MRC Laboratory of Molecular Biology, Hills Road, Cambridge, CB2 2QH, England

INTRODUCTION

In many invertebrates, cell lineages are apparently invariant from
individual to individual. A given precursor cell follows a specific pattern of
cell divisions, and its descendants follow fates that correspond to their
respective positions in the lineage tree. Such a reproducible sequence of
events provides an excellent system for studying how cells come to pursue
particular fates during development. We have been interested to know if a
cell's fate is specified by factors intrinsic to the cell, or if it is
influenced by interactions between the cell and its environment.

Caenorhabditis elegans is a particularly suitable organism for lineage
studies because it is transparent throughout its life cycle, and because it
consists of relatively few cells. Furthermore, C. elegans is a favorable
organism for genetics, so the control of cell lineages can be studied by charac-
terizing mutations that are defective in known lineages.

The cell lineages of C. elegans have been described in the embryo to the
182 cell stage[1] and after hatching[2,3]. Approximately 50 cells resume divisions
post-embryonically. In the somatic tissues, the number of cells (or nuclei) is
increased from about 550 to about 950 in hermaphrodites and to about 1025 in
males. These post-embryonic lineages are essentially invariant from worm to
worm. As the worm enlarges and matures sexually, cells (or nuclei) are added
to previously existing tissues (hypodermis, muscle, gut, and nervous system),
and structures necessary for reproduction are elaborated. The latter include a
gonad in both sexes, a vulva in hermaphrodites, and a tail specialized for
copulation in males.

This paper summarizes the results of laser ablation experiments performed
on cells in the post-embryonic lineages of C. elegans. In particular, we focus
on those experiments that demonstrate a regulative capacity in the cells of
this predominantly invariant system. The post-embryonic lineages have the
practical advantage for these studies that they can be easily traced by direct
observation of the cells as they divide and assume their final fate. The
regulative response, therefore, can be described at a level of cellular detail

that has not been possible in other deletion studies. Our aim in performing these experiments is to infer how cells are controlled during normal development from their behavior in an abnormal situation.

MATERIALS AND METHODS

    C. elegans var. Bristol of wild type was maintained on agar-filled Petri plates seeded with E. coli as described by Brenner[4].

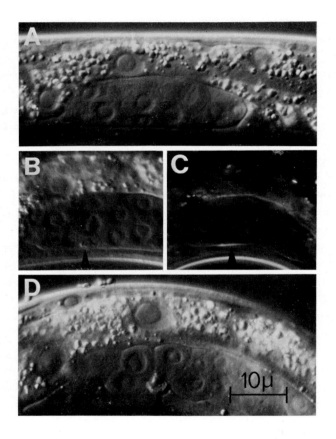

Fig. 1. Nomarski photomicrographs of an anchor cell before ablation (A), within 10 minutes after ablation (B and C), and six hours after ablation (D).

    The details of the laser ablation procedure will be published separately (Sulston and White, in preparation). Briefly, individual worms are anaesthetized, transferred to a thin slab of agar, and covered with a coverslip. A

target cell is identified and centered for ablation at 1000X with Nomarski
optics (Figure 1A). The cell is killed over a period of 5 - 10 minutes (Figure
1B and 1C) by multiple shots of a coumarin 2 dye laser microbeam. A few hours
after the cell ablation, the worm is observed in order to validate the success
of the operation (Figure 1D). Animals that have suffered visible damage to
neighboring cells or that retain the target cell are discarded. Each result
reported here was obtained in at least two, and usually more, individuals.

RESULTS

Ablation of certain cells in the post-embryonic lineages of C. elegans
results in an alteration in the expected lineage of one or more of the remaining cells. Such regulation has been observed among three types of precursor
cells (Figure 2) and their progeny. Within each of these precursor types,
cells are similar in morphological appearance and in prospective fate. Regulation is limited to subsets of the precursors, and each type displays unique
features of regulation.

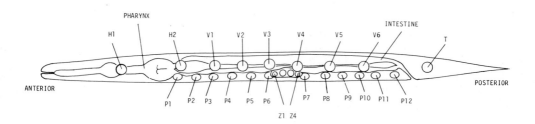

Fig. 2. Locations of three precursor cell types in a hypothetical young worm.
The precursors do not coexist in these positions in a real animal due to
differences between them in timing of divisions and migrations. Precursors of
the ventral hypodermis, P1-P12, are found ventrally. Precursors of the lateral
hypodermis, H1-H2, V1-V6, T are shown on one side only. Precursors of the
gonadal somatic tissues, Z1 and Z4, are found in the mid-ventrally located
gonadal primordium.

Ventral hypodermis

Twelve precursor cells, P1-P12, (Figure 2) give rise to cells of the
ventral hypodermis and neurons in the ventral nerve cord. Regulation occurs in
two groups of ventral hypodermal cells (P3.p-P8.p in hermaphrodites and

P9.p–P11.p in males, where Pn.p is the posterior daughter of Pn). In the intact animal, most Pn.p either become hypodermal cells, or divide once and produce two hypodermal daughters. In hermaphrodites, P5.p, P6.p, and P7.p divide further to make the vulva, and in males, P10.p and P11.p divide further to contribute cells to the copulatory male tail.

For brevity, only the results of ablation experiments pertaining to the male P9.p–P11.p group are presented here (Table 1).

TABLE 1

REGULATION IN THE VENTRAL HYPODERMIS

The first line shows the fates followed by each cell in the intact animal. Subsequent lines show the fates followed by cells after ablation of the cells indicated in the left column.

Cell Ablated	Cell Pn.p and its Fate				
	P8.p	P9.p	P10.p	P11.p	P12.p
–	P8.p	P9.p	P10.p	P11.p	P12.p
P8.p	–	P9.p	P10.p	P11.p	P12.p
P9.p	P8.p	–	P10.p	P11.p	P12.p
P10.p	P8.p	P10.p	–	P11.p	P12.p
P11.p	P8.p	P10.p	P11.p	–	P12.p
P12.p	P8.p	P9.p	P10.p	P11.p	–
P9, P10	P8.p	–	–	P11.p	P12.p
P10.p, P11.p	P8.p	P11.p	–	–	P12.p
P9.p, P10.p, P11.p	P8.p	–	–	–	P12.p

If P11.p is ablated, P10.p assumes the position of P11.p and follows the lineage normally followed by P11.p, and P9.p assumes the position of P10.p and follows the P10.p lineage. If P10.p is ablated, P9.p replaces P10.p, but P11.p is not affected. If P10.p and P11.p are killed P9.p replaces P11.p. Ablation of all three cells, P9.p, P10.p, and P11.p effects no change in lineage of the neighboring cells, and conversely, ablation of neighboring cells P8.p or P12.p effects no response in P9.p, P10.p, or P11.p

The main features of regulation in the male P9.p–P11.p group also apply to the hermaphrodite P3.p–P8.p group:

1) The regulative response involves the precise replacement of one precursor cell for another. The adult animal is therefore missing the progeny of those cells, that are recruited into another lineage and are not replaced

themselves.

2) This replacement occurs according to a hierarchy of fates. In males, P11.p occupies the primary, P10.p the secondary, and P9.p the tertiary position in this hierarchy.

3) Regulation is limited to a small group of cells. These cells are posterior daughters of similar precursor cells and therefore they are similar in ancestry.

Lateral hypodermis

Nine precursor cells of the lateral hypodermis, H1, H2, V1-V6, and T (Figure 2) are found on each side of the newly hatched worm. Regulation in the lateral hypodermis has been studied chiefly in the male where three cells, V5.p, V6.p, and T, normally generate one, five, and three sensory rays respectively for the copulatory apparatus of the male tail. V5 also gives rise to the cells of a special sensillum, the post-deirid.

Two types of regulation have been observed in the lateral hypodermis. The first type is similar in character to the regulation seen in the ventral hypo-dermis, but, in comparison, it is both incomplete and inexact:

1) Regulation occurs by replacement of the specialized structures normally made by the ablated cell (i.e. sensory rays), but is not reproducibly precise. If V6 is ablated, V5 can replace it exactly, or it can make an intermediate number of rays. V4, which normally does not make rays, can be recruited to do so, but V4 never replaces V5 or V6 fully. If V5 is ablated, V4 is recruited to make rays, and V6 remains unaffected.

2) Regulation occurs according to a hierarchy in that the regulating cell always makes more rays than normal.

3) Ray regulation occurs among a small group of cells, V4-V6. Although T also makes rays, no regulation is observed between V6 and T.

The second type of regulation involves a proliferative response without replacement of specialized structures. Several V cells must be ablated to invoke this response. For example, if V4-V6 are ablated, V3 undergoes extra divisions and produces extra hypodermal cells. If V1-V4 are ablated, V5 under-goes extra divisions. In this case, V5 produces supernumerary clusters of presumptive ray cells that do not differentiate into rays.

Gonad

Two precursors, Z1 and Z4, (Figure 2) give rise to the somatic cells of the gonad. Regulation in the gonadal lineages differs from regulation in the hypodermis in that the ability of a cell to alter its lineage correlates directly with a variability in lineage seen in the intact animal. This natural variability involves pairs of cells that follow one of two alternative fates in any given individual. The two members of each pair arise in equivalent branches of the Z1 and Z4 lineages.

The ancestry of two such pairs in the hermaphrodite (cells 1 and 4; cells 2 and 3) is shown in Figure 3a. These four cells, as a group, assume positions

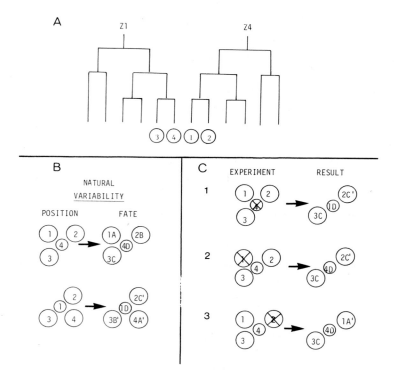

Fig. 3. Ancestry and fate of two cell pairs (cells 1 and 4; cells 2 and 3) in the developing hermaphrodite gonad. a) Members of each cell pair arise in equivalent points in the Z1-Z4 lineage. b) In intact animals, cells 1-4 assume one of two configurations and follow one of two alternative fates. The fate is represented by a letter and the polarity of the cell division pattern with respect to the worm's coordinates is indicated by the absence or presence of a prime (') next to the letter. c) Ablation experiments result in various types of regulation. An X shows the ablated cell. See text for details.

in one of two alternative configurations, and the choice of fate for each of
the four cells corresponds to the configuration of the group (Figure 3b).
Fates A, B, and C are unique with respect to the number of cell divisions, but
are the same with respect to the kinds of cell produced. Fate D involves
differentiation into the anchor cell - a special cell that does not divide and
that appears to induce the vulva.

Ablation experiments show that these cells regulate by following their
natural alternative fate (Figure 3c) in two cases. Three modes of regulation,
however, have been found.

1) If the presumptive anchor cell (fate D) is ablated, the alternative
anchor precursor replaces it (Expt. 1). Since the reciprocal replacement does
not occur (Expt. 2), fate D is primary and fate A is secondary. In the male,
regulation in a homologous pair of cells occurs in the same way.

2) The removal of cell 1, either by regulation (Expt. 1) or by ablation
(Expt. 2), influences cell 2 to follow fate C' rather than B. This alteration
of lineage restores the symmetry of the developing gonad.

3) Ablation of cell 2 influences cell 1 to reverse the polarity of its
division pattern with respect to the worm's coordinates (switch from A to A',
Expt. 3). We call this reversal <u>vectorial regulation</u> (Figure 4). Another
example of vectorial regulation is seen at a different point in the hermaphrodite gonadal lineage.

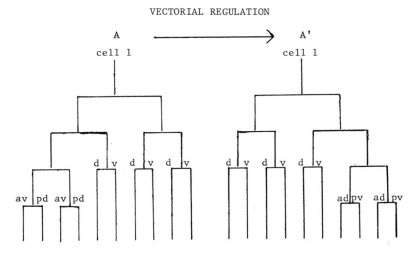

VECTORIAL REGULATION

Fig. 4. Vectorial regulation. The lineage is changed by reversing the pattern
of cell divisions with respect to the anterior-posterior axis of the worm.
Anterior is to the left.

DISCUSSION

Despite the invariance of the post-embryonic lineages in C. elegans, some cells modify their lineages in response to the laser ablation of a neighboring cell. Such a change in the expected behavior of a cell appears to compensate for the deleted cell or cells, and is called regulation.

Three types of regulative response have been observed.

1) In the ventral hypodermis, lateral hypodermis, and gonad, specialized cells are replaced by the recruitment of a neighboring cell. Such replacement occurs according to a hierarchy of fates: if putative cell X is ablated, putative cell Y will replace it, but the converse replacement of cell Y by cell X is never observed. We refer to fate X (the fate typically followed by cell X) as the primary fate, and fate Y as the secondary fate in this hierarchy. In each case, the ablated cell and the recruited cell are similar in ancestry in that they arise in identical branches of the lineages of similar precursor cells.

2) In the lateral hypodermis, a proliferative response has been observed in which neighboring cells undergo extra divisions without replacement of specialized cells.

3) In the gonad, vectorial regulation, a reversal in the polarity of the pattern of cell divisions, without any change in the number or order of cell divisions, has been observed.

The most straightforward interpretation of these regulative responses is that cell-cell interactions influence the lineage a particular cell will follow in the intact animal. Alternatively, the process of ablating a cell might release "determinants", and the neighboring cell might take them up and be reprogrammed. Or, secondary damage to a neighboring cell might destroy some component critical to its determined state and allow reprogramming. Although neither of these latter explanations has been ruled out, both seem unlikely. The specificity and reproducibility with which regulation occurs argue against a random event being the basis of regulation. Furthermore, cells have been observed to regulate in response to the removal of a neighbor, either by ablation of the neighbor or by regulation of the neighbor to a different fate. This argues against the hypothesis that the ablated cell releases determinants to reprogram its neighbor. Our bias, therefore, is that regulative behavior after ablation is indicative of processes that normally influence cell fate.

The various modes of regulation observed in these experiments suggest that lineage patterns can be influenced in a number of ways by cell-cell interactions:

1) The existence of a fate hierarchy indicates that the decision to follow

a secondary or tertiary fate depends on some kind of signal that the higher fates have been assigned.

2) The proliferative response observed suggests that the total number of divisions for a particular cell is subject to influence from its environment.

3) The reversal of the polarity of a cell's lineage suggests that local cell contacts are critical in establishing the orientation of a cell in a group of cells.

Equivalence groups

The form of regulation in which one cell replaces another by assuming its position and lineage is limited to small groups of cells. The cells in such a group are equally competent to follow a primary fate. In the ventral hypodermis, P3.p–P8.p can each follow the P6.p vulval lineage in hermaphrodites, and P9.p–P11.p can each follow the P11.p lineage in males. In the male lateral hypodermis, V5 can be recruited to the V6 lineage, and V4 can approximate the V5 or V6 lineage. In the gonad, either cell 1 or cell 4 (Figure 3) can become the anchor cell in hermaphrodites, and a homologous pair displays a similar regulative response in males. The reciprocal alteration of lineage, in which a cell follows a fate that is lower in the hierarchy, has been seen in the P3.p–P8.p group under two different circumstances. If the gonadal anchor cell is ablated, cells P3.p–P8.p all follow the tertiary fate typical of P3.p, P4.p, and P8.p. And, in a lineage defective (lin) mutant, lin-2 (e1309)X, P3.p–P8.p again all follow the tertiary fate, and no vulva is made (Horvitz and Sulston, unpublished results). We suggest that these groups of cells are equivalent in developmental potential, and call them equivalence groups.

Cells assigned to equivalence groups on the basis of ablation experiments correspond exactly to cells grouped according to two other considerations. First, a comparison of the lineages of P1–P12 in the intact animal reveals differences in lineage detail (e.g. cell deaths, extra divisions) that delineate three groups, P1–P2, P3–P8, and P9–P11 (see [2]). The members of each group share specific lineage features and differ from other Pn. Second, lineage defective mutants alter the lineages of precursor cells differentially. In one mutant, lin-1 (e1026) IV, only P3–P8 are affected. P3.p–P8.p all follow the primary vulval lineage of P6.p resulting in a multivulva phenotype (Horvitz and Sulston, unpublished results). In a second mutant, mab-5 (e1239) III, the V5 and V6 lineages are defective, whereas the T lineage is normal. This mutant honors the V6/T boundary of the lateral hypodermal equivalence group. The delineation of the same groups of cells by several techniques supports the idea that cells in equivalence groups are intrinsically different with respect to their developmental potential from cells outside equivalence groups.

The hypothesis that cells of equivalent developmental potential are set apart in groups raises intriguing questions about the mechanism by which such groups are established and the role played by such groups during development. As far as is known, cells in an equivalence group have a similar ancestry. Each arises in an identical branch of the lineage tree of similar cells (e.g. the posterior branch of the ventral hypodermal precursor cells). Furthermore, in the gonad, the ancestries of the members of an equivalence pair, both in hermaphrodites and males, are equivalent and unique. If the commitment of cells to an equivalence group occurs by a lineage mechanism, the embryonic ancestry of the ventral and lateral hypodermal precursors may reveal differences in the origin of the precursor cells that correspond to equivalence group boundaries.

The developmental significance of equivalence groups is purely a matter for speculation at the present time. One appealing hypothesis is that they are fundamental units of worm assembly analogous to polyclones in fly assembly[5]. One might imagine that distinct groups of cells are founded during embryogenesis that are uniquely responsible for construction of specific regions of the worm's anatomy. Elaboration of this idea, however, must await the isolation and characterization of more mutants that are equivalence group specific.

JEK is a fellow of the Jane Coffin Childs Memorial Fund for Medical Research. This investigation has been aided by a grant from the Jane Coffin Childs Memorial Fund for Medical Research.

REFERENCES

1. Deppe, U., Schierenberg, E., Cole, T., Krieg, C., Schmitt, O., Yoder, B. and von Ehrenstein, G. (1978) Cell lineages of the embryo of the nematode, Caenorhabditis elegans. Proc. Natl. Acad. Sci., 75, 376-380.

2. Sulston, J.F. and Horvitz, H.R. (1977) Post-embryonic cell lineages of the nematode, Caenorhabditis elegans. Develop. Biol., 56, 110-156.

3. Kimble, J. and Hirsh, D. (1979) The post-embryonic lineages of the hermaphrodite and male gonads in Caenorhabditis elegans. Develop. Biol. (in press).

4. Brenner, S. (1974) The genetics of Caenorhabditis elegans. Genetics, 77, 71-94.

5. Crick, F.H.C. and Lawrence, P.A. (1975) Compartments and polyclones in insect development. Science, 189, 340-347.

Cell Lineage, Stem Cells and Cell Determination
INSERM Symposium No. 10
Editor: N. Le Douarin
© 1979 Elsevier/North-Holland Biomedical Press

PATTERN MUTANTS IN *DROSOPHILA* EMBRYOGENESIS

CHRISTIANE NÜSSLEIN-VOLHARD

European Molecular Biology Laboratory, 6900 Heidelberg, P.O. Box 102209, FRG

INTRODUCTION

Our understanding of the mechanisms whereby an initially uniform egg cell develops differentiated organs and tissues in a strict reproducible spatial pattern is still very limited. Various models for pattern formation have been proposed, ranging from the "multiple localized determinants" concept of mosaic development to the more general concept of positional information[1] mediated by concentration gradients of morphogenetic substances. Since all spatial differentiation must be initiated by structural or molecular differences in space, each model should ultimately be explainable in molecular terms and therefore testable using genetic alterations. Mutations in genes coding for substances involved in the process of pattern formation should lead to an altered pattern. Such mutations enable us to dissect this complex process in much the same way as they have been used to uncover biosynthetic pathways and mechanisms of gene regulation in bacterial systems[2].

In this communication, the use of mutants to study pattern formation during *Drosophila* embryogenesis will be described. *Drosophila* is well suited not only because of its excellent genetics, but also because the egg develops into a larva with a rich pattern, amply provided with landmarks for position and polarity making the detection of even small alterations possible. The embryo develops outside the maternal organism in a relatively large egg (500 x 180 μm) which is accessible to microinjection and transplantation. A peculiarity of insect embryogenesis is that the cleavage nuclei are not separated by cell walls until there are about 6000 cleavage nuclei. At this time they get synchronously included into cells forming the first cellular state, the blastoderm, at 3 h of development. At this stage or very soon thereafter, the fate of the cells appears to be quite fixed, at least in the prospective ectodermal region of the embryo and with respect to position along

the antero-posterior egg axis[3,4]. A further difference e.g. to
vertebrate development is that the mesoderm in the insects arises
ventrally, not dorsally, and inductive influences go from ectoderm
to mesoderm, not vice versa[5]: although the first signs of segmentation are seen in the mesoderm, the ectoderm can develop the correct segmented pattern autonomously in the absence of underlying
mesoderm. Fig. 1 shows a fate map of the various regions of the
Drosophila egg at the cellular blastoderm stage.

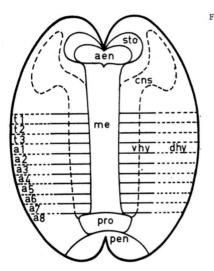

Fig. 1: Blastoderm fate map of a *Drosophila* egg cut open along the
dorsal midline and spread out.
Modified from Poulson[6]. a = abdominal segment, aen = anterior
endoderm, cns = central nervous
system, dhy = dorsal hypoderm,
me = mesoderm, pen = posterior
endoderm, pro = proctoderm,
sto = stomoderm, t = thoracic
segment, v = ventral hypoderm.
The transverse lines indicate
the anterior borders of the segments as determined from laser
irradiation experiments[7].

Although in *Drosophila* mutants have been collected for a long
time, a search for mutants altering the embryonic pattern has only
begun recently. According to genetic criteria, such mutants may be
found among two classes: maternal effect mutants and zygotic mutants. In maternal effect mutants, the embryonic phenotype depends
solely upon the genotype of the female which produced the egg,
while in zygotic mutants it depends on the embryo's own genotype.
Maternal inheritance suggests that transcription of the normal
gene takes place during oogenesis and, directly or indirectly,
yields substances which are stored in the egg to support normal
development. In the zygotic mutants, transcription relevant for
the mutant phenotype, on the other hand, can only take place after

fertilization. In accordance with the separation in time of gene expression in the two mutant classes, the effect on embryonic development is in general earlier and much more dramatic in maternal than in zygotic mutants.

None of the known maternal effect mutants has been shown to affect the location or development of only a single primordium or germ layer[8]. Since these types of mutants have been especially looked for, the failure to find them might be significant and may suggest that the early separation of the egg into the various embryonic primordia at the proper place does not involve specific determinants deposited in the unfertilized egg. The few pattern mutants among the maternal effect lead to global alteration of the embryonic fate map, changing either the entire antero-posterior (*bicaudal*) or dorso-ventral (*dorsal*) pattern of the embryo[9].

MUTANTS AFFECTING THE ANTERO-POSTERIOR PATTERN

Bicaudal mutants. *Bicaudal (bic)* is a recessive maternal effect mutant first described in 1966 by A. Bull[10]. The mutant dramatically affects the antero-posterior pattern of the *Drosophila* embyro: the progeny of mutant females may display two abdominal ends in longitudinal mirror-image symmetry, while head, thorax and anterior abdomen are lacking (Fig. 2). Under normal conditions only few if any of the progeny from *bic/bic* mothers develop a mutant phenotype, while most of them are normal. The penetrance can, however, be raised considerably by genetic and environmental conditions[11]. Best producers are females heterozygous for *bic* and a deletion of the *bic* locus, if kept at high temperature. Under these conditions up to about 40 % of the embryos show a mutant phenotype, regardless the paternal genotype.

An unusual feature of the *bicaudal* mutant is the variability of its phenotype found under all experimental conditions tested[11]. Mutant females always produce a spectrum of phenotypes, in all of which the number of segments is smaller than normal. The most frequent mutant phenotype is the perfect mirror-image duplication of the posterior-most abdominal segments. The number of duplicated segments, however, is variable and ranges from 1-5, the most frequent being 3. Less abundant are asymmetrical duplications in which the posterior part with normal polarity is always larger

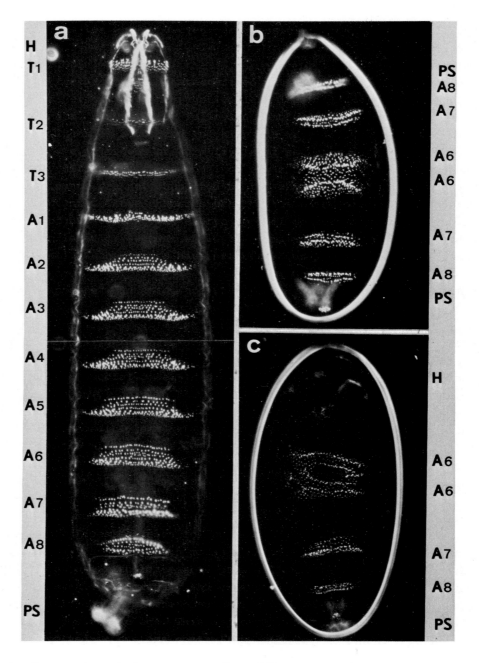

Fig. 2: Ventral cuticular pattern of *Drosophila* wildtype and mutant larvae a) a normal larva, b) a bicaudal larva, c) a Krüppel homozygous larva. A = abdominal segment, T = thoracic segment, H = head, PS = posterior spiracles.

than the anterior part with reversed polarity. In addition, embryos are also found in which the anterior-most pattern elements of a normal larva are missing to various extents, but showing no duplicated patterns. Finally, a various fraction of the eggs develop to normal hatching larvae.

The variability of the phenotype is all the more striking since *bicaudal* has been mapped to a single locus in the *Drosophila* genome (map position 2-67.0)[11]. Gene dosage studies furthermore suggest that the phenotypes are caused by the less than normal amount of a functional gene product. Thus, the *bicaudal* gene product appears to be involved in a pattern controlling system in which minute differences among individual oozytes lead to strikingly different patterns. As to the properties of this system, some further observations on the *bicaudal* phenotypes are informative[9].

1. The entire pattern, not only that in the anterior part of the egg, is changed. This statement is mainly based on the small segment number found in bicaudal embryos (Fig. 2). The fate map (Fig. 1) indicates that the posterior half of a normal *Drosophila* egg gives rise to the entire abdomen with 8 segments, whereas the majority of bicaudal embryos have only 3, and at the most 5 segments in their posterior half.

2. The change in pattern is co-ordinate, in other words, the anterior "knows" what the posterior part is doing. Given the variability in segment numbers, independent decisions in anterior and posterior part would yield mainly asymmetrical embryos with different segment numbers in the two counterparts. This is not the case, since the most frequent bicaudal pattern is that of perfect symmetry.

3. The pattern-controlling system has a polar and a symmetrical stable state. Although there is a continuous range of patterns with increasing number of segments with normal polarity, the symmetrical bicaudal embryos on the one end, and the normal larvae on the other end of the spectrum are the most frequent patterns found, while any intermediate pattern is comparatively rare.

A model which in my opinion may explain those basic features of the aberrant patterns is the model of lateral inhibition of Gierer and Meinhardt[12]. It is based on the assumption that different elements in a spatial pattern are specified by different concentrations rather than different qualities of some principle, e.g. a morphogenetic substance. The normal pattern would be specified by a monotonic concentration gradient of a morphogen, while a bicaudal pattern would arise through a symmetrical gradient (Fig. 3). The general model[12] which has been adapted by Meinhardt to insect embryogenesis[13], describes how such stable concentration gradients could be established by the interaction of two antagonistic substances. A feature of this model, which makes it particularly suggestive for the explanation of the *bicaudal* phenotypes

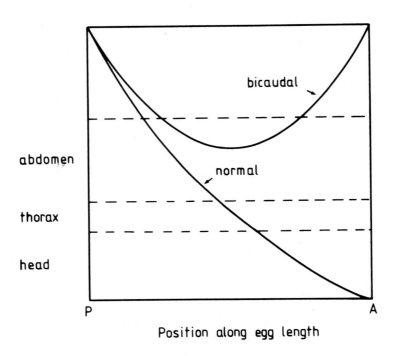

Fig. 3: Hypothetical gradients defining the position along the antero-posterior egg axis (horizontal scale) in normal and bicaudal embryos. The horizontal dotted lines indicate threshold levels for abdomen, thorax and head formation. They are chosen such that the gradient for normal eggs specifies these structures at the positions indicated in the fate map (Fig. 1). The bicaudal embryo is described by a shallow, symmetrical gradient. Only a small portion of the posterior abdomen is specified at the middle of the egg. P = posterior, A = anterior.

is that disturbances of the normal system either are corrected immediately or lead to a symmetrical bipolar concentration gradient as a second, meta-stable state of the system. The model, on the other hand, can not make predictions as to the nature of the pattern forming principles, but only to their type of interaction. It predicts, however, that various kinds of disturbances lead to identical final patterns, which are inherent to the system. It is therefore difficult to assess the role of the *bicaudal* gene product in this system; one may predict, however, that mutants at different loci should produce the same pattern abnormalities as *bicaudal*. Recently we have isolated two further maternal effect mutants which are both not allelic to *bicaudal* but yield exactly the same phenotypes, including their variability.

Other mutants. Among the maternal effect mutants, except for the 3 bicaudal-mutants described above, to my knowledge, none has been shown to specifically affect the antero-posterior pattern. A few zygotic mutants are known which alter parts of the pattern; however, in contrast to *bicaudal*, in these only certain regions are changed while the remainder of the pattern is left intact. Of the zygotic mutants, the most dramatic pattern alteration is seen in *Krüppel*[14]: homozygous embryos have only 3 abdominal segments, one of which is duplicated in reversed pattern, while anterior abdomen and thorax are lacking (Fig. 2c). The head and the posterior terminal region, however, appear normal. Since a maternal effect has been ruled out for this interesting mutant[15], a minimum conclusion we may draw from it's phenotype is that segment number and polarity is not invariably fixed by the time the egg is laid. Mutants which change the specification of individual segments, but leave their total number and polarity intact, are found among the *bithorax* pseudoallele series (see article by G. Morata, this volume) and *Polycomb*[17].

MUTANTS AFFECTING THE DORSO-VENTRAL PATTERN

Dorsal. The maternal effect mutant *dorsal* affects the dorso-ventral pattern of the embryo in a similarly dramatic way as *bicaudal* affects the antero-posterior pattern[9]. As illustrated in the fate map (Fig. 1), the dorso-ventral pattern contains the dorsal and the ventral hypoderm, interspersed with the neurogenic ectoderm, and the mesoderm as pattern elements. The plane of bilateral symmetry cuts through the anlage of the dorsal hypoderm at the dorsal midline and the mesoderm anlage at the ventral midline.

The phenotype of embryos produced by females homozygous for *dorsal* consists of a complete abolition of dorso-ventral polarity, while the outer egg shell polarity is apparently normal. These embryos develop a tube of dorsal hypoderm with many irregular constrictions, filled with unconsumed yolk. Internal organs have never been found in these embryos. *Dorsal* embryos have apparently normal antero-posterior polarity, the segmentation, however, is incomplete and irregular. In contrast to *bicaudal*, the *dorsal* phenotype is fully penetrant and very consistent (Fig. 4).

More insight into the type of pattern forming mechanism affected by *dorsal* is gained by the study of "weak" mutant phenotypes. These are obtained from females homozygous for the less strong *dorsal* allele, *dorsal*[2], or from heterozygous *dorsal*/+ females. In contrast to the variety of phenotypes always found in bicaudal, each given *dorsal* mutant genotype corresponds to a distinct mutant phenotype with but little variation. These weak phenotypes in general consist of partially dorsalized embryos, lacking ventral and ventro-lateral pattern elements to different extents. Embryos from *dorsal*[2] females lack all structures normally derived from the ventral egg half (see fate map, Fig. 1), including mesoderm, endodermal gut, ventral nervous system and ventral hypoderm. From *dorsal*/+ females, comparatively normal looking larvae are obtained, lacking mainly internal organs like mesoderm, parts of the anterior and posterior gut, but also often part of the ventral hypoderm. This latter dominant phenotype is only expressed at high temperature (29°) and is furthermore dependent on the genetic background of the female[9].

The spectrum of defects encountered in these embryos always includes derivatives of all three germ layers and therefore cannot be explained in terms of localized organ- or germlayer determinants. Furthermore, the cause of defects is not a failure of the respective egg regions to develop, but rather a change in the developmental program of ventral and lateral egg regions: ventral egg regions develop structures normally derived from more lateral or even dorsal egg regions.

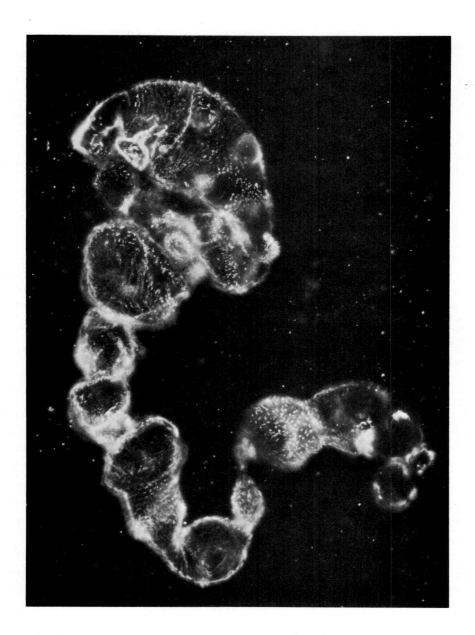

Fig. 4: Differentiated embryo produced by a *dorsal* homozygous female.

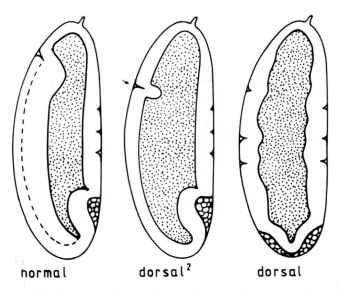

normal   **dorsal²**   **dorsal**

Fig. 5: Schematic drawings of normal and dorsal embryos at gastrulation. Anterior up, ventral egg side left. The dotted vertical line in the normal embryo separates the invaginated mesodermanlage from the outer ectoderm. This anlage is lacking in embryos from *dorsal²* and *dorsal* females (middle and right egg). The arrow in the middle egg points to the invaginating cephalic furrow, which in normal eggs is formed laterally.

Three lines of evidence suggest this:

1. The embryos develop from a normal cellular blastoderm and at no stage of development can massive cell death be detected.

2. The folding and invagination pattern seen at gastrulation in mutant embryos indicates a different programming of the cells from very early on: in *dorsal* embryos, dorsal folds appear also at the ventral and lateral side of the embryo, while in the weak phenotypes no mesodermal invagination is formed and lateral folds extend to the ventral side of the egg (Fig. 5).

3. Fate mapping of the ventral hypodermal anlage with UV-laser-induced local defects[7] indicates that the ventral hypoderm arises midventrally in embryos from *dorsal/+* females[17], a position which in normal embryos forms the mesoderm anlage[6].

In summary, the *dorsal* mutant patterns arise by a change of the entire dorso-ventral fate map: dorsal and lateral anlagen are shifted ventrally at the expense of ventral anlagen. This shift

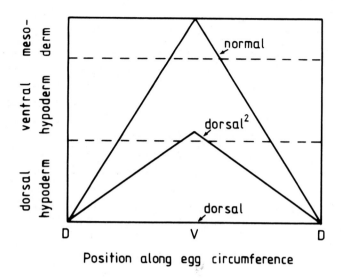

Fig. 6: Hypothetical gradients defining the position along the egg circumference. The horizontal dotted lines indicate threshold levels for mesoderm, ventral, and dorsal hypoderm formation.

appears to be co-ordinate, since an integrated pattern is the result. The changes of the dorso-ventral pattern in mutant embryos may best be described if one assumes that the dorso-ventral pattern of the _Drosophila_ embryo is specified by a graded distribution of a morphogenetic principle. This gradient would be symmetrical, given the bilaterality of the egg (Fig. 6). The weak phenotypes are described by gradients with a slope shallower than normal such that the level the gradient reaches at the ventral midline specifies lateral instead of midventral pattern elements. In the extreme _dorsal_ phenotype, no such gradient may form.

Other mutants. Partially dorsalized embryos are produced in the maternal effect mutant fs(1)K10 (see article by Wieschaus, this volume). This mutant, in contrast to _dorsal_, also changes the outer egg shell polarity and may therefore affect an earlier function in the process of establishment of dorso-ventral polarity than _dorsal_. Among the zygotic mutants, a possible candidate for a pattern mutant is _Notch_ in which mutant embryos show a hypertrophy of the nervous system at the expense of the hypoderm[18]. Other explanations for *Notch*, however, are possible.

CONCLUSIONS

   The sample of well characterised pattern mutants in both the
maternal effect and the zygotic class is still small and certainly
not random. However, the following conclusions may be tentatively
drawn. Theories according to which the many different parts of the
pattern, e.g. organs or germ layers or segments, are specified by
as many different, corresponding, organ or germ layer or segment
determinants are not supported by the phenotypes of maternal effect mutants. These theories predict the existence of maternal effect mutants causing the embryo to fail to form a particular organ
or germ layer or segment while the remainder of the body pattern
is normal. Such mutants have not been found, despite of an extensive search[19,20].

   An apparent exception are the primordial germ cells, for which
prelocalized determinants have been postulated on the basis of
transplantation experiments[4] and maternal effect mutants in which
no primordial germ cells are formed, have been found[20]. Several
lines of evidence, however, indicate that germ cell determination
might be a special case. In bicaudal embryos, primordial germ
cells are only found in the original posterior part, never also in
the duplicated anterior part[9], which indicates that the location
of the primordial germ cells is independent from the patterning of
the somatic tissue.

   The phenotypes of the maternal effect mutants *bicaudal* and *dorsal*
suggest that the informational contents of the egg for patterning
of the somatic tissue is of a rather general and global nature.
Not individual organs or germ layers are affected and the pattern
of defects does not even follow the lines of the respective anlagen on the fate map. Both mutants have been mapped to single loci
and therefore with reasonable probability affect or eliminate primarily single components, the gene products, and yet they lead to
a dramatic change of the prospective fate of the cells in almost
all regions of the egg. This indicates that these gene products
are involved in systems controlling the *entire* pattern in a global
way.

   By these two mutants, we have identified two such pattern con-

trolling systems, one defining the antero-posterior, and the other
the dorso-ventral coordinate of the egg. The pattern alterations
observed in *bicaudal* and *dorsal* are readily described in terms of
gradients of positional values. It appears likely that this formal
description reflects the underlying mechanism, that is that gradients of positional values correspond to concentration gradients
of some morphogenetic principle. A basic feature of this model is
that several structures may be defined by one and the same substance and that spatial differentiation is achieved by quantitative
differences in space.

The establishment of the postulated concentration gradients in
a form stable enough to allow spatial differentiation in a precise
and reproducible way certainly involves more than one component[12].
At present it is not clear which part in the systems *bicaudal* and
dorsal may play. They may directly code for a morphogene, or for
something required for its graded distribution, or for the stability of this distribution, to list some of the possibilities, and
the phenotypes of mutants tell us more about the general features
of the systems than their molecular backgrounds. On the other hand,
maternal effect mutants may help to identify and isolate the mor-
phogenic substances in question, using rescue of mutant embryos by
the injection of wildtype cytoplasm or fractions thereof as an assay.

ACKNOWLEDGEMENTS

I wish to thank Ines Benner for her patience and skill in typing the manuscript.

REFERENCES

1. Wolpert, L. (1969) J. Theor. Biol., 25, 1-47
2. Jacob, F. and Monod, J. (1961) J. Mol. Biol., 3, 318
3. Schubiger, G. and Wood, W.J. (1977) Am. Zool., 17, 565
4. Illmensee, K. (1976) in "Insect Development" (P.A. Lawrence ed.)
   pp 76-98, Blackwell Sci. Publ.
5. Sander, K. (1976) Adv. Ins. Physiol., 12, 125-238
6. Poulson, D.F. (1950) in "Biology of Drosophila" (M. Demerec
   ed.) pp 168-270, Hafner, New York
7. Lohs-Schardin, M., Cremer, C. and Nüsslein-Volhard, C. (1979)

Dev. Biol. in press

8. Zalokar, M., Audit, C. and Erk, I. (1975) Devel. Biol., 47, 419-432

9. Nüsslein-Volhard, C. (1973) in "Determinants of Spatial Organisation" (I. Konigsberg and S. Subtelney ed.), Academic Press pp 168

10. Bull, A.L. (1966) J. Exp. Zool., 161, 221-241

11. Nüsslein-Volhard, C. (1977) Roux's Archives, 179, 159

12. Gierer, A. and Meinhardt, H. (1972) Kybernetik, 12, 30-39

13. Meinhardt, H. (1977) J. Cell Sci., 23, 117-139

14. Gloor, H. (1950) Arch. Julius-Klaus-Stiftung, 25, 38-44

15. Nüsslein-Volhard, C. and Wieschaus, E. in preparation

16. Lewis, E.B. (1979) Nature, 276, 565-570

17. Nüsslein-Volhard, C., Lohs-Schardin, M., Sander, K. and Cremer, C. in preparation

18. Poulson, D.F. (1940) J. Exp. Zool., 83, 271

19. Rice, T. Thesis, Yale 1973

20. Gans, M., Audit, C., Masson, M. (1975) Genetics, 81, 683-704

Cell Lineage, Stem Cells and Cell Determination
INSERM Symposium No. 10
Editor: N. Le Douarin
© *1979 Elsevier/North-Holland Biomedical Press*

THE DISTRIBUTION OF ANLAGEN IN THE EARLY EMBRYO OF DROSOPHILA

WILFRIED JANNING, JÜRGEN PFREUNDT and ROLF TIEMANN
Zoologisches Institut der Universität Münster, Badestr. 9,
D - 4400 Münster

INTRODUCTION

In Drosophila, analyses of genetic mosaics play a prominent rôle in experimental description of normal development by providing information on developmental parameters such as growth factors, determination and cell-lineage. Moreover, it was shown, that data from genetic mosaics can be used to establish fate maps that reflect the relative positions of progenitor cells of larval and adult structures in the early embryo[1-3].

In general, genetic mosaics are created by marking single nuclei (in cleavage stages) or cells with mutant genotypes that express their phenotype autonomously. In the following sections we will discuss fate maps that reveal
1. the relative positions of anlagen in the early embryo, and
2. the distribution of probabilities to form specific structures within anlagen.

GYNANDROMORPH FATE MAPS

The generation of genetic mosaics in which the mutant clones are initiated during cleavage is so far only possible by chromosome loss. Since in Drosophila only aneuploidies of the first (sex) and fourth chromosomes, respectively, survive, and since known marker genes are concentrated on the X-chromosome, gynandromorphs are the mosaics of choice. Most frequently a somatically unstable ring-X chromosome [R(1)2, In(1)w^{vc}] is used to construct gynanders with female XX- and male (mutant) XO-cells (Fig. 1).

The small sample of gynandromorphs shown in Figure 2 illustrates the following general observations and interpretations:
1. Observation: Regarding the distribution of XX- and XO-cells all gynanders are different from each other.

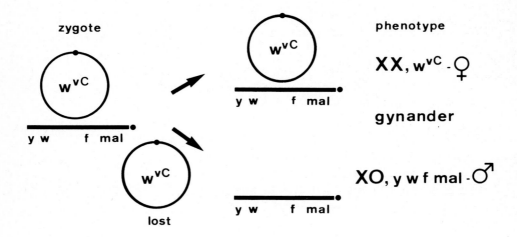

Fig. 1. Schematic representation of the production of gynandromorphs by mitotic loss of an unstable ring-X chromosome (w^{vC}).
The rod-X chromosome carries the marker alleles yellow, white,
forked and maroonlike that express themselves in male XO-cells.

Interpretation: There is no strict determinative development, neither at beginning of cleavage, i.e. orientation of
the spindle axis of the first zygotic division[4], nor at later
developmental stages.

2. Observation: Contiguous patches of either genotype are large.
Interpretation: There is no significant mixing of nuclei or
cells during cleavage, blastoderm formation and growth of
imaginal discs, but there may be small patches of one genotype included in larger patches of the other.

3. Observation: The genotypic dividing lines tend to follow the
longitudinal midline and intersegmental boundaries.
Interpretation: In early stages cells giving rise to imaginal structures on either body side and in different segments
are separated by cells developing into larval or internal
structures. This leads to straight instead of more or less
convoluted borderlines in the adult.

4. Observation: The mean patch size and the mean frequency with
which landmarks are of mutant phenotype are around 0.5.

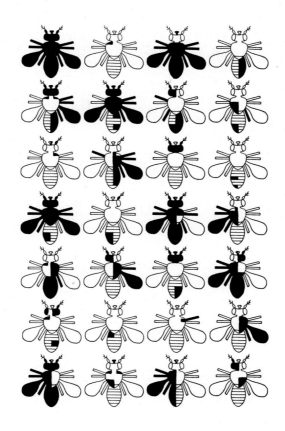

Fig. 2. Outlines of a sample of gynandromorphs generated by loss of an unstable ring-X chromosome. XO areas are shaded.

Interpretation: At the time of clone initiation there are about two nuclei present, i.e. the event takes place at one of the first cleavage divisions.

In 1929 A. H. Sturtevant[1] studying gynandromorphs of Drosophila simulans argued that the frequency with which two landmarks differ in genotype could reflect the distance between progenitor cells in early developmental stages. Fourty years later this idea was taken up by Garcia-Bellido and Merriam[2]. They found, that they could construct a fate map based on frequencies of genotypic separation between landmarks in gynanders. More fate maps were constructed using external and internal[5,6] land-

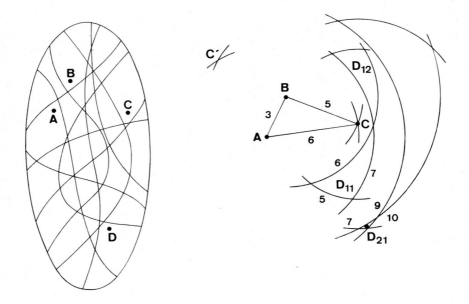

Fig. 3. Demonstration of the principles of fate mapping. See text for explanation.

marks of larva[7] and adult (e.g. Fig. 4a, for review see Janning[8]). The distances between landmarks are given in sturt units[3], whereby 1 sturt is equivalent to a probability of 1% that, among all gynanders scored, two structures will be of different genotypes.

In constructing fate maps we encounter a number of difficulties. These concern:
1. the transformation of distances on the convex egg surface into a two-dimensional map,
2. the unknown course with which the genotypic borderline runs on the surface of the blastoderm, and
3. the degree of mixing of cells during later development.
These complications can be illustrated by the theoretical example shown in Figure 3. On the left of this figure a Drosophila embryo in the blastoderm stage is drawn with ten dividing lines between male and female cells, whereby each dividing line represents that of one gynandromorph. On the surface of the egg

are 4 points (A to D) representing four regions which will develop into different structures of the adult. The frequencies
of genotypic separation between all pairs of points can be used
to construct the relative positions of the points concerned.
In this case A, B and C can be placed by triangulation, but the
position of D cannot be established unequivocally (D_{11}, D_{12}) due
to the convolutions of dividing lines on the blastoderm surface.
If a dividing line passes twice (or any even number of times)
between two points, they are scored as having the same genotype
which leads to an underestimate of the real distance. If we
consider the convolutions, e.g. by additional points between A,
B and C on the one hand and D on the other, D can be mapped at
position D_{21}. Therefore, in the general strategy of constructing fate maps it is essential to use short distances. These
will be found between landmarks of the head, the thorax and the
abdomen. The submaps will then be positioned by a few triangu-
lations using observed distances, though this procedure implies
an underestimate of the real distances.

   Mapping function. The convolutions of the theoretical dividing lines shown in Figure 3 are based upon some general observations in gynandromorph fate mapping:
1. the maximum distance found experimentally is about 50-60
   sturts instead of the expected theoretical maximum of 100
   sturts,
2. map distances are not additive over large distances,
3. fate maps can measure up to 150 sturt units in length.
   These findings resemble strongly the conditions of meiotic
gene mapping where multiple crossovers and interference lead to
an exponential relationship between recombination and map distances[9,10]. Therefore, we looked at the relationship between
observed and actual fate map distances. Plotting the two parameters against each other gave the set of points shown in Figure
5a (based on the fate map of Fig. 4a). As expected, there is no
linear relationship. Linearity up to about 15 sturts may reflect the fact that mainly short distances were used in the mapping procedure and/or that only few convolutions of the dividing
lines occur within short distances. The accumulation of points
at about 35 sturts showing linearity derives from positioning

88

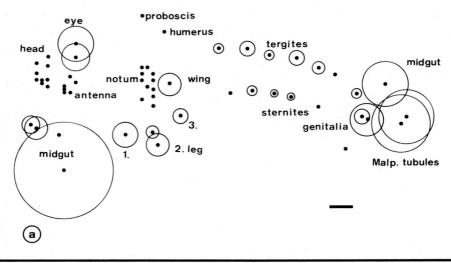

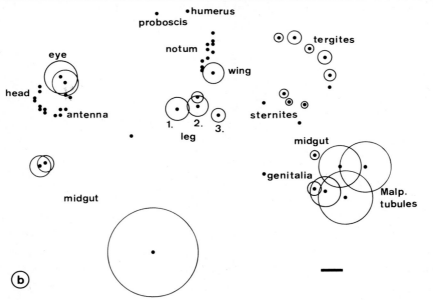

Fig. 4. Gynandromorph fate maps of presumptive adult structures.
Gynanders were produced by ring-X chromosome loss. The diameters
of the circles are proportional to frequencies of mosaicism within the corresponding regions. a) Fate map constructed by triangulation (see Fig. 3). b) Fate map generated by a computer program (see text for explanation). Scale: 10 sturts.

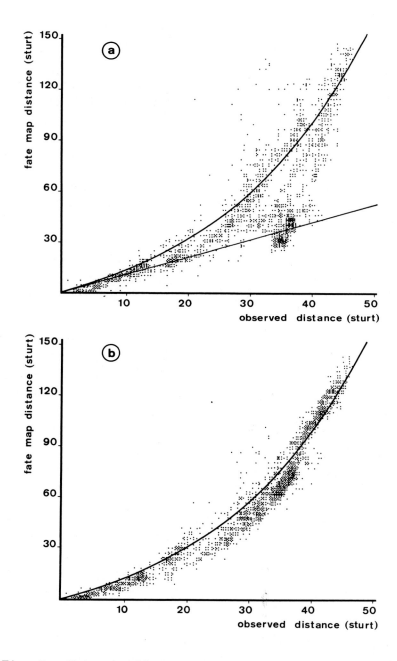

Fig. 5. Fate map distances plotted against observed distances. a) Data from map in Fig. 4a. b) Data from map in Fig. 4b. See text for explanation.

submaps as mentioned above. Among long distances a given observed distance corresponds to a wide range of fate map distances and vice versa.

To describe mathematically the relationship between observed
and fate map distances by a mapping function we arbitrarily
chose the exponential function $f(x) = a(e^{x/a} - 1)$, where $\underline{a}$ was
estimated to be 25. There are, of course, other functions with
which the same relationship could be described[11].

The mapping function can now be used to construct fate maps
that are better adapted to the internal parameters of fate mapping (see Fig. 3). A computer program was established in which
observed distances are converted into distances estimated from
the mapping function and then compared with corresponding distances in the original map (Fig. 4a). The error between all
pairs of distances is minimized by successive iterations using
a modified Newton method. (The PL/I computer program is available on request from the authors.)

After 15 iterations, plotting of fate map distances against
observed distances results in good adaptation to the mapping
function (Fig. 5b). The corresponding fate map (Fig. 4b) shows
some modifications as compared to the original fate map (Fig.
4a). In general, internal structures are more ventral and the
dorsal band of cuticular anlagen is more pronounced. We believe
that this map is in better accordance with embryological data[12].

Fate maps and development. In principle, gynandromorph fate
maps and fate maps established by descriptive embryology[12] show
the same spatial distribution of anlagen. We shall now ask what
stage of development is represented by fate maps that are based
on gynander data. An answer could be given if we would know the
time in development when genotypic separations are fixed between
cells or groups of cells from which the landmarks scored are
derived. Therefore, we will subdivide our question as follows:
1. When in development are the genotypic dividing lines fixed?
2. When does restriction of developmental potentialities take
   place?
These questions imply that gynandromorph fate maps do not provide information on the time when determination of different
anlagen occurs.

In answering the first question we can say that it is the blastoderm stage when for the first time in development cells are formed, and in a gynandromorph a borderline will now separate cells of two different genotypes. During subsequent development, morphogenetic movements, region specific growth rates and other events will change the course of the dividing line. Final fixation of this line will be different for different cell types: it will occur early in development for larval tissues[13], and late for imaginal cells which proliferate up to metamorphosis[14,15].

The second question is more difficult to answer. Again, different groups of cells become determined at different times. Experiments performed to reveal the potentialities of cells in the blastoderm stage[16-22] suggest that around this stage the cells are divided into groups giving rise to segments, and in the case of the thorax to anterior and posterior compartments within a segment[23-25]. Within imaginal discs, successive clonal restrictions seem to occur during subsequent development[24,26]. In discs of the late third instar, fragmentation and transplantation show that the arrangement of landmarks is the same as in the adult after differentiation.

Going back to our main question what stage of development is represented by gynandromorph fate maps we can now argue:

the fate maps reflect at least the relative positions of progenitor cells of segments and compartments at blastoderm.

If we could superimpose this fate map on a blastoderm we could point to cells giving rise to different segments.

The compartment hypothesis postulates that all cells of a compartment exhibit the same genetic activity[23]. That means that in principle any cell can differentiate any structure of the compartment. Thus, the positions of small landmarks, e.g. bristles, shown in gynandromorph fate maps cannot represent the positions of real blastoderm cells from which they are derived. Nevertheless fine structure fate maps can be obtained from gynander data[27-29]. Obviously, sturt distances between pairs of landmarks within a compartment are measured between cells after they had been determined to differentiate these landmarks, and the dividing lines became fixed between them. For imaginal

disc derivatives this is around the end of third instar. This
statement becomes clearer if we consider that one type of dividing line in the blastoderm will most probably result in a
variety of different lines in the adult, depending on the degree
of indeterminacy of the developing system[8].

However, we must not forget that the mature disc is composed
of clones which date back to founder cells in the blastoderm
stage. If at this early stage a genotypic dividing line cuts
through a group of founder cells, then the corresponding clones
in the mature disc are also genotypically separated. But there
is no strict cell-lineage within compartments, which means that
there are no unique sets of cuticular structures differentiated
by each clone. Therefore, the fine structure maps reflect the
relative positions of "probabilities to form specific landmarks" in the blastoderm. For elucidation we consider what
would happen to cells in the proliferating disc with respect to
their location. If growth is isodiametric the "probability fate
map" would show the same arrangement of landmarks as found after
determination in the disc. But if there were differences in
proliferation rate or morphogenetic movements (which both would
change the course of the dividing lines) the "probability fate
map" and the positions of corresponding landmarks in the adult
would differ, reflecting exactly these changes between blastoderm and final differentiation. In Figure 7 the arrangement
of notum bristles in the adult fly and the corresponding fine
structure map obtained from gynandromorphs (distances were
measured in sturtoid-units[30], see below) are shown for comparison. The strong similarity between the two figures is evident and implies that little changes occurred during proliferation in this subcompartment[27].

To ascertain that this fine structure map could be a blastoderm map in the sense mentioned above we tried to establish
fate maps based upon clones which were initiated at blastoderm
or even later in development.

BLASTODERM AND FIRST INSTAR FATE MAPS
The most powerful technique to label genetically single cells
at nearly any time in development is X-ray induced mitotic re-

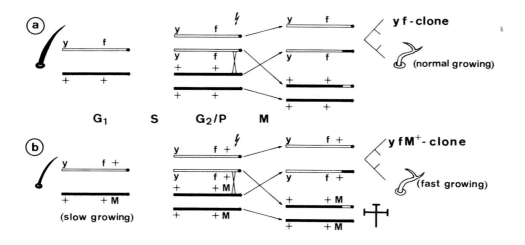

Fig. 6. Schematic representation of X-ray induced mitotic recombination. Irradiation of heterozygous cells in G2/P phase
of the cell cycle may cause recombination leading to homozygous
cells after next mitosis. a) Clones marked with yellow and
forked are easily distinguished from wildtype background. b) Mitotic recombination in slow-growing cells heterozygous for a
Minute mutation [M(1)o^Sp] results in fast-growing M^+- clones[33].

TABLE 1

CLONE FREQUENCY AND CLONE SIZE IN THE NOTUM AFTER X-RAY INDUCED
MITOTIC RECOMBINATION

Series[a]	Number of half-nota scored	Number of clones	Mean clone size (bris-tles/clone)	Clone frequen-cy (%)	Frequency of large clones (%)[b]
+ 3	26 236	332	2.5	1.2	3.3
M 3	12 110	373	5.1	3.1	37.8
+ 24	26 952	330	2.5	1.2	4.9
M 24	11 868	444	3.8	3.7	22.5

[a] Abbreviations: + and M for the two clone types shown in Figures 6a and 6b, respectively. 3 and 24 for irradiation
(1000 R) at blastoderm and first instar (3 ±0.5 and 24 ±0.5
hours after egg laying, respectively).
[b] 7 - 11 bristles/clone

combination[31] (Fig. 6). The disadvantage of this method is that
the usual dose of 1000 R may kill about 50% of the cells of a
disc[32]. Nevertheless, the remaining cell groups recover and
form normal structures.

In the notum with 11 landmark bristles we produced two types
of clones: normal growing y f - clones in normal heterozygous
females (Fig. 6a), and fast growing y f - clones in Minute -
heterozygotes[33] (Fig. 6b).

In Table 1 the results are summarized. The clone frequency
which depends on the fraction of sensitive cells at the time of
irradiation is about three times higher in the Minute than in
the non-Minute genotype. The reason for this difference is
unknown[34]. Some proliferation between 3 and 24 hours is indicated by the increase in clone frequency and decrease in mean
clone size in the Minute genotype. In the normal genotype the
mean spot size is 2.5 bristles/clone at both stages with a large
fraction of clones with only one marked bristle. For this reason we did not find a change in mean clone size or frequency.
In all series we found clones with up to 11 marked bristles in
various combinations of landmarks. From these data we calculated sturtoid distances (d)[30] between all pairs of the 11 landmarks:

$d = 100 \ (n_{01} + n_{10})/n_{01} + n_{10} + 2n_{11}$ (0 = wildtype, 1 = mutant).
Fate maps (Figs. 8 and 9) were established using the computer
program with variation of parameter a (see above).

In both, the blastoderm and first instar fate maps the distribution of landmark bristles is generally the same as in the gynandromorph fate map (Fig. 7), but the similarity is more pronounced in the maps based on fast growing clones (Figs. 8b, 9b).
This demonstrates clearly that there are no gross morphogenetic
movements within the anlage during growth from blastoderm to
first instar nor to final differentiation.

But there are also differences between the maps depending on
the following conditions of this technique of fate mapping:
1. Inclusion of different sets of landmarks in clones is required. If there were a strict cell-lineage, clonally unrelated groups of landmarks would be separated by the maximum
   distance of 100 sturtoids and could not be placed relative

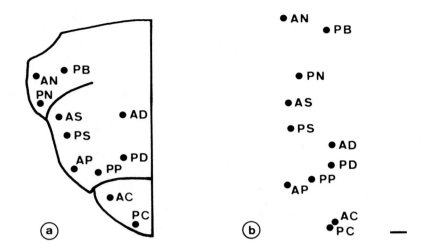

Fig. 7. Bristles of the notum. a) Arrangement of bristles in
the adult. b) Gynandromorph fate map. Scale: 2 sturtoids.
Bristles: PB, presutural; AN, PN, anterior and posterior noto-
pleural; AS, PS, anterior and posterior supraalar; AP, PP, anterior and posterior postalar; AD, PD, anterior and posterior
dorsocentral; AC, PC, anterior and posterior scutellar.

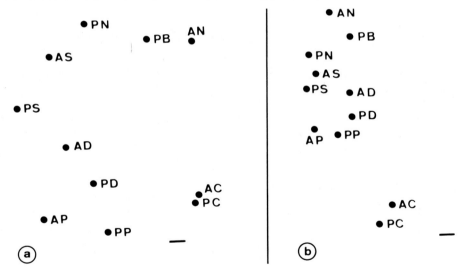

Fig. 8. Blastoderm fate maps of the notum, based upon a) normal
growing and b) fast growing clones (see Fig. 6). Clones were
started one cell division after blastoderm. Scale: 10 sturtoids.
Abbreviations as in Fig. 7.

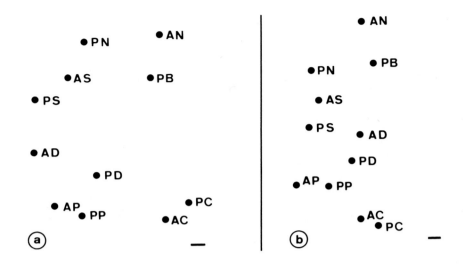

Fig. 9. First instar fate maps of the notum, based upon a) normal growing and b) fast growing clones (see Fig. 6). Clones were started one cell division after irradiation of 24-hours-stages. Scale: 10 sturtoids. Abbreviations as in Fig. 7.

to each other.

2. Variation in clone size should be sufficient so that the largest clones cover the whole area examined. Otherwise, the distances between landmarks never included in the same clone will reach the maximum of 100 sturtoids, too. Variation in clone size may result from differences in growth rate that occur normally or are caused by the X-ray treatment.

These conditions are fulfilled in all four series of experiments, but with differences in mean clone size and frequency of large clones (Tab. 1). In the Minute series the fast growing clones produced a high frequency of large clones resulting in a wide range of sturtoid distances. The mean clone size of normal growing clones on the other hand is much smaller with a low fraction of large clones. Therefore, intermediate and large distances are more similar to each other and near the maximum distance of 100 sturtoids. This is the reason why the corresponding fate maps are c-shaped (Figs. 8a, 9a).

In the blastoderm fate map based on fast growing clones, the distance between scutal and scutellar bristles is remarkably larger than in all other fate maps presented. Within the notum this reflects a developmental restriction that is very frequently respected by fast growing clones[24,35]. In the first instar fate map, the compartment boundary is not visible because mean clone size and fraction of large clones are too small.

In summary, we believe that the method of mosaic fate mapping can portray anlagen at different developmental stages and can reveal developmental parameters, such as morphogenetic movements, growth rate differences and cell mixing within anlagen.

ACKNOWLEDGEMENTS

We thank Dr. Rolf Nöthiger for valuable comments on the manuscript, Miss Regina Münster for expert technical assistance and the Deutsche Forschungsgemeinschaft for support (Ja 199/6 and 8).

REFERENCES

1. Sturtevant, A.H. (1929) Z. Wiss. Zool., 135, 323-356.
2. Garcia-Bellido, A., Merriam, J.R. (1969) J. Exp. Zool., 170, 61-76.
3. Hotta, Y., Benzer, S. (1972) Nature, 240, 527-535.
4. Parks, H.B. (1936) Ann. Entomol. Soc. Am., 29, 350-392.
5. Janning, W. (1974) Wilhelm Roux' Archiv, 174, 349-359.
6. Kankel, D.R., Hall, J.C. (1976) Develop. Biol., 48, 1-24.
7. Janning, W. (1976) Wilhelm Roux's Archives, 179, 349-372.
8. Janning, W. (1978) Results and Problems in Cell Differentiation, vol. 9, Springer, Berlin-Heidelberg-New York, pp. 1-28.
9. Haldane, J.B.S. (1919) J. Genet. 8, 299-309.
10. Morgan, T.H., Bridges, C.B., Schultz, J. (1935) Carnegie Inst. Wash. Yearbook, 34, 284-291.
11. Flanagan, J.R. (1976) Develop. Biol., 53, 142-146.
12. Poulson, D.F. (1950) Biology of Drosophila, Wiley, New York, pp. 168-274.
13. Szabad, J., Schüpbach, T., Wieschaus, E. (1979) Develop. Biol. (in press).
14. Nöthiger, R. (1972) Results and Problems in Cell Differentiation, vol. 5, Springer, Berlin-Heidelberg-New York, pp. 1-34.

98

15. Gehring, W.J., Nöthiger, R. (1973) Developmental Systems: Insects, vol. 2, Academic Press, London-New York, pp. 211-290.

16. Chan, L.-N., Gehring, W. (1971) Proc. Natl. Acad. Sci., 68, 2217-2221.

17. Bownes, M. (1975) J. Embryol. Exp. Morph., 34, 33-54.

18. Wieschaus, E., Gehring, W.J. (1976) Develop. Biol., 50, 249-263.

19. Lawrence, P.A., Morata, G. (1977) Develop. Biol., 56, 40-51.

20. Illmensee, K. (1978) Results and Problems in Cell Differentiation, vol. 9, Springer, Berlin-Heidelberg-New York, pp. 51-69.

21. Lohs-Schardin, M., Sander, K., Cremer, C., Cremer, T., Zorn, C. (1979) Develop. Biol., 68, 533-545.

22. Lohs-Schardin, M., Cremer, C., Nüsslein-Volhard, C. (1979) Develop. Biol. (in press).

23. Garcia-Bellido, A. (1975) Cell Patterning, Ciba Found. Symp., 29 (NS), 161-178.

24. Garcia-Bellido, A., Ripoll, P., Morata, G. (1976) Develop. Biol., 48, 132-147.

25. Steiner, E. (1976) Wilhelm Roux's Archives, 180, 9-30.

26. Garcia-Bellido, A., Merriam, J.R. (1971) Develop. Biol. 24, 61-87.

27. Ripoll, P. (1972) Wilhelm Roux' Archiv, 169, 200-215.

28. Wieschaus, E., Gehring, W.J. (1976) Wilhelm Roux's Archives 180, 31-46.

29. Baker, W.K. (1978) Genetics, 88, 743-754.

30. Gelbart, W.M. (1974) Genetics, 76, 51-63.

31. Becker, H.J. (1976) The Genetics and Biology of Drosophila, vol. 1c, Academic Press, London-New York, pp. 1019-1087.

32. Haynie, J.L., Bryant, P.J. (1977) Wilhelm Roux's Archives, 183, 85-100.

33. Morata, G., Ripoll, P. (1975) Develop. Biol., 42, 211-221.

34. Ferrus, A. (1975) Genetics, 79, 589-599.

35. Murphy, C., Tokunaga, C. (1970) J. Exp. Zool., 175, 197-220.

THE MOUSE TERATOCARCINOMA. A MODEL TO STUDY THE DETERMINATION AND SEGREGATION OF CELL LINES

Cell Lineage, Stem Cells and Cell Determination
INSERM Symposium No. 10
Editor: N. Le Douarin
© *1979 Elsevier/North-Holland Biomedical Press*

PROPERTIES OF SOME MONOCLONAL ANTIBODIES RAISED AGAINST MOUSE
EMBRYONAL CARCINOMA CELLS

Rolf KEMLER, Dominique MORELLO and François JACOB
Service de Génétique cellulaire du Collège de France et de
l'Institut Pasteur, 25 rue du Dr. Roux, 75015 Paris (France)

INTRODUCTION

Antisera prepared by immunizing animals with embryonal carcinoma cells (EC, i.e. stem cell of teratocarcinoma) make it possible
to detect surface structures on cells of early mouse embryo. With
antisera against a nullipotent embryonal carcinoma cell, the F9
line, two major results have been obtained. 1) a syngeneic anti-
F9 serum has allowed the detection of a surface structure, probably related to the T/t locus of the mouse[1,2]. 2) A rabbit anti-
F9 serum allows the detection of a cell surface structure, the
masking of which by Fab fragments blocks the transition from
morula to blastocyst[3].

It is not clear yet whether the two sera detect the same membrane antigen. Such complex antisera contain a large variety of
heterogeneous antibody populations, even in the case of the syngeneic antisera[4]. It was therefore decided to use the experimental
approach introduced by Köhler and Milstein[5] and to isolate hybrid
cell lines producing monospecific antibodies against surface
structures of embryonal carcinoma cells. To obtain a high diversity of hybrid cell lines secreting monoclonal antibodies against
a wide variety of surface antigens, mouse myeloma cells were fused
with spleen cells of rats previously immunized with mouse embryonal carcinoma cells. This report describes the properties of some
of the monoclonal antibodies obtained by this technique.

MATERIALS AND METHODS

Animals. Random bred rats, OFA, were obtained from Ifra-Credo,
France.

Cells. The origin and nature of different EC lines used are
summarized in Table 1 and 2. F9-41, a nullipotent EC cell[6] shows
a slight endodermal differentiation under certain *in vitro* condi-

tions[7]. Mouse myeloma cell line P3/X63-Ag8 was isolated originally by Dr. C. Milstein. X63-Ag8 secretes an IgGl(κ). It is HPRT$^-$ (hypoxanthine-guanine phosphoribosyl-transferase) and dies in selective HAT (hypoxanthine-aminopterin-thymidine) medium. Mouse lymphocytes and sperm were prepared as described elsewhere[4]. Sheep red blood cells were kept sterile at 4°C and washed three times in PBS (phosphate buffered saline) before use. Preimplantation embryos were obtained from super-ovulated 129/Sv virgin females and freed off their zona pellucida as described[3]. At blastocyst stage, inner cell masses (ICM) were isolated by immunosurgery[8]. For endoderm differentiation, ICM were cultured for a period of about 48 hours in Eagle's medium with 15 % foetal calf serum (FCS)[9].

Antisera. Rats were immunized with F9 cells starting with a subcutaneous and intramuscular injection of 2 x 10[7] cells in incomplete Freund's adjuvant. After four weeks, the animals received weekly 1.5 x 10[7] cells in Hank's medium intraperitoneally for one month. Three days after the last injection, the rats were bled and spleen cells were used for fusion. Purified rabbit antibodies specific for rat IgM and IgG, 1 mg/ml PBS each, were kindly provided by Dr. J.C. Antoine, Institut Pasteur. Purified rabbit F(ab)$_2$ anti-rat Fab, 1 mg/ml were a gift from Dr. A.F. Williams, MRC, Oxford, England. Fluoresceinated antisera against rat (Nordic), mouse and rabbit (Institut Pasteur) immunoglobulins were dialyzed, preabsorbed and stored in aliquots at -20°C as described[2].

Cell fusion. Spleen cells were removed from rats three days after the last immunization, isolated and washed three times in Hank's medium. Myeloma cells (2.5 x 10[7]) washed in Hank's medium were mixed with lymphocytes (1 x 10[8]). After centrifugation, supernatant was removed as completely as possible and 2.0 ml of polyethylene-glycol (PEG, MG : 4,000, Roth KG, Karsruhe, Germany, 20 g PEG dissolved in 28 ml Hank's medium containing 15 % dimethylsulfoxide (DMSO)) were added. After 1 min. at 37°C, the PEG solution was diluted by adding every 5 seconds one drop of Hank's medium over a period of 5 min. The cells were centrifuged, resuspended in HAT medium and cultured in tissue culture clusters (Costar), each well containing between 2 and 3 x 10[6] lymphocytes. HAT medium was changed once a week and hybrid clones appeared usually after 2 or 3 weeks.

Subcloning. Hybrid cells were subcloned in HAT medium 20 % FCS, containing 1 % methyl-cellulose (Herculus Inc.). Subclones were isolated and grown on a feeder layer of a X-irradiated fibroblast cell line (STO)[10].

Cytotoxicity test. Cytotoxicity tests were done as described by Artzt et al.[6]. For screening of hybrid culture supernatants, a microcytotoxicity test was carried out according to Mittal[11].

Absorption. After concentration by ultrafiltration (Amicon) and precipitation with 40 % ammonium sulphate, monoclonal antibodies were absorbed on different cell types by incubating one volume of cells with one volume of culture supernatants (at appropriate dilution), 1 h at 4°C. After centrifugation, 10 minutes at 4,000 g, the absorbed antibodies were stored until use at -80°C.

Immunofluorescence staining. Tests were usually performed as a "triple sandwich technique" using purified anti-rat IgM or IgG antibodies (5 - 10 µg/ml) as a second layer. The fluorescence staining was done on viable cells with standard conditions as described by Damonneville et al.[4].

Radioactive binding-assay. Rabbit $F(ab)_2$ anti-rat Fab was iodinated with ^{125}I as described by Jensenius and Williams[12]. The radioactive binding-assay was done in round bottom microtiter plates, $3 - 5 \times 10^4$ target cells were incubated 45 min. at room temperature with 50 µl of (undiluted or diluted) supernatant from hybrid clone cultures. After three washings in Hank's medium containing 4 % immunoprecipitated FCS plus 0.2 % NaN_3, the cells were resuspended in 50 µl ^{125}I $F(ab)_2$ anti-rat Fab (200,000 cpm) for 45 min. at room temperature, washed again three times and transferred to tubes for counting. Each point in the assay was performed in triplicates. The maximal binding of the added counts was between 10 and 20 per cent of the counts added.

Controls. In immunofluorescence staining, cytotoxicity test and radioactive binding assay, controls were 1) concentrated culture supernatants (see Absorption) from X63-Ag8 cells and 2) concentrated supernatants from a hybrid cell line which had no activity against F9 cells.

RESULTS

Production and detection of antibody-secreting hybrids. Cell
fusion of lymphocytes from immunized rat with mouse myeloma cells
seems to be very efficient. In about 80 % of the costar wells,
hybrids were found to grow. By testing culture supernatants in
a microcytotoxicity test, a high fraction of wells turned out
to be active on F9 cells. In one experiment, 1 well out of 4 ; in
another one, 1 well out of 2.5 contained activity against F9 cells.
From a total number of 93 wells, 28 have been found to produce
antibodies against F9 cells. Five positive wells were chosen and
their cell population subcloned twice in 1 % methyl-cellulose.
From each subclone, culture supernatant was concentrated about 100
times (see Materials and Methods). They are referred furtheron
as ECMA 1 to 5 (Embryonal Carcinoma Monoclonal Antibody).
Results of cytotoxic activities are summarized in Fig. 1. ECMA

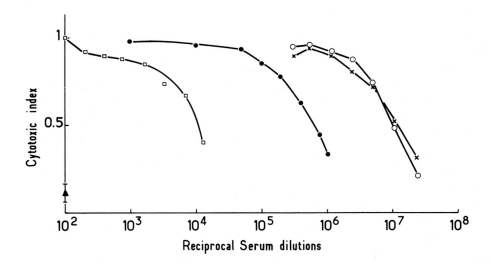

Fig. 1. Cytotoxic activities of ECMAs against F9 cells.
● : ECMA 1; o : ECMA 2 ; x : ECMA 3 ; ◻ : ECMA 5 ; ▲ : culture
supernatants from X63-Ag8 cells (culture supernatants from a
negative hybrid cell line give similar results). ECMA 4 shows
no cytotoxic activity at all.

1 to 3 had high activity against F9 cells with cytotoxic titers of $1/10^6$ and more. ECMA 5 had a comparably lower titer ($1/4.10^3$) and ECMA 4 showed no cytotoxic activity at all. For comparison, total rat serum taken at time when cell fusion was performed had a cytotoxic titer of $1/10^4$. Concentrated culture supernatants from X63-Ag8 cells and from a negative hybrid cell line had a cytotoxic index lower than 0.1. The activity of each ECMA was also measured in a radioactive binding assay (Fig. 2) ECMA 4 showed the lowest binding activity. Controls from culture supernatants of X63-Ag8 cells and of a negative hybrid cell line ranged between 300-1200 cpm.

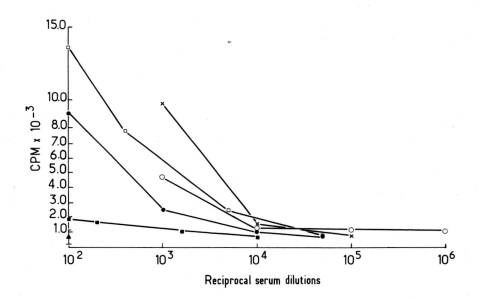

Fig. 2. Activities of ECMAs against F9 cells in a radioactive binding-assay.
● : ECMA 1 ; o : ECMA 2 ; x : ECMA 3 ; ■ : ECMA 4 ; □ : ECMA 5 ;
▲ : background counts obtained with concentrated culture supernatants of X63-Ag8 cells (culture supernatants from a negative hybrid cell line give similar results).

TABLE 1

ANTIGENS DETECTED BY ECMAS ON VARIOUS CELL TYPES[a]

Cell type	Mouse strains	Ref.	ECMA:Embryonal Carcinoma Monoclonal Antibody				
			1 (IgM)[b]	2 (IgM)	3 (IgM)	4 (IgG)	5 (IgM)
PCC4 Aza, EC, Multipotent	129/Sv	13	+[d]	+	+	+	-
C17-S1-1191, EC[c]	C$_3$H	14	-	+	+	n.t.	-
LT-1, EC, nullipotent	LT	15	-	+(40)[e]	+(15)	+(100)	-
Differentiated derivatives of EC cells							
PYS-2 : parietal yolk sac	129/Sv	16	-	-	-	+(100)	-
3/A/1-D-3:mesenchyme-like	"	17	+	+	-	+	+
3/TM 1:trophoblastoma	"	18	-	+(70)	-	n.t.	-
PCD/2:myoblast	"	19	-	+(25)	+(5)	+(100)	n.t.
PCD/3:fibroblast	"	20	-	+	-	n.t.	n.t.
SRBC : sheep red blood cells			-	-	-	n.t.	+
Lymphocytes	129/Sv		+	+	-	-	+
Sperm	129/Sv		+	+	+	-	+

a Tests were done by absorption or indirect immunofluorescence (see Materials and Methods)
b Immunoglobulin class
c Subclone of C17-S1, EC cell restricted to nervous differentiation (H. Jakob, pers.com.)
d + : Activity removed by absorption. e Percent of positive cells in immunofluorescence tests.

In order to determine the immunoglobulin class each hybridoma produces, ECMAs were tested with anti-immunoglobulin-isotype-specific antibodies in a triple immunofluorescence test. Four hybridomas were found to produce IgM and only one IgG antibodies.

Activity against different cell lines. The activity of each ECMA against various cell types was studied by absorption followed by measure of residual activity against F9 cells in a cytotoxicity test or radioactive binding assay. When necessary, the fraction of reactive cells was determined in an indirect immunofluorescence test. The results obtained with ECMA 1 to 5 are summarized in Table I. From these results, the following conclusions can be drawn :

a) EC cells : ECMA 2, 3 and 4 react with all EC cell lines tested, whatever their origin (129/Sv, LT or C3H). ECMA 1 reacts with EC cells from 129/Sv mice but not from C3H or LT. F9 cells are the only EC cells which ECMA 5 reacts with.

b) Differentiated derivatives from EC cells : a number of differentiated derivatives of EC cells were tested for their reactivity with ECMAs. The pattern of reactivities appears to be different for the five ECMAs. ECMA 2 and 4 react with most of the lines tested. ECMA 1 and 5 react only with the 3/A/1/-D-3 line, a mesenchymal like derivative. ECMA 3 reacts only with a minor subpopulation of PCD/2, a myoblast derivative.

c) Sperm : ECMA1, 2, 3 and 5, but not ECMA 4 react with sperm cells from 129/Sv mice.

d) Lymphocytes : ECMA 1, 2 and 5 (but not 3 and 4) react with lymphocytes (129/Sv mice).

e) Sheep red blood cell (SRBC) : ECMA 5 is the only one which reacts with SRBC.

From these results, it can be concluded that each of the five ECMAs detects a different antigenic specificity.

Distribution of surface antigens during *in vitro* differentiation of EC cells. EC cell line PCC3/A/1 is able to differentiate *in vitro* under certain culture conditions[13]. The expression of antigens detected by each ECMA can therefore be followed during *in vitro* differentiation. PCC3/A/1 cells were grown under conditions allowing differentiation. At various times, cells were harvested and the fraction of cells reacting with each ECMA was

measured in an indirect immunofluorescence test.   The results of
these experiments are given in Table 2.   ECMA 4 labels 100 %
of the cells at any time during differentiation.   ECMA 1 and 5
label only a minor subpopulation at any time during differentiation.

TABLE 2

EXPRESSION OF ANTIGENS DETECTED BY ECMAS DURING *IN VITRO* DIFFEREN-
TIATION OF EC CELLS

Cell line		ECMA				
		1	2	3	4	5
		(IgM)[a]	(IgM)	(IgM)	(IgG)	(IgM)
PCC3/A/1[b]	24 h	2.5[c]	70	70	100	1
	48 h	n.t.	70	50	100	6
	8 d	4	6	3	100	10
	13 d	1	1	2	n.t.	10

[a] Immunoglobulin class each ECMA produces
[b] EC differentiates *in vitro* under certain culture conditions[13]
[c] Percentage of labelled cells in indirect immunofluorescence tests

In contrast, ECMA 2 and 3 label 70 % of EC cells.   This percentage decreases rapidly as differentiation proceeds.   Concentrated
culture supernatants from X63-Ag8 cells and a negative hybrid cell
line did not label more than one cell in two thousands at any
time.

Expression of antigens on preimplantation embryos.   The
expression of antigens detected by ECMAs was tested on 129/Sv
preimplantation embryos in an indirect immunofluorescence test
(Table 3).   For each ECMA, more than a hundred embryos at
different stages were tested.

ECMA 2 and 3 were negative on unfertilized eggs, but reacted
clearly with two cell-embryos.   They were strongly positive on
morulae (up to a dilution of $1/4.10^3$).   At the blastocyst stage,

TABLE 3

EXPRESSION OF ANTIGENS DETECTED BY ECMAS ON PREIMPLANTATION
EMBRYOS[a]

	ECMA				
	1 (IgM)[b]	2 (IgM)	3 (IgM)	4 (IgG)	5 (IgM)
Non-fertilized eggs	n.t.	−	−	n.t.	n.t.
Two-cell embryos	−	+	+	n.t.	n.t.
Morulae	−	+	+	−	−
Blastocysts	+	+	+	−	−
ICM	+	+	+	−	−
ICM, with endodermal differentiation	+	+	+	−	n.t.

[a] ECMAs were tested in an indirect immunofluorescence test at
concentrations 100-1000 times higher than those giving clear
staining on F9 cells.

[b] Immunoglobulin class each ECMA produces

both trophectodermal cells and cells of the inner cell mass (ICM)
were labelled, but at considerable lower dilutions (1/50) for
ICM cells. After two days of culture under conditions allowing
endodermal differentiation, staining of ICM became significantly
stronger (Fig. 3). ECMA 1 began to label embryos only at blastocyst stage. Both ICM and a few trophectoderm cells were then
found positive. Finally, ECMA 4 and 5 were negative on all
preimplantation stages tested.

DISCUSSION

In a first attempt to obtain monoclonal antibodies against a
large variety of cell surface antigens, rats were chosen for immunization with mouse EC cells. This procedure is supported by the
results described here. The antigens detected by each of the 5
ECMA studied seem to have different cell distribution. Although

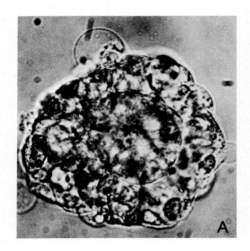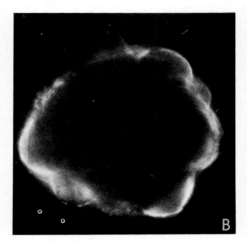

Fig. 3.   Immunofluorescence with ECMA 3 on cultured ICM.
Tests were done in a "triple sandwich-technique" (see Materials and
Methods).   ECMA 3, 1/200 dilutions. A : phase ; B : fluorescence.

more detailed investigations with other cell types and characterization by immunoprecipitation are needed, preliminary results can
be summarized as follows :

   a) ECMA 1 reacts with EC cells of the 129/Sv genotype and only
with a mesenchymal-like derivative of teratocarcinoma.   Its activity is absorbed by sperm and lymphocytes of various genotypes.
ECMA 1 does not label embryos before blastocyst stage.

   b) ECMA 2 reacts with all EC cells tested, as well as with the
majority of their differentiated derivatives.   Its activity is
also absorbed by sperm and lymphocytes.   ECMA 2 labels embryos
from 2-cell stage on.

   c) ECMA 3 is positive on all EC cells.   The only differentiated
cell types which absorb its activity are a myoblast-like cell line
and sperm.   ECMA 3 labels embryos from 2-cell stage on.

   d) ECMA 4 was found positive on all *in vitro* grown cell lines
derived from teratocarcinoma where it labels always 100 % of the
cells.   In contrast, it does not react with any *in vivo* cell tested,
such as lymphocytes, sperm or preimplantation embryos.   This

difference suggested that ECMA 4 could detect a component of the serum used in the culture medium. Yet its activity is not absorbed on copolymerized fetal calf serum.

e) ECMA 5 reacts with no other EC cells than F9. It labels also a mesenchymal-like teratocarcinoma derivative. Its activity is absorbed by sperm, lymphocytes and SRBC. It does not label preimplantation embryos.

ECMA 2 and 3 turn out to be the most interesting for the study of early stages of embryonic development. Both react not only with EC cells of various genotypes and with sperm but also with all stages of preimplantation embryos. Both disappear almost completely during *in vitro* differentiation of EC cells.

They differ, however, since the antigen detected by ECMA 2 is expressed on a wide spectrum of differentiated cells. Preliminary results indicate that the surface antigen detected by ECMA 2 is expressed on a minor subpopulation of adult lymphocytes (D. Morello, unpublished observations). For the present time, the antigen detected by ECMA 3 appears to be the only one having a distribution similar to that described for the "F9 antigen" characterized by a syngeneic anti-F9 serum. However, in contrast with anti-F9 syngeneic serum, ECMA 3 reacts with a minor subpopulation ($\simeq$ 5 %) of PCD/2 cells, a myoblast derivative of EC cells. Since syngeneic anti-F9 serum turned out to be more complex than originally thought, the activity of this serum has to be investigated in more detail.

Monoclonal antibodies reacting with surface structures on embryonic carcinoma cells and embryos have already been described by Stern *et al.*[21], Knowles and Solter[22] and Goodfellow *et al.*[23]. ECMA 5 has some similarities with the monoclonal antibody described by Stern *et al.*[21] since its activity is also absorbed by SRBC. They differ, however, in that the latter but not ECMA 5 reacts with preimplantation embryos.

Four of the five hybridomas are IgM producers. Since spleen cells from hyperimmune rats were used for fusion, the high frequency of IgM producing clones is remarkable and interesting in itself. There are several explanations.

1) The major determinants of F9 cells during hyperimmunization of rat or mouse immunizations are detected by IgM as it has been

described for syngeneic immunization with F9 cells[4].

2) IgM-producing plasma cells fuse more easily, or persist longer in the spleen, than IgG producing cells do.

3) In our procedure, the first selection of active hybridomas used a microcitytoxicity test against F9 cells, thus favorising the detection of IgM producing clones.

The results reported in this paper support the use of xenogenic immunization since five hybridomas, taken at random from 28, turned out to produce antibodies against different antigenic structures. None of them seems to recognize a mouse specific antigen, i.e. an antigen present on all mouse cell types.

Xenogenic antisera detect a wider range of surface antigens than allo- or syngeneic antisera do. As long as they are not present on all mouse cell types but exhibit a specific distribution, many of these antigens are likely to be useful as markers for the study of development. Because of their extreme complexity, however, conventional xenogenic antisera can hardly be used in such a study. In contrast, xenogenic monoclonal antibodies, each of which detects a single specificity provide the tool required for such an analysis.

ACKNOWLEDGEMENTS

This work was supported by grants from the Centre National de la Recherche Scientifique (LA 269), the Institut National de la Santé et de la Recherche Médicale (C.R.A.T. n° 76.4.311), the Délégation Générale à la Recherche Scientifique et Technique (A.C.C. n° 77.7.0966) and the André Meyer Foundation.

REFERENCES

1. Artzt, K., Bennett, D. and Jacob, F. (1974) Proc.Nat.Acad. Sci.USA, 71, 811-814.

2. Kemler, R., Babinet, C., Condamine, H., Gachelin, G., Guénet, J.L. and Jacob, F. (1976) Proc.Nat.Acad.Sci.USA , 73, 4080-4084.

3. Kemler, R., Babinet, C., Eisen, H. and Jacob, F. (1977) Proc.Nat.Acad.Sci.USA, 74, 4449-4452.

4. Damonneville, M., Morello, D., Gachelin, G. and Stanislawski, M. (1979) Europ.J.Immunol., in press.

5. Köhler, G. and Milstein, C. (1975) Nature, 256, 495-497.

6. Artzt, K., Dubois, P., Bennett, D., Condamine, H., Babinet, C. and Jacob, F. (1973) Proc.Nat.Acad.Sci.USA, 70, 2988-2992.

7. Sherman, M.I. and Miller, R.A. (1978) Develop.Biol., 63, 27-34.

8. Solter, D. and Knowles, B.B. (1975) Proc.Nat.Acad.Sci.USA, 72, 5099-5102.

9. Hogan, B. and Tilly, R. (1978) J.Embryol.Exp.Morph., 45, 93-105.

10. Martin, G.R. and Evans, M.J. (1975) Proc.Nat.Acad.Sci.USA, 72, 1441-1445.

11. Mittal, K.K. (1977) Vox Sang., 34, 58.

12. Jensenius, J.C. and Williams, A.F. (1974) Europ.J.Immunol., 4, 91-97.

13. Nicolas, J.F., Dubois, P., Jakob, H., Gaillard, J. and Jacob, F. (1975) Ann.Microbiol.(Inst.Pasteur), 126A, 3-22.

14. McBurney, M.W. (1976) J.Cell.Physiol., 89, 441-445.

15. Stevens, L.C. and Varnum, D.S. (1974) Develop.Biol., 37, 369-380.

16. Lehmann, J.M., Speers, W.C., Swartzendruber, D.E. and Pierce, G.B. (1974) J.Cell.Physiol., 84, 13-28.

17. Nicolas, J.F., Jakob, H. and Jacob, F. (1978) Proc.Nat.Acad. Sci.USA, 75, 3292-3296.

18. Nicolas, J.F., Avner, P., Gaillard, J., Guénet, J.L., Jakob, H. and Jacob, F. (1976) Cancer Res., 36, 4224-4231.

19. Boon, T., Buckingham, M.E., Dexter, D.L., Jakob, H. and Jacob, F. (1974) Ann.Microbiol.(Inst.Pasteur), 125 B, 13-28.

20. Kelly, F. and Boccara, M. (1976) Nature, 262, 404-411.

21. Stern, P., Willison, K., Lennox, E., Galfre, G., Milstein, C., Secher, D. and Ziegler, A. (1978) Cell, 14, 775-783.

22. Knowles, B.B., Aden, D.P. and Solter, D. (1978) Current Topics in Microbiol. and Immunol., 81, 51-53.

23. Goodfellow, N., Levinson, J.R., Willams II, V.E. and McDewitt, H.O. (1979) Proc.Nat.Acad.Sci.USA, 76, 377-380.

Cell Lineage, Stem Cells and Cell Determination
INSERM Symposium No. 10
Editor: N. Le Douarin
© *1979 Elsevier/North-Holland Biomedical Press*

CELL LINEAGES OF THE MOUSE EMBRYO AND EMBRYONAL CARCINOMA CELLS; FORSSMAN
ANTIGEN DISTRIBUTION AND PATTERNS OF PROTEIN SYNTHESIS

M.J. EVANS[1], R.H. LOVELL-BADGE[1], P.L. STERN[2], and M.G. STINNAKRE[3].
University of Cambridge, Department of Genetics, Downing Street, Cambridge
CB2 3EH (1)
Uppsala Universitets, Biomedicinska Centrum, Avdelningen for Immunologi
Box 582, S75123 Uppsala, Sweden (2)
Institut de Recherche de Biologie Moleculaire, Tour 43, 2 Place Jussieu,
Paris 5, France (3)

INTRODUCTION

Cells are often recognised and classified by the complex criteria of their
morphology, their position in recognisable tissues within the organism,
their relationship to other cells and tissues and their behaviour. These
criteria, in addition to being sometimes poorly defined, are often less useful
in experimental situations, such as after isolation or in culture where the
normal tissue relationships of the cell no longer provide an identification.
These difficulties of identification of cell type are particularly evident
where differentiating cell lineages are being studied in isolation from the
whole organism.

Serological reagents are extremely useful in the definition, recognition
and experimental manipulation of specific types of cell and a variety of
antisera showing reactions against surface components of early mouse embryo
cells have been described[1]. It is additionally interesting that some of these
antigens could have a developmentally functional importance[2].

The activity of conventional antisera consists of a large range of
immunoglobulin molecules reacting with a range of determinants on possibly
more than a single antigenic target. Their action in any particular
situation can only be fully interpreted in the light of careful appropriate
controls which may be difficult to carry out with the small amounts of tissue
available from early mammalian embryos. Moreover it may be difficult to
prepare such antisera repeatably. On the other hand monoclonal antisera
secreted by lines of hybrid cells, prepared by the fusion of primed spleen
cells with a myeloma cell line, consist of molecules of a single type of
active immunoglobulin reacting against one specific antigenic determinant and
they are consistently produced by the clonal, hybrid cell line[3].

We report here the use of one such reagent, monoclonal antiserum M1/22.25 which recognises a specificity of the Forssman antigen[4]- (a cell surface glycolipid), and have investigated its expression by cell lineages of the early mouse embryo and by those of the foetal gonad.

The homology between embryonal carcinoma cells and one of the pluripotent cell lineages of the embryo may be considered in the light of the cells' reaction with M1/22.25, but this comparison makes use of one single small aspect of the cell phenotype whose expression need not necessarily be representative for this purpose. We have, therefore, also compared the phenotype of these cell lineages and embryonal carcinoma cells by the use of two-dimensional electrophoresis of their total cellular proteins; thus allowing an objective comparison between cell types based upon the expression of poly-peptides from many different genes.

MATERIALS AND METHODS

The methods used are more fully described elsewhere[5,6,7]. All embryos were isolated from an inbred stock of 129 Sv Ev mice. The day of a mating plug was considered as day 0 of pregnancy. Allowance was made in interpretation of the results for litters varying in their developmental age by up to $\pm \frac{1}{2}$ day. Embryos were isolated and germ layers dissected after trypsin treatment. The isolated tissue layers were further dissaggregated when required by a second trypsin treatment. $10\frac{1}{2}$ day and later embryos were dissected directly using tungsten needles. $12\frac{1}{2}$ day and older embryonic gonads were sexed by their appearance and the presence of the spermatic blood vessel. Earlier embryos were sexed by orcein staining of the amnion[8]. Alkaline phosphatase staining of unfixed cells was carried out in an isotonic saline (0.075M Tris/HCl buffer pH 8.6 0.8% NaCl, 0.05% napthol ASMX phosphate 2% dimethylformamide and 0.01% fast blue BB diazo salt). Δ 5-3β hydroxysteroid dehydrogenase staining was as described by Wattenberg[9]. For double staining the immunofluorescence staining had to preceed the histochemical staining. Immunfluorescence staining used a single batch of M1/22.25 directly conjugated to fluorescein. Cells were suspended in $\frac{1}{4}$ diluted M1/22.25-F1 for $\frac{1}{2}$ hour at 0°C washed twice and examined with a Zeiss photomicroscope III equipped with epifluorescent illumination. Cells were observed with phase contrast as well as epifluorescence and only live cells were scored. Cytotoxicity assays used $\frac{1}{2}$ diluted Guinea-pig comple-ment (L.I.P. Ltd., U.K) at 37°C for $\frac{1}{2}$ hour. Cell death was observed by trypan blue staining.

For ^{35}S labelling tissues were isolated as above and incubated for 3 hours in methionine-free Eagles MEM+5% foetal calf serum to which was added

[35]S methionine at 4mCi per ml (>600 Ci/m mol). Germ cells were flushed from the gonadal ridge by teasing in phosphate-buffered saline and incubated for 3 hours as above. Immediately after incubation they were applied to the top of a pre-formed Percoll gradient in Eagles medium and centrifuged for 3 minutes at approximately 500g. The Percoll gradient was prepared by centrifugation of 0.4ml of a mixture of Percoll and Eagles medium of density 1.077 at approx. 10,000g for 1 hour in a microfuge. Labelled tissues or cells were lysed with a total of 20μl lysis buffers and two-dimensional electrophoresis was carried out accordingly to a modified procedure[6] based on that described by O'Farrell[10]. The pH gradient in the focussing gel was 4.5-7.5 and the SDS gels were 10% acrylamide. 10^5-10^6 cpm were loaded per gel and proteins detected by autofluorography.

RESULTS

<u>Expression of Forssman antigen on cells of embryos between $4\frac{3}{4}$ and $7\frac{3}{4}$ days</u>

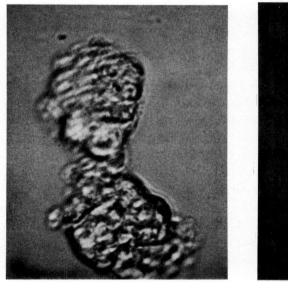 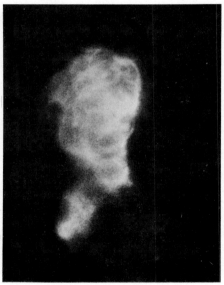

Phase Contrast   Immunofluorescence

Fig. 1. Partly dissected 5 day embryo; indirect immunofluorescence M1/22.25. Both the primary endoderm and the epiblast show Forssman antigen expression but the extra embryonic ectoderm is negative

Inner cell mass cells isolated from $3\frac{1}{2}$-$4\frac{1}{2}$ day embryos express Forssman antigen as has already been reported by Willison and Stern[11]. The inner cell mass differentiates into primary endoderm on its luminal surface and subsequently the internal cells change into an embryonic ectoderm. For the purposes of clarity of discussion in this paper the term epiblast will be adopted for these internal cells until the time when they elongate around the proamniotic cavity at the beginning of day 6. When these two tissues are isolated from $4\frac{3}{4}$ - $5\frac{1}{2}$ day embryos they are both very strongly Forssman antigen positive as seen by indirect immunofluorescence. The extra-embryonic ectoderm, which is derived from the trophoblast[12], is Forssman antigen negative during this period and subsequently; Figure 1.

By $5\frac{3}{4}$-6 days the intensity of the immunofluorescence observed on the epiblast is much reduced but both the parietal and visceral endoderm remain strongly positive. By $6\frac{1}{2}$ days and later through to $7\frac{3}{4}$ days all trace of immuno-fluorescence is absent from embryonic ectoderm cells.

When 6-$7\frac{3}{4}$ day egg cylinder stages are dissected into embryonic and extra-embryonic regions and the germ layers further dissected and examined either as tissue sheets or cell suspensions by M1/22.25 immunofluorescence or cytotoxicity, those dissects containing endodermal cells have significantly greater proportions of antigen-positive cells. The antigen-expressing cells have an endodermal morphology; these cells being generally larger and with more granular cytoplasms than the ectodermal cells. For example in one such experiment $7\frac{1}{2}$ day separated disaggregated embryonic ectoderm had no antigen-positive cell by immunofluorescence whereas embryonic endoderm had 76% Forssman antigen-positive cells. The cells which are non-fluorescent in embryonic endoderm preparations have a morphology consistent with them being contaminating embryonic ectoderm. The same cell preparations were examined by cytotoxicity. 70% of the embryonic ectoderm was alive after incubation with M1/22.25 and guinea pig complement whereas only 13% of the cells of the endodermal dissect survived. All these latter were small cells with a smooth cytoplasm, suggesting that they were contaminating ectodermal cells. In the later egg cylinders examined, embryonic mesoderm was present but was not separated from the ectoderm. The immunofluorescent results would suggest that these cells are also Forssman antigen negative. Both parietal and visceral endoderm continue to express the antigen.

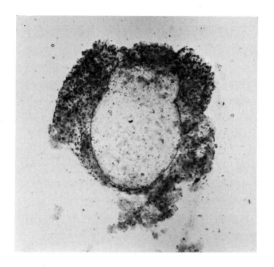

Fig. 2. Embryonic portion
of 6½ day egg cylinder
M1/22.25 cytotoxicity;
dead cells stained with
trypan blue. The survival
of the embryonic ectodermal
cells is not dependent upon
the integrity of the embryo
(as shown here) for diss-
aggregated ectoderm cells
are also not killed.

Expression of Forssman antigen by embryonal carcinoma cells and their
differentiated derivatives

Immunofluorescent staining of embryonal carcinoma cells grown as a
homogeneous undifferentiated population on killed fibroblast feeder layers
shows > 90% positive cells. The primary endodermal cells which differentiate
when these cells are allowed to form embryoid bodies in vitro are also
Forssman antigen positive (Figure 3).

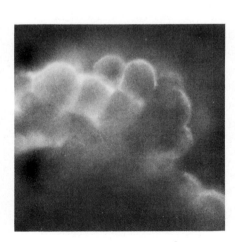

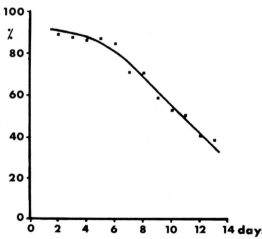

Fig. 3. M1/22.25 Fluorescence of
embryoid body endoderm

Fig. 4.   Reduction in proportion of
Forssman +ve cells as EC cells
differentiate in suspension.

As further differentiation is allowed to proceed in suspension, leading
to the formation of a cystic embryoid body with ectodermal and mesodermal cell
types, the proportion of Forssman antigen positive cells decreases (Figure 4)
and antigen negative cells appear with a phase-contrast appearance similar
to that of embryonic ectodermal cells.

Expression of Forssman antigen by cells of gonadal tissues

Between 11 and 14 days the gonadal ridges contain increasing proportions
of Forssman antigen positive cells. This is consistent with the population
of the gonadal ridges by germ cells migrating into them from the area of
the hind gut endoderm via the dorsal mesentery and their proliferation before
their differentiation. The germ cells are easily identified by their
distinctive morphology and high levels of alkaline phophatase. The extremely
bright immunoflourescence available with M1/22.25 allows double staining
for the Forssman antigen and alkaline phosphatase activity. Table 1
shows that at 12 days there is a good correlation between these markers.
After this time it is known that alkaline phosphatase is a less specific
marker for germ cells because other cells in the genital ridge develop this
activity. Before day 15 the majority of the Forssman antigen positive cells
have a distinct germ cell morphology (Figure 5) but after this time cells
other than germ cells in the gonad express the Forssman antigen. These
cells are small granular cells and there are two main cell populations in
the testis which they might represent; Leydig cells or Sertoli cells. It
is possible to identify Leydig cells by histochemical staining for Δ 5-3β-
hydroxysteroid dehydrogenase. Double staining for this enzyme and M1/22.25
fluorescence shows that Leydig cells do not constitute the non-germ cell
Forssman positive population on day 16. All stages of gonocyte differentiation and mature sperm in the post-partum mouse testis are Forssman
antigen negative but new born testis contains 40% antigen positive cells.
Only 3% of the cells are Leydig cells and these are Forssman antigen negative.
The only cells present in sufficient numbers to account for the results are
Sertoli cells and we conclude that these cells and their foetal precursors
probably account for the Forssman antigen positive cell populations. We
have also shown (data not included here) that the tissue distribution of
Forssman antigen expression is not significantly different from normal
in W^v/W^v homozygote male mice where the testis is devoid of germ cells.

Table 1

Comparison of Forssman antigen expression with alkaline phosphatase staining and phase contrast appearance of cells from germinal ridges.

Embryo age in days	Sex	Alkaline phosphatase +ve cells		Total Forssman +ve cells with germ cell morphology
		% FA +ve	% FA −ve	
11	♂ + ♀	26	74	91
12	♂ + ♀	83	17	−
12	♂	83	17	95
12	♀	77	23	92
13	♂	64	36	90
13	♀	40	60	97
14	♂	−	−	83
14	♀	−	−	91
15	♂	−	−	3
15	♀	−	−	63
16	♂	−	−	16
16	♀	−	−	33

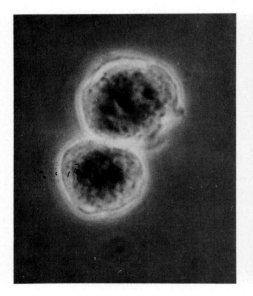 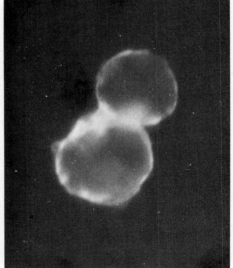

Phase contrast   M1/22.25 Fluorescence

Fig. 5. Appearance of germ cells isolated from 12 day gonadal ridges

Two dimensional separations of total cell proteins

Isolation of germ cells

We did not obtain a homogeneous population of germ cells from 12 day
ridges by the methods described by Heath[9]. By either alkaline phosphatase
or M1/22.25 staining or morphological appearance only approximately 50% of
the cells were germ cells. Consequently we resorted to a purification of
these cells after labelling them during culture _in vitro_ for 3 hours. It
was possible to prepare small scale gradients of Percoll and obtain a reliable
purification of ^{35}S labelled germ cells: Figure 6.

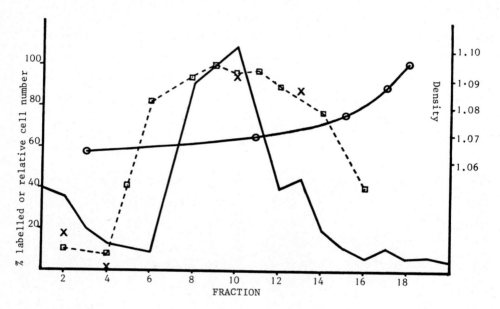

Fig. 6. Separation of germ cells on a Percoll gradient total volume 0.4ml;
———— cell number in an arbitary small volume withdrawn from each
fraction; ---◻--- % of alkaline phosphatase +ve cells; X % of M1/22.25 +ve
cells; —◯— density of solution.

Protein separations

Of the separations obtained at least four gels each from $7\frac{1}{2}$ day ectoderm
and endoderm and the embryonal carcinoma samples and eight gels of 12 day
germ cells have been closely compared. Results for the 5 day embryonic portion
(i.e. epiblast and endoderm together) and the $6\frac{1}{2}$ day dissects are based on
comparison of fewer gels and with particular emphasis upon the spots seen

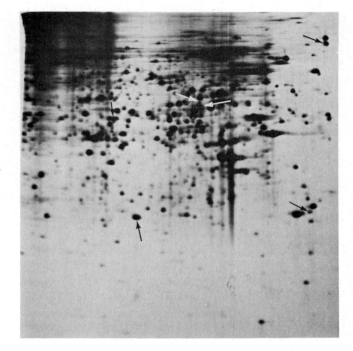

Fig. 7. Two
dimensional separ-
ation of total
protein of Embryonal
carcinoma cell
PSMB as a pure
EC cell mono-
layer.

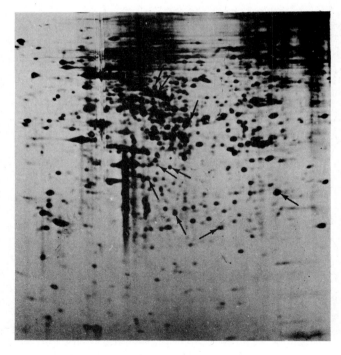

Fig. 8. Two
dimensional separ-
ation of total
protein of the
embryonic endo-
derm from a $7\frac{1}{2}$
day embryo.

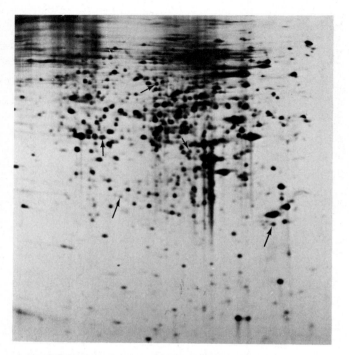

Fig. 9. Two
dimensional
separation of
total protein of
the embryonic
ectoderm from a
7½ day embryo

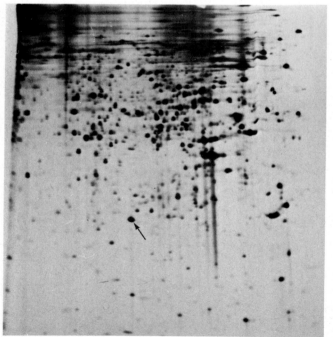

Fig. 10. Two
dimensional
separation of
total protein of
purified germ
cells from 12½
day germical
ridge.

to be of interest from the other comparison. For this reason they should be regarded as preliminary as other minor differences might emerge as a result of a more comprehensive analysis of more gels.

Out of over 1000 spots resolved on the autofluorographs only 19 showed consistent variation between all the samples studied. These spots are arrowed in figures 8-11. Their presence or absence in all the cell samples is set out in Table 2. Figure 12 provides a key to the spot numbers.

Eighteen out of the nineteen spots showing differences are conspicuous by their absence from the germ cells including four that are present in all the other cell types. Spots number 8 to 15 would appear to be characteristic of endodermal cells as they are only found in samples containing endoderm. Spot 1 is only found in samples with undifferentiated embryonal carcinoma cells and spots 2 and 3 are only found in samples of embryonal carcinoma cells and their early differentiating products, and 5 day embryos.

Table 2. Distribution of the 19 Polypeptides showing cell specific differences.

SPOT	PSMB	PSMB CLUMP	5 DAY EMB	E.B.	6 DAY ECT	6 DAY END	7 DAY ECT	7 DAY END	G.C.
1	+	±	-	-	-	-	-	-	-
2	+	+	±	±	-	-	-	-	-
3	+	+	±	±	-	-	-	-	-
4	+	+	±	+	±	+	-	+	-
5	+	+	+	±	±	+	-	+	+
6	-	±	-	±	+	+	+	+	-
7	-	±	+	+	+	+	+	+	-
8	-	±	±	+	-	±	-	+	-
9	-	±	+	+	-	+	-	+	-
10	-	-	±	+	-	±	-	+	-
11	-	-	+	+	-	+	-	+	-
12	-	-	+	+	-	+	-	+	-
13	-	-	±	±	-	+	-	+	-
14	-	-	-	-	-	±	-	+	-
15	-	±	-	-	-	-	-	+	-

Key

PSMB - a pluripotential cell line - pure undifferentiated EC cells.

PSMB clump. Cell aggregates labelled during the first 3 hours of their suspension.

5d Emb. The embryonic portion of a 5½ day embryo both epiblast and endoderm present.

EB's. Embryoid bodies formed from PSMB clumps after 4 days of differentiation.

In addition, spots 16, 17, 18 and 19 are not present in G.C.

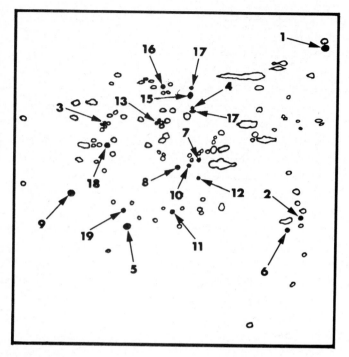

Fig. 11. Key to
numbering of
spots seen in
Figs. 8-11 and
Table 2.

DISCUSSION

A number of different monoclonal antibodies reacting with the cell surface
of embryonal carcinoma cells and early embryos have already been described[13,14],
and it is clear that many others are likely to be produced. They will be
particularly useful in an analysis of cell surface changes associated with
mouse embryonic development, especially when their antigenic target has been
identified. Their use should help to resolve the apparent complexities of
action of current conventional antisera[15]. Embryonal carcinoma cells provide
a convenient antigen and target cell for preparing and/or screening monoclonal
antisera likely to react with early embryo cells, but it may be that some
antigens of greater interest for analysis of early embryonic development only
appear as a result of differentiation and are not present on embryonal carcinoma
cells. The cells from the first few days of cystic embryoid body differentiation would provide a large source of cells equivalent to those of the embryo
during early postimplantational development. M1/22.25 was not raised delib-
erately as a reagent against embryonal carcinoma cells, and it is probable
that as specific monoclonal reagents become available other unexpected antigens
may be found to have interesting cell distributions during early development.

Cell surface antigens are often thought to provide cell lineage markers although there does not seem to be any *a priori* reason why this should be the case. In order to fulfil this rôle the antigen needs to be displayed upon the precursor cell and upon some only of its differentiated products. Cell types not associated with this lineage should not display the antigen. Within the restricted scope of the mouse embryo up to 7¾ days of development the Forssman antigen does indeed provide a cell lineage marker; (Figure 12). It is present on cells of the morula and these give rise to trophectoderm and inner cell mass cells both of which are Forssman antigen positive but it is lost from the trophectoderm cells at about the time of implantation. The inner cell mass gives rise to the primary endoderm and the epiblast both of which are Forssman antigen positive. When the epiblast later forms the embryonic ectoderm the antigen expression is lost. The extra embryonic ectoderm which is a derivative of the trophectoderm[12] remains antigen negative as does the mesoderm, a derivative of the embryonic ectoderm. If this interpretation of the Forssman antigen as a marker of cell lineage is valid, it might be expected that the definitive endoderm derived from the embryonic ectoderm would be antigen negative despite its endodermal phenotype. Its Forssman antigenic status is not known. The distribution of the Forssman antigen in the gonadal tissues is not consistent with cell lineage. It is present on the primordial germ cells but is lost at 15 days and thereafter reappears on other unrelated cell types in the gonad.

The primordial germ cells are first clearly distinguishable in the posterior area of the primitive streak at the base of the allantois[16]. If they have a common origin with embryonic ectoderm and if their expression of the Forssman antigen is taken to provide information of lineage within the early embryo it suggests that they become segregated before the time of conversion of the epiblast into embryonic ectoderm.

On the same basis of their Forssman antigenicity taken together with their pluripotentiality, embryonal carcinoma cells might be homologous with inner cell mass cells, epiblast cells or primordial germ cells. Comparisons of embryonal carcinoma cells with inner cell mass cells have been made by Dewey *et al*[17] and although it is very difficult to compare their results with ours[6, 7] the clear conclusion in each case is that the two cell types are quite distinct. Dewey et al found 60 differences whereas we found 27 qualitative and 25 quantitative differences. The results presented here and elsewhere[6] show that embryonal carcinoma cells are much more similar to embryonic ectoderm and that the changes in protein synthesis patterns which take place as embryoid body

formation occurs closely parallel   those seen in the normal embryo.
Primordial germ cells are also similar to embryonic ectoderm but lack those
polypeptides which might be considered to be concerned with differentiation
of the epiblast or embryonal carcinoma cell as well as four other spots. It
will be interesting to have two dimensional separations of the proteins of
pure populations of 5 day epiblast cells for comparison.

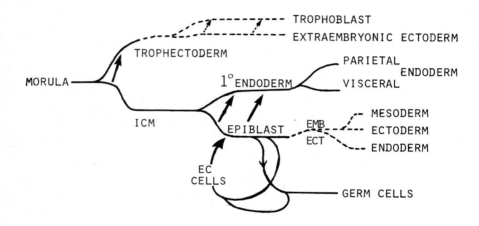

Fig. 12. Cell lineages: Forssman antigen positive lineages are drawn
with a full line, negative with a dotted line.

There is some evidence that both in the case of ICM/Trophectoderm and
Epiblast/Endoderm steps of cell determination the inner cells retain their
ability to re-form outer cells for a short period[18,19,20]. This suggests that
these cell determinations should not be viewed as dichotomous cell decisions
but as stem cell situations as shown in Figure 12 which not only presents a
lineage diagram of Forssman antigen expression but also attempts to incorporate
our suggestion for the relationship to these lineages of primordial germ cells
and embryonal carcinoma cells.

Informative cell markers are distinct differences between cells. Monoclonal
antibodies are ideal reagents for this purpose. It is also reproducible
differences between cell phenotypes which are sought in an analysis of two
dimensional protein patterns. Gel electrophoresis results might be used to
identify polypeptides against which it would be useful to prepare monoclonal
reagents.

ACKNOWLEDGEMENTS

We are grateful to the Cancer Research Campaign, the Medical Research Council and the Wellcome Trust for the provision of grants that have made this work possible. Miss K. Whitley is thanked for her careful typing of the manuscript.

REFERENCES

1. Erickson, R.P. (1977) in Immunobiology of the gametes. Ed. Cambridge University Press pp. 85-114.

2. Kemler, R., Babinet, C.C., Eisen, H. and Jacob, F. (1977) Proc. Natl. Acad. Sci. USA 74, 4449-4452.

3. Kohler, G. and Milstein, L. (1975) Nature (London) 256, 495-497.

4. Stern, P.L., Willison, K., Lennox, E., Galfre, G., Milstein, L., Secher, D., Ziegler, A. and Springer, T. (1978) Cell 14, 775-783.

5. Stinnakre, M.G., Evans, M.J., Willison, K.R. and Stern, P.L. Submitted to J. Embryol. Exp. Morphol.

6. Lovell-Badge, R.H. and Evans, M.J. Submitted to J. Embryol. Exp. Morphol.

7. Lovell-Badge, R.H. (1978) Ph.D. Thesis, Univeristy of London.

8. Forias, E., Kajii, T. and Gardner, L.I. (1967) Nature (London) 214, 499-500.

9. Wattenberg, L.W. (1958) J. Histochem. Cytochem. 6, 225-232.

10. O'Farrell, P.H. (1975) J. Biol. Chem. 250, 4007-4021.

11. Willison, K.R. and Stern, P.L. (1978) Cell 14, 785-793.

12. Gardner, R.L. and Papaioannou, V.E. (1975) Early Development of Mammals. Ed. Balls, M., Wild, A.E. 2nd symposium of the British Society for Developmental Biology, Cambridge University Press pp. 107-132.

13. Solter, D. and Knowles, B.B. (1978) Proc. Natl. Acad. Sci. USA 75, 5565-5569.

14. Goodfellow, P.N., Levinson, J.R., Williams, V.E. and McDevitt, H.O. (1979) Proc. Natl. Acad. Sci. USA 76, 377-380.

15. Jacob, F. (1977) Immunol. Rev. 33, 3-32.

16. Ozdzenski, W. (1967) Zool. Pol. 17, 367-379.

17. Dewey, M.J., Filler, R. and Mintz, B. (1978) Develop. Biol. 65, 171-182.

18. Handyside, A.H. and Johnson, M.H. (1977) J. Anat. 124, 236.

19. Pedersen, R.A., Spindle, A.I. and Wiley, L.M. (1977) Nature (London) 270, 435-437.

20. Evans, M.J., Lovell-Badge, R.H. and Stern, P.L. (1976) Teratology 14, 367.

Cell Lineage, Stem Cells and Cell Determination
INSERM Symposium No. 10
Editor N. Le Douarin
© 1979 Elsevier/North-Holland Biomedical Press

CELLULAR INTERACTIONS BETWEEN EMBRYONAL CARCINOMA CELLS

Jean-François NICOLAS
Service de Génétique cellulaire du Collège de France et de
l'Institut Pasteur, 25 rue du Dr. Roux, 75015 Paris, France

INTRODUCTION

All differentiated tissues of multicellular organisms derive
from a unique cell : the fertilised egg. During embryonic development, the cells pass through different developmental states
during which the choice of the genetic programme they will express
is progressively made. Some of the events involved in this phenomenon happen at the level of groups of cells, as shown by clonal
analysis in both insects[1, 2] and allophenic mice[3]. Such observation is compatible with an interdependent behaviour of embryonic
cells. This has, therefore, suggested hypotheses involving either
chemical or physical gradients and/or communication between
cells[4, 5]. The experimental analysis of such problems remains
difficult, in particular in mammals.

The model system of differentiation established using embryonal
carcinoma cells (EC)[6] allows a new approach to these problems.
EC cells which present many similarities to multipotential cells
of the embryo[6, 7] are available in culture[8]. Certain EC cell
lines can differentiate in vitro ; from such cultures differentiated EC derivatives can be obtained and maintained in the laboratory[9]. Such lines are especially useful for immunological and
biochemical analysis.

Here we shall analyse some properties related to membrane components of EC cells : the metabolic cooperation between cells and
the action of a xenogeneic anti-EC serum on cell-cell interactions.

DIRECT COMMUNICATION BETWEEN EC CELLS

Various types of cell junctions have been described. One of
them, gap junction, enables both electrical coupling and the
exchange of small molecules, including metabolites[10], to occur.
In order to determine the ability of EC cells to establish such

direct communication, metabolic cooperation between EC cells
devoid of hypoxanthine-phosphorybosyl-transferase (HPRT⁻), and
wild type cells has been investigated.

Metabolic cooperation in HAT medium

HAT medium allows the growth of HPRT⁺, but is toxic to HPRT⁻
cells. In such medium, however, HPRT⁻ cells can be rescued by
co-culture with HPRT⁺ cells. This rescue involves the transfer
of metabolites from HPRT⁺ to HPRT⁻ cells[11]. Because EC cells lyse
rapidly when exposed to toxic conditions, it is possible to estimate the fraction of dead cells simply by measuring the radioactivity released into the supernatant by cells previously labelled
with a tracer (^{14}C-thymidine). Thus, in HAT medium the measurement
of radioactivity specifically released by HPRT⁻ EC cells (lytic
index) in the presence of increasing numbers of HPRT⁺ cells
allows an accurate estimate of metabolic cooperation occurring
between cells[12].

All EC cells - whatever their properties (nulli- or multipotent) and their origin (murin or human) - efficiently rescue
HPRT⁻ EC cells (Figure 1). Under the same conditions, differentiated cell lines are ineffective in rescuing EC cells (Figure 1,
Table 1 ; see also Nicolas et al.[12, 13]).

Metabolic killing in 6-thioguanine medium

In the presence of 6-thioguanine, HPRT⁻ cells survive whilst
HPRT⁺ cells are killed. In such medium, however, the transfer of
metabolites from HPRT⁺ cells to contiguous HPRT⁻ cells results in
the death of the resistant cells[14]. Measurement of HPRT⁻ EC cell
lysis in the presence of an increasing number of HPRT⁺ cells gives
an estimate of the efficiency of communication between cells
(Nicolas, unpublished). Results similar to those obtained in HAT
medium are obtained when HPRT⁻ cells are tested against EC and
differentiated HPRT⁺ cells (Figure 2).

In these two systems, both HPRT⁻ and HPRT⁺ cells were put in
selective medium six hours after plating, to allow the establis-
ment of intercellular contacts. Supernatants were harvested two
days later.

The results of these experiments suggest the existence of
communicative junctions between EC cells. This has been confirmed
by direct examination using freeze etching electron microscopic

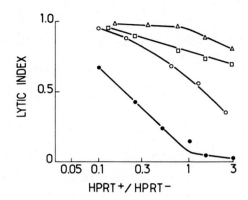

Fig. 1 Metabolic cooperation in HAT medium between various HPRT[+]
cells and PCC4 HPRT-.   2.10[5] PCC4 HPRT- cells were mixed with
increasing numbers of : mouse EC cells, LT-1-2A (●——●) ;
human teratoma cells, Tera I-E-13 (o——o) ; human teratoma
cells, Huttke (□——□) and human carcinoma cells, HeLa D 98
(△——△). HPRT- cells were previously labelled with ^{14}C thymidine as in Nicolas et al.[12]. Lytic index was calculated as in
Nicolas et al.[12].

TABLE 1

METABOLIC COOPERATION AND METABOLIC KILLING BETWEEN PCC4 HPRT[-] AND
VARIOUS CELL LINES

| HPRT[+] cell line | Cell type | Lytic index[a] | |
		Hat medium	6-thioguanine medium
PCC4	Mouse, EC	0.05	—
LT-1	Mouse, EC	0.06	0.85
3/A/1-D-1	Mouse, mesenchyme	0.92	0.02
3/A/1-D-3	Mouse, fibroblast	0.96	0.17
Tera I-E 13	Human, teratoma[b]	0.25	0.60
Huttke	Human, teratoma[b]	0.70	0.73
HeLa D 98	Human, carcinoma[b]	0.80	0.01

[a] Conditions as in Nicolas et al.[12]. HPRT[+]/PCC4 HPRT[-] ratio : 3.
[b] For details on these cell lines see Muramatsu, T., Avner, P.,
   Fellous, M., Gachelin, G. and Jacob, F., submitted to J. of
   Cancer and Nicolas et al.[13].

134

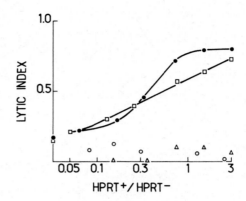

Fig. 2 Metabolic killing in 6-thioguanine medium. 2.10^5
PCC4 HPRT⁻ cells were mixed with increasing number of : mouse EC
cells LT-1 (●——●) ; human teratoma cells, Huttke (□——□) ;
mouse fibroblast, 3/A/1 D-1 (o——o) ; human carcinoma cells,
HeLa (D 98) (△——▲).

techniques. All EC cells establish numerous gap junctions and
some like PCC4 also produce tight junctions[15].

The fact that HPRT⁻ EC cells are not rescued in HAT medium by
differentiated cells and are not killed in 6-thioguanine medium,
can be explained by assuming that EC cells do not establish
junctions with differentiated cells, even when such differentiated
cells are known to form junctions between themselves. In mixed
culture, EC cells may form junctions much more easily with other
EC cells than with differentiated cells. This hypothesis is in
agreement with results of experiments involving different EC cell
lines. The efficiency of cooperation is higher in homologous
conditions (LT + LT HPRT⁻ ; PCC3 + PCC3 HPRT⁻) than in heterologous conditions (LT + PCC3 HPRT⁻) (Figure 3). The variation in
cooperation efficiency may reflect, in part, differences in recognition.

ACTION OF RABBIT ANTI-EC SERUM ON EC CELLS
It has been shown that monovalent IgG fragments from rabbits
immunised against EC cells (F9 cells) impair the compaction of
morulae (i.e. the close apposition of the blastomeres) and the
formation of the blastocyst[16]. To obtain additional information

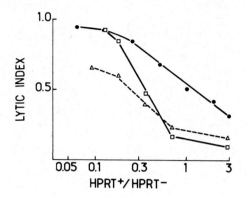

Fig. 3 Homologous and heterologous metabolic cooperation between
EC cells. 2.10[5] HPRT[-] cells were mixed with increasing number of
HPRT[+] cells : LT-1 HPRT[-] + LT-1 HPRT[+] (□——□) ; PCC3 HPRT[-] +
PCC3/A/1 HPRT[-] (△---△) ; PCC3 HPRT[-] + LT-1 HPRT[+] (●——●).
Lytic index was calculated as in Nicolas et al.[12]

on the mode of action of this antiserum, its effects on adhesion
and junction formation in EC cells have been studied[17].

Action on cell adhesion

The action of anti-F9 Fab fragments on adhesion has been
studied at two levels. Firstly, on EC cells aggregation by
plating isolated cells in the presence of Fab fragments and
following cell clumping as a function of time. Secondly, by
looking at the effect of the serum on already clumped cells (de-
compaction effect). The effects observed vary according to the
EC cell line examined. Some like PCC4 are very sensitive to the
two effects (Figure 4). Others, though sensitive to the effect
on aggregation are incompletely decompacted. LT-1 and PCC7-S are
insensitive to both effects.

Action on cell junctions

The action of the antiserum on cell junctions has been followed
by measuring metabolic cooperation. Figure 5 shows that in the
presence of 5 µl/100, the lytic index increased from 0.2 to 0.74,
a value very close to that of the control obtained by mixing
γ-irradiated PCC4 HPRT[-] cells and HPRT[+] cells. The Fab fragments
totally inhibit metabolic cooperation between PCC4 cells. These
observations have been extended by electron microscopic studies.
Addition of the antiserum to PCC4 cultures causes the rapid

136

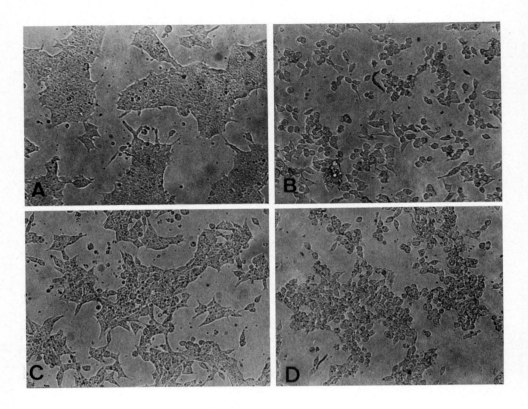

Fig. 4 Action of Fab anti-F9 fragments on EC cells. A : Isolated
F9 cells plated without Fab fragments. Photographed 18 hrs after
plating. B : Isolated F9 cells plated with 4 µl/100 of Fab fragments (300 γ/ml). Photographed 18 hrs after plating. C : Isolated PCC4 cells plated without Fab fragments. Photographed 18 hrs
after plating. D : Clumps of PCC4 cells as in C, in presence of
4 µl/100 of Fab fragments for 30 min.

rounding up of the cells and the disappearance of both tight and

gap junctions. After half an hour, numerous gap junctions are

found as vesicles in the cytoplasm previously communicating

cells. After thirty hours, only such internalised gap junctions

are observed. No junctions can be seen even in those regions

where the cells remain in contact[15]. These various effects are

not observed with two other Fab preparations against embryonic

liver and brain even though these sera react with EC cells in

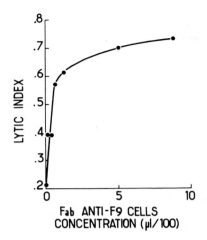

Fig. 5   Effect of rabbit anti-EC Fab fragments on metabolic cooperation between PCC4 HPRT⁻ cells and PCC4 HPRT⁺ cells (in HAT medium).   Abscissa : number of microliters of Fab solution
(300 γ/ml) added to the cells.   Ordinate : lytic index calculated
as in Nicolas et al.[12]

indirect immunofluorescence tests.

The presence of material able to absorb the decompacting activity of the anti-EC serum has been investigated : the remaining
activities of sera absorbed with cells from various lines was
tested on previously aggregated PCC4 cells.   Some embryonic non
EC cell lines (an endodermal line and a trophoblastoma) were found
to absorb this activity whilst others (an embryonic fibroblast and
a mesenchymal cell line) do not[17].

DISCUSSION

As could be expected, Fab fragments from rabbit anti-F9 serum
exert on EC cell an effect similar to that observed on preimplantation embryo[16] : in both cases, they prevent cells from aggre-
gating, and even decompact already aggregated cells.

The question can be raised of whether or not monovalent anti-
F9 Fab fragments exert their effect at one particular state of
embryonic development.   Since EC cells are likely to corres-

pond, not to morula cells, but rather to ICM cells[6], the factors
of aggregation sensitive to the Fab effect are not cell state-
specific. This suggests the existence of a mechanism used for
cell adhesion during early embryonic development.

As reported in this paper, work with EC cells also allows
investigation of the effect of Fab fragments on junctional complexes. By a mechanism which is still rather unclear, Fab fragments lead to disorganisation of intercellular junctions and even
to internalisation of gap junctions.

Furthermore, it turns out that all EC cell lines do not exhibit
identical behavior. Some EC cell lines are insensitive to the
action of the Fab fragments although they aggregate. This
suggests that different structures are involved in the adhesion
of these cells. Furthermore EC cell lines differ from one another
in their efficiency to rescue PCC4 HPRT$^-$ cells. These two observations indicate that these cell lines have different membrane
properties. Whether this results from the fact that they correspond to various states of differentiation of the multipotential
cells of the normal embryo remains to be established.

Some differentiated cell lines absorb the decompacting activity of the serum. This is probably due to the presence of molecules similar to those present on EC cells or to the persistence
of the same structure on certain type of cells.

That communication between EC cells, as detected by metabolic
cooperation exhibits a certain degree of specificity and that the
disappearance of these junctions can be obtained by interaction
of cell membrane with certain molecules may have embryological
implication.

ACKNOWLEDGEMENTS

I would like to thank P.R.A. Avner and M. Fellous for the gift
of the human cell lines used in these studies ; and also P.R.A.
Avner, H. Condamine, F. Jacob, H. Jakob, F. Kelly, R. Kemler and
J. Wood for stimulating discussions and for reading the manuscript.

This work was supported by grants from the Centre National de
la Recherche Scientifique (LA 269), the Institut National de la

Santé et de la Recherche Médicale (C.R.A.T. n° 76.4.311), the
Délégation Générale à la Recherche Scientifique et Technique
(A.C.C. n° 77.7.0966) and the André Meyer Foundation.

REFERENCES

1. Gehring, W., Mindek, G. and Hadorn, E. (1968) J.Embryol.Exp.
    Morphol., 20, 307-322.

2. Garcia-Bellido, A. (1975) In "Cell Patterning", Ciba
    Foundation Symposium, pp. 161-182.

3. Gearhart, J.D. and Mintz, B. (1972) Develop.Biol., 29,
    27-37.

4. Crick, F.H.C. and Lawrence, P.A. (1975) Science, 189, 340-
    347.

5. Kauffman, S.A., Shymko, R.M. and Trabert, K. (1978) Science,
    199, 259-270.

6. Jacob, F. (1978) Proc.R.Soc.Lond.B, 201, 249-270.

7. Mintz, B. and Illmensee, K. (1975) Proc.Nat.Acad.Sci.USA,
    72, 3585-3589.

8. Nicolas, J.F., Dubois, P., Jakob, H., Gaillard, J. and
    Jacob, F. (1974) Ann.Microbiol.(Inst.Pasteur), 126 A, 3-22.

9. Nicolas, J.F., Avner, P., Gaillard, J., Guénet, J.L.,
    Jakob, H. and Jacob, F. (1976) Cancer Research, 36, 4224-
    4231.

10. Gilula, N.B., Raymond Reeves, O. and Steinback, A. (1972)
    Nature, 235, 262-265.

11. Subak-Sharpe, J.M., Burk, R.R. and Pitts, J.D. (1966)
    Heredity, 21, 342-343.

12. Nicolas, J.F., Jakob, H. and Jacob, F. (1978) Proc.Nat.
    Acad.Sci.USA, 75, 3292-3296.

13. Nicolas, J.F., Avner, P.R.A. and Fellous, M., In preparation.

14. Hooper, M.L. and Slack, C. (1977) Develop.Biol., 55, 271-
    284.

15. Dunia, I., Nicolas, J.F., Jakob, H., Benedetti, E.L. and
    Jacob, F. (1979) Proc.Nat.Acad.Sci.USA, In press.

16. Kemler, R., Babinet, C., Eisen, H. and Jacob, F. (1977)
    Proc.Nat.Acad.Sci.USA, 74, 4449-4452.

17. Nicolas, J.F., Kemler, R. and Jacob, F., In preparation.

Cell Lineage, Stem Cells and Cell Determination
INSERM Symposium No. 10
Editor: N. Le Douarin
© *1979 Elsevier/North-Holland Biomedical Press*

INTERACTIONS BETWEEN MOUSE EMBRYOS AND TERATOCARCINOMAS

V.E. PAPAIOANNOU

Department of Zoology, South Parks Road, Oxford, OX1 3PS, U.K.

INTRODUCTION

Teratocarcinomas are unusual tumours propagated and perpetuated by unusual stem cells, the embryonal carcinoma (EC) cells. These cells are capable of indefinite proliferation if the tumour is transplanted from host to host or if the cells are continuously subcultured in tissue culture. Throughout many generations of proliferative cell divisions the majority of EC cells retain their peculiar set of covert phenotypic options, that is, they retain the capacity to differentiate into foetal and adult tissues derived from all three traditional embryonic germ layers. The potential of EC cells is strikingly similar and perhaps equivalent to certain multipotent cells of the early embryo, whereas the difference in the behaviour of these two cell types is in some aspects of the control of proliferation and the expression of potential. A teratocarcinoma tumour or even to some extent a differentiated teratocarcinoma culture can resemble an embryo in the quality but not in the relative quantity of different cell types, nor in its cellular organization. The persistence of the EC stem cell in teratocarcinomas is quite unlike the developmental progression of its early embryonic equivalent which gradually becomes restricted as its potential is realized in a foetus.

An examination of interactions between these two stem cells may shed light on the mechanisms of control of proliferation and differentiation. This paper is an attempt to summarize and evaluate many experiments which have as their common basis the combination of embryonic cells and embryonal carcinoma cells.

STEM CELLS OF THE EMBRYO AND TERATOCARCINOMAS

In the adult animal, stem cells are features of renewing cell populations such as haematopoietic cells or intestinal crypt cells. They retain a relatively undifferentiated phenotype and are capable of self-renewal or of yielding daughter cells of different phenotypes. Their proliferation and differentiation have the effect of maintaining particular cell populations in equilibrium by countering the loss of the terminally differentiated cells. In the embryo on the other hand, cell populations are developing, growing, and changing, not maintaining equilibrium. In the early mammalian embryo cell

populations with the properties of self-renewal and potential for further
differentiation are mostly short lived and transitory. As development proceeds,
these populations of cells become more and more restricted in their potential
and although they still maintain the morphological characteristics of undifferentiated cells, their covert differentiation progressively limits the range of
phenotypic options open to their daughters. Eventually, in the later stages of
embryogenesis, systems are formed which in the adult are characterized by the
presence of stem cells with very limited potential.

For example, most of the trophectoderm cells of the mouse blastocyst
terminally differentiate into the trophoblast giant cells which are no longer
capable of division. During the first part of gestation the number of giant
cells increases rapidly and it is a population of diploid, dividing trophoblast
cells in the core of the ectoplacental cone which provides daughters that
differentiate into giant cells and also daughters that remain as dividing stem
cells. The extraembryonic ectoderm of the egg cylinder, incidentally, is in
the same cell lineage, derived from the polar trophectoderm[1], and the cells may
act as stem cell precursors of this tissue as well. Toward the end of
gestation the giant cells begin to degenerate and are not renewed, indicating
the cessation of stem cell function.

Similarly, some of the progeny cells of the inner cell mass (ICM) form
primitive endoderm which then expands by cell division, while others retain an
undifferentiated phenotype and are called the primitive ectoderm. There is
perhaps a short period of time over which the primitive ectoderm serves as a
stem cell population for endoderm and also continues to renew itself. Certainly
the primitive ectoderm retains endoderm forming capacity for several days after
the initial differentiation of endoderm[2] before the covert potential of these
"undifferentiated" cells becomes restricted by the progression of development.

One could also consider the ectoderm as a stem cell population for the
formation of mesoderm which occurs over a somewhat less restricted period of
time. Mesoderm formation begins at the first appearance of the primitive
streak and the ectoderm is still capable of mesoderm production at least until
the headfold stage[3]. There are several other instances of these transitory stem
cell populations in the early embryo[4] and if any of these were maintained longer
than usual, the result would certainly be abnormal morphogenesis. The close
control of the proliferation of these cells is an essential ingredient in the
establishment of embryonic cell lineages and the orderly process of embryogenesis. If EC stem cells correspond to some early stem cell in the embryo then
the persistence of EC stem cells is a major departure from normal embryonic

processes.

The spontaneous occurance of teratocarcinomas from foetal germ cells in the male testes and from parthenogenetically developing eggs in the female ovary, as well as the experimental induction by ectopic transplantation of early embryos or genital ridges, attests to the close relationship of embryonic and embryonal carcinoma stem cells. In addition to the similarities in developmental potential already mentioned, EC cells share morphological, antigenic, and biochemical properties with early embryonic cells (see Graham[5] for review). The pattern of protein synthesis in EC cells differs from cleavage, morula, and blastocyst stage cells[6], but closely resembles that of the primitive embryonic ectoderm[7], the progenitor of all the foetal cell lineages[1].

As EC stem cells differentiate either within a tumour or in culture, there is evidence that they irreversibly lose their stem cell characteristics, a feature shared with other stem cells, notably embryonic stem cells. Tumourigenicity is also lost in the immediate differentiated products of EC cells in most situations. It is possible to establish differentiated cell lines in culture directly from solid or ascitic teratocarcinomas and although these lines retain a certain proliferative potential as differentiated cells, they have lost the ability to grow progressively in adult hosts except in a few cases where secondary transformation events have been implicated (see Graham[5] and Martin[8] for reviews). The special circumstance of differentiated cells growing as tumours in chimaeras will be discussed more fully in the next section but in this case it is certainly possible that secondary changes in the EC cells had occurred during the long culture period and that the formation of malignant, differentiated cells was not a primary property of the EC cells.

Differentiating cultures of EC cells are becoming increasingly studied as models of embryonic cell differentiation, providing access to large numbers of cells which are proceeding through the same developmental step. Changes in gene expression, biochemical and surface properties and other signs of differentiation can be more easily documented using EC cell cultures than the embryo itself. Combinations of EC and embryonic cells should extend the usefulness of EC cell models by indicating the controls that embryonic cells can exert on EC cells, or vice versa, to influence or direct the choice of developmental pathway taken by the stem cells.

EMBRYO - EMBRYONAL CARCINOMA CELL CHIMAERAS

The most spectacular combinations of EC and embryonic cells have been the adult chimaeric mice produced by the introduction of EC cells into the blastocyst followed by a return of the injected embryo to the uterus for development[9-15]. In some of these embryos the EC cells participated in normal development, producing functional differentiated cell progeny as evidenced by the presence of differentiated cells such as melanocytes (Fig. 1A). These chimaeras are particularly interesting because of their potential use as transmitters to the mouse germ line of mutant genes selected in EC cell cultures. Three chimaeras have indeed produced functional EC derived gametes[12,16] but these were chimaeras with noncultured EC cells and as yet, cultured EC cells have not produced a germ line chimaera.

Table 1 summarizes the blastocyst injection experiments including those with EC cells direct from solid or ascitic tumours, those using cultured EC cells, and finally those using EC derived differentiated cells. Also included are experiments involving EC injection into vesicles of pure trophectoderm. It would seem from the results of the injections analysed at term or midgestation that the EC cells or their daughters have three possibilities once inside the embryo. Either they die, or they behave as normal cells and participate with the embryonic cells in producing normal tissue, or they behave as malignant cells. It is clear from the table that only a small proportion of the injected blastocysts develop as chimaeras, many fewer than would be expected if the injected cells were synchronous embryonic cells[17,18], and that some lines are better than others in this respect, particularly amongst the in vitro lines. This could indicate that most EC cells put into blastocysts die soon after injection. However, this has not yet been directly demonstrated and, although a variety of genetic markers have been used with varying sensitivity, it is not inconceivable that a very low EC contribution could go undetected. Different isozymes of the ubiquitous enzyme glucose phosphate isomerase (GPI) are the most commonly used markers and although 2-5% of a minor component can be detected in tissue homogenates, most of the analysis is done only on samples of tissues, not the entire tissue. These negative results then, cannot be interpreted with certainty as the death of the EC cells although this may be true in many cases.

A second possibility is that of normal differentiation within the embryo with the concomitant loss of malignancy. Most of the chimaeras listed probably represent this EC cell fate. Some of the EC cell markers used allowed direct detection of differentiated cells such as the pigment markers in all experiments, β-galactosidase[19] and liver proteins[12]; more often the marker was GPI which indicated varying contributions of EC progeny to tissues that remained normal for the life of the animal and were probably normally differentiated, nonmalignant cells.

The distribution of EC progeny in chimaeras is worth noting. If cells from a normal, age matched, genetically marked ICM are injected into a blastocyst, the resulting chimaeras can show a range of proportions of the two tissue types as illustrated for coat pigmentation in Figure 1B. However, within any one chimaeric animal there is usually a reasonable correlation between different tissues in the relative proportions of the two cell types (see McLaren[20] for review). On the contrary the EC contributions to tissues in chimaeras is often sporadic and there are not necessarily correlations even between developmentally related tissues. For example, mosaic male N in the study of Illmensee and Mintz[11] showed a 75% EC contribution in lungs but none in any other tissue. Similarly, mouse T120 in the study of Papaioannou et al.[14] showed high levels of chimaerism in all tissues tested except brain, liver, hair follicles and spleen which were entirely host type.

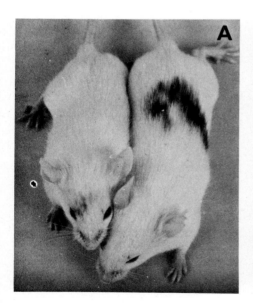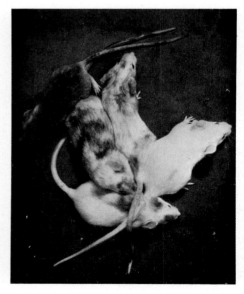

Figure 1. A. Chimaeric mice produced by the injection of C17 EC cells into genetically albino blastocysts. B. Chimaeric mice produced with normal embryonic tissue from albino and pigmented strains.

TABLE 1   SUMMARY OF BLASTOCYST AND VESICLE INJECTION EXPERIMENTS

Tumour or EC line	Origin			Analysis at Term				
	Tumour	Embryo Age	Strain	Host blasto-cyst	No. anal-ysed	No. chim-aeras	No. tum-ours	No. tum-ours with EC
IN VIVO								
OTT6050		6½ day	129	Swiss	60	1	0	
OTT6050		6½ day	129	C57BL	164	31**	6	1+?
LT72484		Spontan-eous	LT/Sv	CBAT6/T6	74	8**	3	?
IN VITRO								
PSA1 NG2⧸	OTT5568	3½ day	129	C57	44	10	0	
TK⁻	OTT6050	6½ day	129	C57	31	3	0	
S1KR OSB	OTT5568	3½ day	129	AG/Cam	44	1	0	
PCC3/A/1	OTT6050	6½ day	129	AG/Cam	86	4	1	0
C17	17	6½ day	C3H	CFLP	77	13	8	1
OC15S1	OTT6050	6½ day	129					
C86	86	7½ day	C3H	CFLP	74	6	6	6
C86S1A1⧸	86	7½ day	C3H					
C145b*	145b	6½ day	C3H	CFLP PO, A2G	201	0	0	
F1/9*	F1(C3Hx 129)/9	6½ day	F1(C3Hx 129)	CFLP	18	0	0	
1009*⧸		Spontan.	RI	SJL	137	0	0	
PCC4	OTT6050	6½ day	129					
PSA1 NG2⧸	OTT5568	3½ day	129					
PC13TG8⧸	OTT6050	6½ day	129					
R5/3⧸	OTT6050	6½ day	129					
DIFFERENT-IATED LINES								
C145 Endo 1	145b	6½ day	C3H					
OC15S1 End	OTT6050	6½ day	129					

* Euploid lines by banding;   ** Includes germ line chimaeras;   ⧸ HGPRT⁻ lines.
Unpublished work presented is that of the author and the following collaborators:
a) C.F. Graham;   b) R.L. Gardner;   c) S.J. Gaunt;   d) C. Babinet and J.F. Nicolas.

Tumour or EC line	Analysis at Midgestation			Analysis In Vitro			References
	Host blasto-cyst	No. anal-ysed	No. chim-aeras	No. blasto-cysts injected	No. vesicles injected	EC growth	
OTT6050							9
OTT6050							11-13, 16
LT72484							16, 22
PSA1 NG2[✝]							10
TK[-]							22
S1KR OSB							14, 15
PCC3/A/1							
C17							
OC15S1	F₁(CFLPxPO) F₁(C57xCBA) CBA	21	2				a
C86	CFLP	13	3-5				14, 15
C86S1A1[✝]	CFLP				18	0	b
C145b[*]	CFLP, 129 PO, A2G	404	5	34		4	21
F1/9[*]	CFLP, C57	71	0	20		0	c
1009[*✝]	SJL	15	0	38		4	d
PCC4	F₁(C57xCBA)				28	6	d
PSA1 NG2[✝]				75		16	
PC13TG8[✝]	CFLP			24		10	c
R5/3[✝]	CFLP			30		8	c
					20	3	
C145 Endo 1	CFLP, A2G	55	0				a
OC15S1 End	F₁(CFLPxPO) F₁(C57xCBA) CBA	26	0				a

Different cell lines certainly exhibit different capabilities in making chimaeras and it is also possible that the developmental potential within a chimaera is cell line specific. If one examines the patterns of colonization, there are certain tissues more frequently chimaeric than others but these differ between cell lines. For example, 8 out of 10 chimaeras made with single OTT6050 cells were chimaeric in lungs[11], 7 out of 9 PSA1 NG2 chimaeras were chimaeric in brain[10], and 7 out of 13 from C17 were chimaeric in the eyes, including all 5 normal chimaeras[15]. This last observation, however, may simply reflect a greater sensitivity in detecting eye pigment compared with detecting isozymes. With OC15S1 and C145b EC cells, colonization was detected only in parietal endoderm or yolk sac, and this could indicate that the cells differentiated into endoderm soon after injection or that they were already undergoing a transition to endoderm-like cells at the time of injection[21].

In summary, with the limited number of chimaeras available for analysis it is impossible to characterize fully the cell lines in terms of their potential. It is clear, however, that this potential differs from line to line and is sometimes distinct from embryonic cell potential. There is also some suggestion that there are developmental patterns characteristic of particular EC cell lines. The

negative results obtained with differentiated cells derived from EC lines (C145 Endo 1 and OC15S1 End, V. Papaioannou and C.F. Graham, unpublished) are compatible with the differentiated products of EC cells having limited potential.

Finally, the third possibility is that EC cells retain their malignancy in spite of their position within the developing embryo. This path is probably represented by the chimaeras which formed well differentiated teratocarcinomas following injection of EC cells from in vivo[22] and by the six chimaeras made from in vitro C86 cells[14]. These latter all developed at least one tumour which was usually detectable at birth and grew rapidly. The size of the tumours at birth was compatible with exponential growth from the time of cell injection into the blastocyst and this might indicate either that the embryonic cues were not sufficient to normalize the EC cells, due perhaps to secondary genetic changes that occurred in the EC cells in vitro, or that communication between embryo and EC cells was defective.

The tumours which developed in C17 chimaeras were usually differentiated cell tumours such as fibrosarcomas or rhabdomyosarcomas[15] and these must represent a modification of the EC cell malignancy. The tumours did not arise until the animals were adults and may have sprung from EC derived cells that were far beyond the original EC stem cell developmental stage. It is possible that the

developing embryo imposed a particular developmental regime on the cells
sufficient to direct their differentiation but not to suppress their malignancy
indefinitely. The pancreatic adenocarcinoma which arose following OTT6050
injection[11] may also fall into this category although it was eventually
described as a "cryptic teratocarcinoma"[19].

One of the great frustrations with this analysis of chimaeras is that any
conclusions must remain highly speculative due to the separation of the initial
combination of EC and embryonic cells and the analysis, in both time and the
variety of changes that have occurred in the developing embryo. Even when
potential chimaeras are analysed at midgestation the limitations of detection of
the markers in small tissue samples greatly reduces the information that can be
obtained so that the only additional information concerns the distribution of
EC progeny in foetal membranes and the confirmation by examination of implantation sites that the EC cells do not kill the embryos.

EMBRYO - EMBRYONAL CARCINOMA CELL COMBINATIONS IN VITRO

We have recently embarked on a line of experimentation that should give us
some information on which of the three paths just discussed a given EC cell will
follow once inside an embryo and also provide us with some indication of how an
embryo exerts control over an EC cell. Particular experiments involve the
examination of the behaviour in vitro of injected blastocysts or trophectoderm
vesicles, and also an examination of the extent of metabolic coupling between EC
and embryonic cells, a means of communication possibly concerned with controlling
and directing stem cell proliferation.

Many of the EC lines used in these studies have been tested for their ability
to form chimaeric animals (C145b, F1/9, 1009 and PSA1 NG2, see Table 1). In
addition, an azaguanine resistant subline of C86, C86S1A1, was injected into
vesicles and two other cell lines, PC13TG8, a metabolic cooperation competant
line [23], and R5/3, its cooperation defective derivative[24] were also used. The
various experiments have been done with somewhat different questions in mind so
the experimental procedures have not all been identical. Nonetheless it seems
worth summarizing the results to date to help indicate the areas for further
investigation.

Growth in blastocysts

A few disaggregated cells or small cell clumps were injected into whole
blastocysts in a manner similar to that used for the chimaera experiments but
these were allowed to heal and then were put into culture conditions favourable

150

both for EC cell growth and for blastocyst outgrowth. Occasionally cells could be seen on the outside of healed, reexpanded blastocysts. These were most likely EC cells that had escaped the blastocoelic cavity before healing occurred; these embryos were usually discarded. Figure 2 illustrates the appearance of injected blastocysts before culture. Cultures were examined frequently over periods of several days to several weeks and although blastocyst attachment and initial outgrowth was indistinguishable from controls, the appearance and growth of cells with EC morphology was a variable feature.

No cells of EC morphology appeared in outgrowths of F1/9 injected blastocysts and in only a few outgrowths from 1009 and C145b injected blastocysts (although in 2 of these cases from the latter cell line external EC cells were detected before culture[21]). The EC cells were first distinguishable growing in a monolayer at the edge of the blastocyst outgrowth.

EC cell growth was a much more common feature in outgrowths of blastocysts injected with the other 3 cell lines, PSA1 NG2 (C. Babinet, personal communication), PC13TG8 and R5/3 (V. Papaioannou and S.J. Gaunt, unpublished). With PC13TG8 injected blastocysts, like 1009 and C145b, cells with typical EC morphology were evident after several days of culture at the edge of the blastocyst outgrowth. If left undisturbed these EC cells soon overgrew the embryonic cells (Figure 3A). PSA1 NG2 and R5/3 cells behaved somewhat

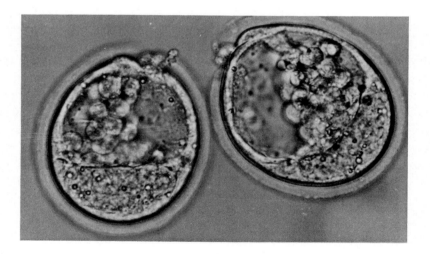

Figure 2. Blastocysts approximately one hour after injection of clumps of C145b cells. EC cells are clearly visible in the blastocoelic cavity.

differently and appeared to proliferate within the ICM of the blastocyst outgrowth. The presence of PSA1 NG2 derived cells was confirmed by GPI analysis
of some of the outgrowths and the presence of R5/3 EC cells was confirmed by
disaggregation of the outgrowths followed by replating when cells of typical
EC morphology were recovered. Characteristic of the R5/3 outgrowths was also
what appeared to be an unusual proliferation of trophectoderm which formed
giant cells (Figure 3B). These were shown to be of embryonic cell origin since
they did not survive culture in thioguanine. Occasionally but less frequently
a similar proliferation of trophectoderm was seen in control blastocyst outgrowths under these culture conditions so until larger numbers have been
analysed it is not possible to distinguish what part

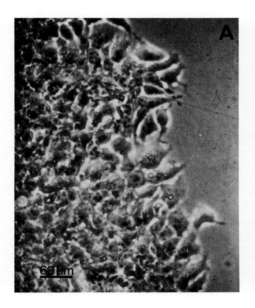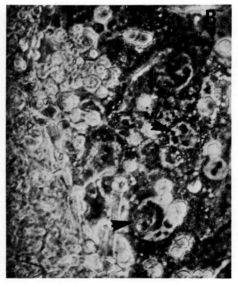

Figure 3. A. Edge of an outgrowth from a PC13TG8 injected blastocyst after
13 days of culture. Only cells of EC morphology are visible. B. Edge of an
outgrowth from an R5/3 injected blastocyst after 13 days showing a number of
giant trophoblast nuclei (arrows).

the R5/3 cells play in this phenomenon. It is clear however that some EC cell
lines persist and proliferate in short term culture after injection into
blastocysts including the in vitro line with the best record of making chimaeras,
PSA1 NG2. Other cell lines show no or very limited proliferation perhaps due to
immediate terminal differentiation or death. In the case of C145b this lack of
growth is also reflected by a loss of tumourigenicity when injected blastocysts
are transplanted to ectopic sites[21].

Growth in vesicles

Of the two distinct tissues of the blastocyst, the ICM and the trophectoderm,
it is the ICM which contains all the cells in the foetal lineage while the
trophectoderm produces only trophoblast and the extraembryonic ectoderm[1]. It is
also some of the cells of the ICM that EC cells most resemble. An interaction
between ICM and trophectoderm cells has been implicated in maintaining the
proliferation of some of the trophectoderm cells which otherwise cease division
and become giant[25]. It seemed interesting to see to what extent EC cells might
substitute for ICM cells in this particular interaction. Also it was of
interest to compare the EC injected blastocysts with EC injected trophectoderm
vesicles to see what effect on EC growth could be attributed to the presence of
the ICM.

Trophectoderm vesicles were prepared and injected as described by Gardner et
al.[25] or by a modification which allowed injection and cutting in one step.
Usually a small clump of cells was injected. As with injected blastocysts, the
vesicles attached and initially outgrew normally. Healed, reexpanded vesicles
with cells remaining outside are not included in the results reported here.

Vesicles injected with C86S1A1 were allowed to grow 3-4 days before selective
medium (HAT) was added to kill the EC cells. This was done to allow easier
counting of the trophoblast cells. Before the addition of selective medium
there were no cells with EC morphology visible in the outgrowths, and after
culture for two days in selective medium the number of trophoblast cells did not
appear to be different from control vesicle outgrowths although it was lower
than in control intact blastocyst outgrowths. This cell line, at least during
this short culture period did not appear to have proliferated or to have
affected the proliferation of trophectoderm cells (V. Papaioannou and R.L.
Gardner, unpublished).

In an experiment with the metabolic cooperation defective R5/3 EC cells, in
outgrowths from 3/16 injected vesicles there was evidence of EC cell proliferation. In each case cells with EC morphology were growing on the edge of the

giant cell growth. There was no evidence of enhancement of trophectoderm
proliferation as was suggested by injection of this line into intact blastocysts.
Similar results were obtained with line PCC4 (Table 1).

Metabolic cooperation between EC and embryonic cells

It seemed important to establish to what extent metabolic cooperation between
cells, or the lack of it, might be involved in EC - embryo interactions. For
this purpose the two HGPRT⁻ cell lines PC13TG8 and its derivative R5/3 seem
ideal since the latter can serve as a control line being incapable of metabolic
cooperation[24]. Gaunt and Papaioannou[26] have tested pre- and post- implantation
embryonic tissue for the ability to cooperate with these two lines in vitro.
Morulae, outgrowing blastocysts, isolated ICMs and 7 different cell types from
the 8th day embryo were cocultured with EC cells in the presence of ³H-
hypoxanthine. Only HGPRT⁺ cells, that is, the embryonic cells, and cells
metabolically coupled with them should show grains following autoradiography.

All tissues were negative for metabolic cooperation with R5/3 cells as
expected. With PC13TG8, on the other hand, metabolic cooperation was selectively
established and the results were consistent with the view that the trophectoderm
and its derivatives, the ectoplacental cone cells and extraembryonic ectoderm,
do not metabolically couple with EC cells. However, early morulae cells prior
to trophectoderm differentiation as well as the cells of the ICM and ICM cell
lineage, the embryonic endoderm, mesoderm and ectoderm and the extraembryonic
mesoderm and endoderm readily couple with EC cells.

A few PC13TG8 and R5/3 injected trophectoderm vesicles were also grown in
conditions that would allow the recognition of cells in metabolic coupling
similarly to the experiment just described. In 4/5 outgrowths from PC13TG8
injected vesicles unlabeled cells could clearly be seen in the centre of the
giant cell outgrowth after 3 days of culture, indicating metabolic cooperation
had not been established. This is consistant with the results of coculture of
EC and blastocysts which indicated that trophectoderm and EC do not cooperate.
In the four R5/3 injected vesicle outgrowths there were no unlabeled cells
visible, nor were there any cells with EC morphology; all were normal looking
trophoblast giant cells. Since these EC cells are defective in metabolic
cooperation, we must conclude that they had died and disappeared by the 3rd day
in culture. Obviously generalization is difficult with such small numbers but
an extention of these experiments should help correlate metabolic cooperation
with different effects in embryo - EC cell combinations. In particular, the
establishment of differences between cell lineages within the embryo in their
ability to metabolically couple with EC cells [26] may have important implications

for the control and direction of EC stem cells introduced into the embryo and likewise for the control of differentiation within the embryo itself.

ACKNOWLEDGEMENTS

I wish to thank the Medical Research Council for financial support and Joan Brown and Teresa Clements for preparing the manuscript. Special thanks are due to my collaborators who have allowed me to quote unpublished results and to Stephen Gaunt and Chris Graham for commenting on the manuscript.

REFERENCES

1. Gardner, R.L. and Papaioannou, V.E. (1975) The Early Development of Mammals. Eds. M. Balls and A.E. Wild, Cambridge University Press, Cambridge, pp. 107-132.

2. Pedersen, R.A., Spindle, A.I. and Wiley, L.M. (1977) Nature 270, 435-437.

3. Svajger, A. and Levak-Svajger, B. (1976) Experientia 32, 378-380.

4. Papaioannou, V.E., Rossant, J. and Gardner, R.L. (1978) Stem Cells and Tissue Homeostasis. Eds. B.I. Lord, C.S. Potten, and R.J. Cole, Cambridge University Press, Cambridge pp. 49-69.

5. Graham, C.F. (1977) Concepts in Mammalian Embryogenesis. Ed. M.I. Sherman, M.I.T. monograph pp. 315-394.

6. Dewey, M.J., Filler, R. and Mintz, B. (1978) Dev. Biol. 65, 171-182.

7. Martin, G.R., Smith, S. and Epstein, C.J. (1978) Dev. Biol. 66, 8-16.

8. Martin, G.R. (1975) Cell 5, 229-243.

9. Brinster, R.L. (1974) J. Exp. Med. 140, 1049-1056.

10. Dewey, M.J., Martin, D.W., Martin, G.R. and Mintz. B. (1977) Proc. Natl. Acad. Sci. USA 74, 5564-5568.

11. Illmensee, K. and Mintz, B. (1976) Proc. Natl. Acad. Sci. USA 73, 549-553.

12. Mintz, B. and Illmensee, K. (1975) Proc. Natl. Acad. Sci. USA 72, 3585-3589.

13. Mintz, B., Illmensee, K. and Gearhart, J.D. (1975) Teratomas and Differentiation, Eds. M.I. Sherman and D. Solter, Academic Press, Inc. London. pp. 59-82.

14. Papaioannou, V.E., McBurney, M.W., Gardner, R.L. and Evans, M.J. (1975) Nature, 258, 70-73.

15. Papaioannou, V.E., Gardner, R.L., McBurney, M.W., Babinet, C. and Evans, M.J. (1978) J. Embryol. exp. Morph. 44, 93-104.

16. Cronmiller, C. and Mintz, B. (1978) Dev. Biol. 67, 465-477.

17. Gardner, R.L. (1978) Excerpta Medica International Congress Series No. 432. Birth Defects. pp. 153-166.

18. Papaioannou, V.E. and Gardner, R.L. (1979) J. Embryol. exp. Morph. (in press).

19. Dewey, M.J. and Mintz, B. (1978) Dev. Biol. 66, 550-559.

20. McLaren, A. (1976) Mammalian Chimaeras, Cambridge University Press, Cambridge.

21. Papaioannou, V.E., Evans, E.P., Gardner, R.L. and Graham, C.F. (1979)
    J. Embryol. exp. Morph. (submitted).

22. Illmensee, K. (1978) Genetic Mosaics and Chimaeras in Mammals. Ed.
    L.B. Russell, Plenum Press, New York. pp. 3-25.

23. Hooper, M.L. and Slack, C. (1977) Dev. Biol. 55, 271-284.

24. Slack, C., Morgan, R.H.M. and Hooper, M.L. (1978) Exp. Cell Res. 117,
    195-205.

25. Gardner, R.L., Papaioannou, V.E. and Barton, S.C. (1973) J. Embryol. exp.
    Morph. 30, 561-572.

26. Gaunt, S.J. and Papaioannou, V.E. (1979) J. Embryol. exp. Morph.
    (submitted).

Cell Lineage, Stem Cells and Cell Determination
INSERM Symposium No. 10
Editor: N. Le Douarin
© *1979 Elsevier/North-Holland Biomedical Press*

GENE EXPRESSION IN CHIMERIC MICE

KARL ILLMENSEE

Department of Biology, University of Geneva, CH-1224 Geneva (Switzerland)

INTRODUCTION

Considerable progress in clonally propagating teratocarcinoma cell lines
has opened new possibilities of selecting for somatic mutations *in vitro*[1].
It has therefore been proposed that teratocarcinomas might provide us with a
unique kind of cell which can be selected *in vitro* for a given somatic mutation
and then cycled through mice via blastocyst injection for further *in situ*
analysis[2]. Following such an experimental scheme, teratocarcinoma cells deficient for hypoxanthine phosphoribosyltransferase (HPRT) apparently retained
their developmental potential to a remarkable extent[3]. It thus seemed promising to us to find out whether foreign genetic material could be introduced
into teratocarcinoma cells via somatic cell hybridization in order to study
xenogeneic gene expression during differentiation and to assay for the ontogenetic appearance, coexistence and regulation of the foreign gene products
in various tissues during development.

XENOGENEIC GENE EXPRESSION

Human x mouse hybrid cells

In collaboration with Dr. C. Croce (Wistar Institute), the combination of
cell hybridization techniques with our biological system has recently opened
up a new line of research. In his laboratory, cultured mouse teratocarcinoma
cells first were selected for thymidine kinase (TK) deficiency. After microinjection into mouse blastocysts[4], the TK deficient cells became integrated
during normal organogenesis and contributed substantially to several internal
tissues, thus demonstrating their suitability as a gene carrier. The TK deficient mouse teratocarcinoma cells were then fused *in vitro* with HPRT deficient
human fibrosarcoma cells using inactivated Sendai virus. Only the interspecific hybrid cells can grow in hypoxanthine/aminopterin/thymidine (HAT) selective medium. On the contrary, TK- and HPRT-deficient parental cells, which

Selected in part from a paper presented at the Symposium on Differentiation
and Neoplasia, Minneapolis, 1978.

lack the enzymes required for the incorporation of thymidine and hypoxanthine respectively, do not survive in this medium. Under these selective conditions, the viable hybrid cells, which quickly lose human but not mouse chromosomes, retain at least human chromosome 17 that carries the locus for TK. This particular chromosome also carries a second known gene that is closely linked to TK and coded for galactokinase (GLK). The latter enzyme, with its characteristic electrophoretic mobility quite different from the equivalent mouse enzyme, serves as another useful biochemical marker for detecting the presence and normal expression of the human gene product in the hybrid cells.

After subcutaneous implantation into athymic *nude* mice, the human x mouse hybrid cells formed predominantly undifferentiated tumors. In contrast, when injected into genetically marked mouse blastocysts, the malignant hybrid cells became integrated during embryogenesis and participated in orderly differentiation of the coat and seven internal organs. Although the hybrid cells contributed up to 60% in some tissues of chimeric mice as judged from enzyme analysis, the human-specific gene product of GLK has only been detected in the heart of one chimera and the kidneys of another; both tissues, by the way, showed the highest participation of hybrid cells in the enzyme tests[5]. The failure to disclose human GLK in the other mosaic organs might have resulted from (1) use of assay techniques not sensitive enough for the recovery of minor enzyme activity, (2) loss of human chromosome 17 during *in situ* cell divisions in the absence of selective pressure to retain this chromosome, or (3) tissue-specific restriction in gene activity.

Rat x mouse hybrid cells

In order to facilitate a more extensive analysis of foreign gene expression *in vivo*, it would be desirable to utilize a hybrid cell line containing several xenogeneic chromosomes, thereby allowing the search for a number of different gene products. In this respect, interspecific hybrid cells between TK deficient mouse teratocarcinoma and HPRT deficient rat hepatoma[6] that had retained almost all of the mouse chromosomes and various numbers of rat chromosomes, seemed ideal for blastocyst injections (Fig. 1). While the cell hybrids usually formed malignant tumors in athymic *nude* mice, at least some of these tumor cells were still capable of reverting to a normal phenotype in chimeric mice[7]. In contrast to previous results, tissue contributions of the rat x mouse hybrid cells remained limited to the liver and a few other organs of endomesodermal origin, probably due to the rat hepatoma cell parent. Very recently, we

produced several fetal chimeras which once again contained rat x mouse hybrid
cells in their liver and a few other cell-lineage related organs (e.g. intestine, lungs), thus confirming our previous observations that this particular
hybrid cell preferentially channels into the liver pathway. Such a preference

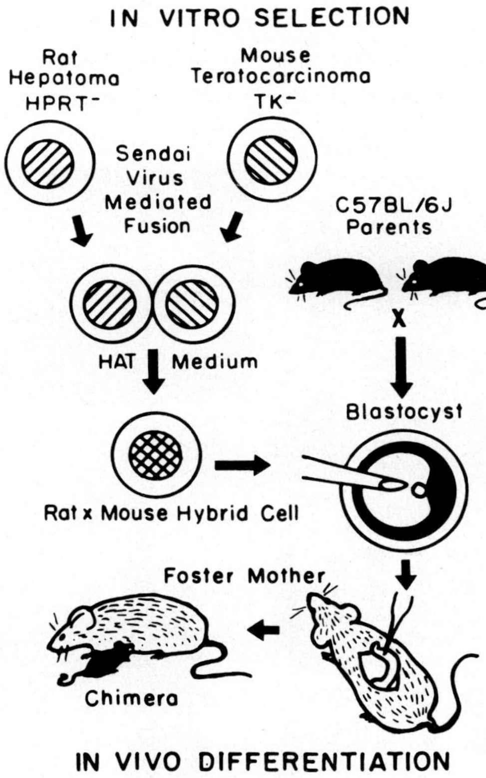

Fig. 1. Experimental scheme of cycling rat x mouse hybrid cells through mice
via blastocyst injection. TK deficient mouse teratocarcinoma cells and HPRT
deficient rat hepatoma cells were fused using inactivated Sendai virus and
selected in HAT medium, in which only the hybrid cells could survive. These
cells were then injected singly into C57BL/6 blastocysts carrying several
genetic markers, thereby enabling any *in situ* differentiation of the cell
hybrids. After microinjection, the blastocysts had to be surgically implanted
in pseudopregnant foster mothers to allow development to term. The experimental
offspring were analyzed for hybrid-cell contributions in their tissues [7]

160

for a particular developmental pathway may permit specific cell-lineage analysis which usually remains obscured by the random integration of injected normal cells during development[8].

Reversion of malignancy appeared more surprising because, on the one hand, the hybrid cells formed undifferentiated tumors in adult hosts and, on the other hand, differentiated normally into liver, lung, kidney, gut, and fat pad during *in situ* organogenesis. A comparable situation occurred with the human x mouse hybrid cells, which produced undifferentiated tumors in *nude* mice but contributed normally to a number of different tissues in chimeric mice. It therefore seems as if the prospective potential of the malignant hybrid cells

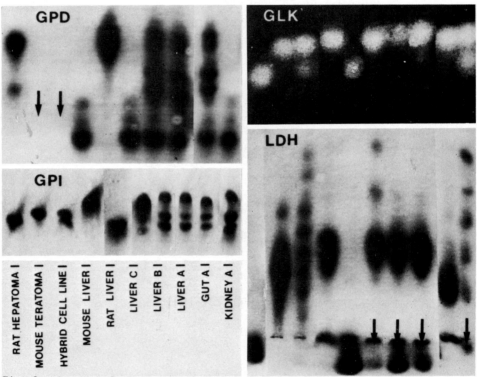

Fig. 2. Starch gel electrophoresis of rat- and mouse-specific enzyme variants of glycerolphosphate dehydrogenase (GPD), glycosephosphate isomerase (GPI), galactokinase (GLK), and lactate dehydrogenase (LDH). Cell extracts from liver, gut, and kidneys of chimeric mice A, B and C reveal rat x mouse hybrid cell contributions. Note the absence of GPD activity (arrow) in the hybrid cells and the rat hepatoma and its appearance in the liver B and A as well as in gut A. The formation of rat - mouse heteropolymers in these mosaic tissues documents functional cooperation of the interspecific gene products. The appearance of adult rat LDH-5 (arrow), not detectable in the hybrid cells, indicates differential modulation of the xenogeneic genes during *in vivo* development[7].

remains limited in the adult host and will only be fully revealed in the environment of the embryo.

But what happened to the rat chromosomal genes in the chimeric mice ? Because the rat x mouse hybrid cells retained several rat chromosomes, it was possible to detect nine different rat-specific enzymes in the various mosaic tissues. The appearance *in vivo* of rat gene products not detectable in the hybrid cells *in vitro* and the formation of heteropolymers with the corresponding mouse enzymes indicates a functional expression of the rat genes during mouse development. The synthesis of adult-specific enzyme variants further demonstrates the proper modulation of the xenogeneic genes during organogenesis (Fig. 2). Extending this kind of analysis to other genes (including X-chromosomal ones) should reveal their developmental stage-specificity and ultimately give insight into the processes that control gene activity during mammalian differentiation.

ACKNOWLEDGEMENTS

I should like to thank Drs. C.M. Croce, P.C. Hoppe, and L.C. Stevens for continuous collaboration. The receiving of various mouse strains from the Jackson Laboratory and the Füllinsdorf Institute is greatly appreciated. Our current research is supported by grants FN 3.183-0.77 and 3.183-1.77 from the Swiss National Science Foundation and by an appropriation from the G. and A. Claraz Foundation.

REFERENCES

1. Sherman, M.I. and Solter, D. eds. (1975) Teratomas and Differentiation. Academic Press, New York.

2. Mintz, B., Illmensee, K. and Gearhart, J.D. (1975) In: Teratomas and Differentiation, eds. Sherman, M.I. and Solter, D. Academic Press, New York, pp. 59-82.

3. Dewey, M.J., Martin, D.W., Martin, G.R. and Mintz, B. (1977) Proc. Natl. Acad. Sci. USA 74, 5564-5568.

4. Illmensee, K. (1978) In: Genetic Mosaics and Chimeras in Mammals, ed. Russell, L.B. Plenum Publ., New York, pp. 3-25.

5. Illmensee, K., Hoppe, P. and Croce, C.M. (1978) Proc. Natl. Acad. Sci. USA 75, 1914-1918.

6. Litwack, G. and Croce, C.M. (1979) Cell Physiol., in press.

7. Illmensee, K. and Croce, C.M. (1979) Proc. Natl. Acad. Sci. USA 76, 879-883.

8. Gardner, R.L. (1978) In: Birth Defects, eds. Littlefield, J.W. and DeGrouchy, J. Excepta Medica, Princeton, pp. 154-166.

Cell Lineage, Stem Cells and Cell Determination
INSERM Symposium No. 10
Editor: N. Le Douarin
© *1979 Elsevier/North-Holland Biomedical Press*

EMBRYONIC HEMOGLOBIN PRODUCTION BY TERATOCARCINOMA-DERIVED CELLS IN *IN VITRO* CULTURES.

CLAUDE A. CUDENNEC, ANNIE DELOUVEE and JEAN-PAUL THIERY
Institut d'Embryologie du CNRS et du Collège de France, 49bis, Avenue de la Belle-Gabrielle, 94130 Nogent-sur-Marne (France)

The first population of red blood cells which arises during the prenatal life of the mouse occurs in the yolk sac between the 7th and the 14th day of gestation. The erythrocytes formed in this extraembryonic site are morphologically and biochemically different from those of the adult. They appear as large nucleated erythrocytes synthesizing embryonic types of hemoglobin (Hb)[1,2,3]. These cells represent a transient population of red blood cells which is progressively replaced by cells arising from fetal liver hematopoiesis from the 10th day of development. The latter are small non-nucleated cells containing only adult Hb[1,2,4]. At the end of gestation, fully-developed bone-marrow becomes the preferential site of hematopoietic cell production.

Teratocarcinoma is generally considered as an interesting model system for the study of mammalian ontogenesis[5]. We have previously described the formation of blood islands in organ cultures of the PCC$_3$/A/1 teratocarcinoma cell line[6]. The red blood cells of these hematopoietic foci were shown to share morphological features of yolk sac primitive erythrocytes. We present here biochemical evidence that the spontaneous erythropoiesis of the PCC$_3$/A/1 line corresponds to normal yolk sac erythropoiesis.

MATERIAL AND METHODS.

Mice : 129/Sv mice were used in this study since the teratocarcinoma OTT 6050 originates from this strain of mice[7]. Adult blood cells were collected by sectioning the tail end. Mice at 6 to 8 weeks of age were used for mating. One male and 5 females were caged together overnight. The day of the vaginal plug was considered as day 0 of gestation.

Cultures : The established cell line PCC$_3$/A/1[8] was maintained in an undifferentiated state by serial transplantation at 2.10^6 cells per ml in tissue culture dishes (NUNC) in DMEM supplemented with 15% fetal calf serum (selected batches). Confluent cultures were used in this study to set up primary organ cultures as described elsewhere[6]. Secondary organotypic cultures consisted of 1-mm^3 fragments of tissues excised from 10-day-old primary organotypic cultures and subsequently transferred onto new Millipore filters (figure 1).

<u>Sample preparation</u> : Fragments of 7-day-old secondary organotypic cultures
containing blood foci were picked off and pooled in 0.25 M sucrose (Merck)
containing 1% (^{V}/$_w$) Trasylol (Sigma) and 0.1% KCN. Tissue aggregates were
disrupted by gentle pipetting. The cell suspension was spun 10 min at 1000rpm
and the supernatant discarded. The pellet was then lyophilised and stored at
-20°C. Red blood cells of adult mice and embryos were collected in saline,
centrifuged and washed in 0.25 sucrose + Trasylol + KCN, and then lyophilised.

   Cell pellets of about 0.1μl in volume were incubated for 30 min in 1μl of
lysis buffer[0.5% Nonidet P40 (BDH) ; 2% Ampholine mix (LKB) (15% pH 5-7 +
70% pH 7-9 + 15% pH 9-11) ; 20% sucrose ; 1% Trasylol]. The lysate was centrifuged in a Beckman microfuge for 1 min. The supernatant was loaded on an isoelectric focusing gel.

<u>Identification of hemoglobin</u> : Appropriate concentration of haptoglobin (a gift
of Drs.Rosa and Tsapis) known to bind irreversibly to Hb[9] [1μl of stock solution binds 25μg of hemoglobin] was added to the teratocarcinoma blood sample
and incubated for 45 min at room temperature. In this case the ampholine range
was pH 3.5 to 10 both for the sample solution and the polyacrylamide gel.

<u>Isoelectrofocusing slab gel</u> : Micro slab gels (25 x 37 x 0,15 mm) were prepared
according to Schwartz and Neukirchen (personal communication). Two microscope
slides previously washed with B1 detergent and rinced with distilled water,
were assembled with spacers and combs, made of Kodak X-ray film without emulsion
(150 μm thick) ; the micro slab gel was sealed with melted paraffin. The gel
solution was introduced by capillarity between the two slides. It was composed
of 7% Acrylamide, 0.4% Bisacrylamide (BIORAD), 4% Ampholine mixture pH 7-9
(LKB), 0.5% Nonidet P40 (BDH), 10% Sucrose (Merck). This solution was degassed
for at least 15 min under vacuum, finally ammonium persulfate (0.04% final
concentration) and N, N, N', N'-tetramethylethylenediamine (TEMED) (0.04% final
concentration) were added. Polymerisation was carried out in a moist
chamber under nitrogen for 2 hours. Gels were either used immediately or kept
in the cold for up to two days.

   One μl samples were loaded with fine glass capillaries and overlaid with a
10% sucrose solution containing 1% Ampholine mixture pH 7-9 and 0.5% Nonidet-
P40. The gel bottom was introduced in the lower reservoir filled with freshly
degassed 0.02M sodium hydroxide solution containing 6% sucrose.The top of the gel
was connected with a Whatman 3MM chromatography paper to the upper reservoir
containing 0.01M phosphoric acid and 6% sucrose. The microgel was cooled by
applying a copper sheet connected to an ice bath.

Isoelectric-focusing was carried out for approximately 45 min. at 40V
(400 µA down to 200 µA) and 45 min at 80V (400 µA down to 150 µA).One slab
gel plate was then removed and the gel adhering to the other plate was succes-
sively immersed in 1% 3,3'-dimethoxybenzidine (Eastman-Kodak) in methanol
for 4 min, 3% hydrogen peroxide in 70% ethanol for 2min and finally washed
in distilled water. Gels were subsequently dried out on a glass coverslips
and photographed with Collodium -Guilleminot film.

Electron microscopy : Fragments of secondary organotypic cultures were fixed
with 3% glutaraldehyde in cacodylate buffer (0.1M, pH 7.4) for 20 min at
room temperature and then post-fixed with 1% osmium tetroxide in the same
buffer for 1 h at 4°C. After alcohol dehydration, samples were embedded in
Epon 812. Ultrathin sections were obtained using a Reichert Ultramicrotome
OMU 2, double-stained with uranyl acetate and lead citrate and observed in a
Hitachi HS9 Electron Microscope.

RESULTS

A - Morphological studies

Previous *in vitro* or *in vivo* experiments showed the teratocarcinoma $PCC_3/A/1$
cell line to be a multipotential line[10]. As described by Nicolas et al.[11],con-
fluent cultures of this line are able to differentiate into a wide variety of
embryonic tissues, derived from the three primitive embryonic germ layers,
including muscle, cartilage, skin, nerve and endodermal vesicles. Attempts
made to detect erythropoietic differentiation using hemoglobin (Hb) as a marker
were unsuccessful. Nevertheless when placed in an *in vivo* environment these
cells appear to be able to differentiate into a large variety of tissues including blood cells[12].

Our previous data showed that this line was able to express a potentiality
to differentiate blood cells even *in vitro* if the cells were grown in mass
culture on a Millipore filter at the interphase air-CO_2/medium[6]. Blood foci
were easily visualized in living cultures, due to the red coloration of hemo-
globin-containing cells.

We present here a procedure to increase the frequency of appearance of
visible blood foci in organotypic culture (figure 1). Ten days after seeding
onto the Millipore filter (PO : Primary organotypic culture) teratocarcinoma
cells form a thick disc of tissue(about 1mm thick). These cultures were cut
into fragments of about 1/2 mm^3 in volume . Each of them represented 1/50 of
the total volume of the primary culture and was individually transferred onto

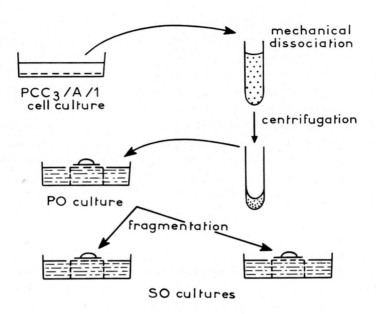

Fig. 1. Culture procedure used to allow erythroïd capabilities to be expressed by the cells of the PCC₃/A/1 teratocarcinoma line (PO culture : Primary Organotypic culture ; SO culture : Secondary Organotypic culture).

 a new Millipore filter (SO : secondary organotypic culture). In this case, blood foci appeared in 90% of the cultures, most of them between the 6th and 9th day after seeding (see figure 2).

   Irrespective of the type of organotypic culture prepared, hematopoietic cell populations arising from teratocarcinoma were similar and occurred in the vicinity of hollow vesicles. Figure 3 shows an electron micrograph of a blood focus taken from a 7-day-old SO culture. Blood cells were located in the inter-cellular space near the wall of a hollow vesicle. This wall consisted of an epithelium of columnar cells with microvilli decorating the cell pole directed toward the vesicle lumen. Hematopoietic cells were sometimes seen in close con-tact with these epithelial cells but, more often, seemed to be free of contact with surrounding tissues.

   All these features recall the structure of the normal mouse embryo yolk sac when this organ is hematopoietically active (i.e. : from day 7 to day 14 of

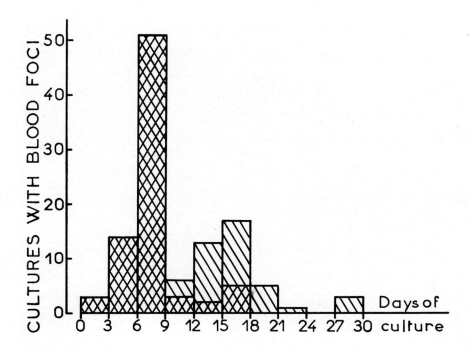

Fig. 2. Time of appearance of blood foci in organotypic cultures of PCC3/A/1 (data collected from one set of 90 cultures of each type). Only 50% of PO cultures ⬜ but 90% of SO cultures ⬛ differentiate blood islands. In addition, blood foci appear sooner in SO cultures than in PO cultures.

gestation). Nevertheless the blood cells of teratocarcinoma cultures were not located in the lumen of vessels, as is the case in the yolk sac, but in intercellular spaces of the upper part of organotypic cultures.

Smears were prepared from blood foci of these cultures and stained by benzidine and hematoxylin. Benzidine-positive cells were always nucleated, which, in addition to the above-described histological features, strongly suggests that they belong to the primitive generation of erythrocytes of the mouse embryo.

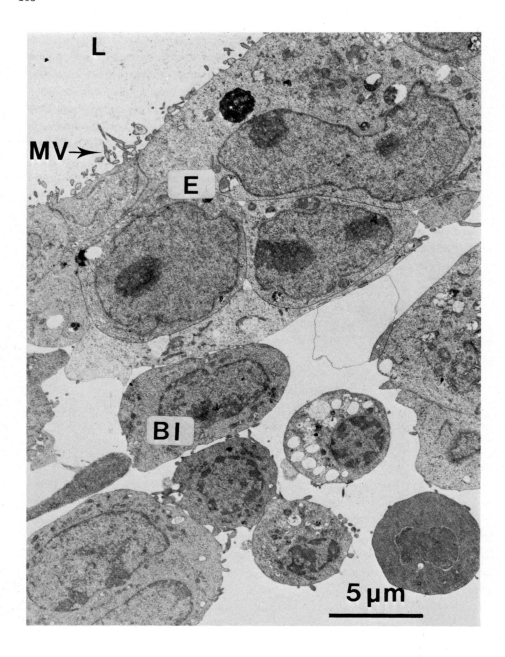

Fig. 3. Electron micrograph of a blood foci from SO culture of PCC$_3$/A/1. Blood island (BI) differentiates in the vicinity of hollow vesicles. (L : lumen of the vesicle ; E : endodermal-like epithelium ; MV : microvilli).

B - Biochemical analysis

Isoelectric focusing under native conditions is the most resolutive technique available to characterize the different types of hemoglobins (Hb) (for a review see[13]). In the mouse, it is known[2] that the adult Hb is composed of one major band accompanied by at least one minor band, whereas the embryonic form is made up of 3 major components. So far, the nomenclature of these various Hb has not been established and in this paper we will refer to their isoelectric point.

Blood samples contained usually between several hundred and a thousand red cells and represented only 10% of the total cell population harvested from the organotypic teratocarcinoma culture. We had therefore to devise a microelectrophoretic system allowing the specific detection of Hb. Our isoelectric focusing polyacrylamide gel electrophoresis technique described above is suitable for such a low cell number. The lower limit of detection corresponds to the material extracted from 100 cells.

Pseudo-peroxide activity of Hb was used as a specific method of detection, since the ^{59}Fe incorporation procedure was too drastic for stem cells in our *in vitro* system.

Figure 4 (centre) shows a typical electrophoregram of Hb prepared from teratocarcinoma organ culture blood cells. On either side are reference samples of Hb from adult 129 mouse peripheral red blood cells and from erythrocytes collected from 10-day-old 129 mouse embryos (This strain of mouse was chosen since PCC_3/A/1 teratocarcinoma line originated from it).

The focusing patterns of the two preparations are different. The major component of the adult Hb has an isoelectric point of 7.5 whereas the three major components of the embryonic Hb focus at pH 7.15, pH 7.70 and pH 8.05.

It appears that Hb prepared from teratocarcinoma organ culture blood cells comprises three major components which have the same isoelectric points as the embryonic Hb of the normal counterpart.

Other benzidine-positive bands may result from the presence in teratocarcinoma sample preparation of other peroxidases such as catalases and myoglobin. Further evidence that these benzidine-positive bands correspond to Hb was provided by the haptoglobin binding experiment. Haptoglobin is a serum protein known to bind with a very high affinity to Hb[9]. The complex can be detected by its peroxidase activity and focuses at pH 4 under native isoelectric focusing conditions.

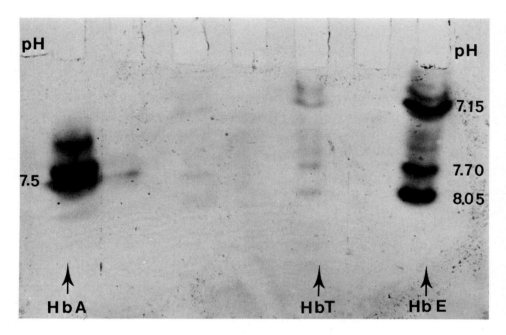

Fig. 4. Isoelectric focusing of hemoglobin synthesized by teratocarcinoma derived cells under organ culture conditions. Teratocarcinoma sample (HbT) was placed between adult 129/sv hemoglobin (HbA) and hemoglobin prepared from 10-day-old 129 embryos (HbE).
(Isoelectric focusing performed on polyacrylamide gel in the pH range 7-9. The actual size of the gel is 3 x 2 cm).

The gel presented on figure 5 clearly demonstrates that the addition of haptoglobin to a teratocarcinoma blood sample shifts the benzidine-positive activity to the acid side. No other peroxidase activity could be detected in the pH range 4-9, indicating that the only peroxidase-positive activity in the teratocarcinoma sample was due to Hb.

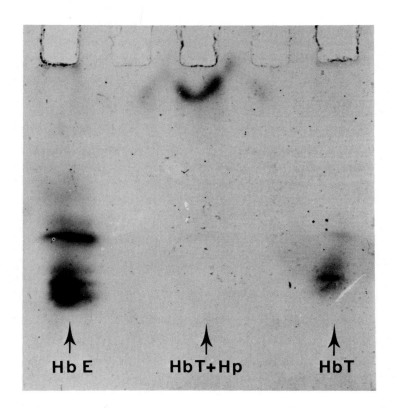

Fig. 5. Isoelectric focusing of teratocarcinoma hemoglobin before (HbT) and after treatment with haptoglobin (HbT + Hp) compared to an embryonic hemoglobin sample (HbE).
(Isoelectric focusing performed on polyacrylamide gel in the pH range 3-10).

DISCUSSION

Biochemical characterization of hemoglobin produced in organotypic terato-carcinoma cultures corroborates previous morphological observations and clearly demonstrates that conditions provided by the mass culture in contact with the atmosphere allow the differentiation of primitive erythrocytes from teratocar-cinoma $PCC_3/A/1$ line. In contrast, histiotypic immersed cell type cultures are unfavourable for such development, probably because both the tridimensional arrangement of cells and a high oxygenation of tissues are decisive factors for the differentiation of blood cells.

We have reported elsewhere[14] & Cudennec and Johnson, submitted for publica-tion) data indicating that blood foci contain, in addition to fully-differen-tiated cells, stem cells able to undergo further hemopoietic differentiation, and particularly into definitive-type erythrocytes. Therefore the conditions offered by the organotypic culture appear to be inadequate to allow expression of the full hemopoietic potentialities of teratocarcinoma stem cells.

Organotypically cultured teratocarcinoma, sensitive to extrinsic conditions, could become a useful model system to search for the factors involved in the differentiation of stem cells towards primitive and definitive erythrocytes of the mouse embryo. It may also shed some light on the mechanisms responsible for the switch from primitive to definitive erythropoiesis occurring in intra-embryonic sites by the 10th day of development.

ACKNOWLEDGEMENTS

This work was supported in part by a grant from the Fondation pour la Recherche Médicale Française and the Centre National de la Recherche Scientifique (ATP n° 3213).

We wish to thank Pr. Uli Schwartz and Dr. Robert Neukirchen (Max Planck Institute für Virusforschung, Tübingen, West Germany) for their help in setting up the microgel technique.

REFERENCES

1. Craig, M.L. and Russell, E.S. (1964) Devel. Biol. 10, 191-201.

2. Barker, J.E. (1968) Devel. Biol. 18, 14-29.

3. Gilman, J.G. and Smithies, O. (1968) Science, N.Y. 160, 885-886.

4. Fantoni, A., Bank, A. and Marks, P.A. (1967) Science, N.Y. 157, 1327-1329.

5. Graham, C.F. (1977) in : Concepts in mammalian embryogenesis. Ed. M.I. Sherman. MIT Press Cambridge, MA. pp. 315-394.

6. Cudennec, C.A. and Nicolas, J.F. (1977) J.Embryol.exp.Morph. 38,203-210.

7. Stevens, L.C. (1958) J. Nat. Cancer Inst. 20, 1257-1276.

8. Jakob, H., Boon, T., Gaillard, J., Nicolas, J.F. and Jacob, F. (1973) Ann. Immunol. (Institut Pasteur) 124B, 269-282.

9. Emes, A.V., Latner, A.L., Martin, J.A. and Mulligan, F. (1976) Biochim. Biophys. Acta, 420, 57-68.

10. Nicolas, J.F., Avner, P., Gaillard, J., Guénet, J.L., Jakob, H. and Jacob,F. (1976). Cancer Res. 36, 4224-4231.

11. Nicolas, J.F., Dubois, P., Jakob, H., Gaillard, J. and Jacob, F. (1975). Ann. Microbiol. (Institut Pasteur) 126A, 3-22.

12. Papaioannou, V.E., Gardner, R.L., McBurney, M.W., Babinet, C. and Evans, M.J. (1978). J. Embryol. exp. Morph. 44, 93-103.

13. Righetti, P.G. and Drysdale, J.W. (1976). Laboratory techniques in bioche-mistry and molecular biology. Vol. 5, part II Isoelectric focusing Ed. T.S. Work and E. Work, North-Holland Publishing Company, pp.337-590.

14. Cudennec, C.A. and Salaün, J. (1979). Cell Diff. 8, 75-82.

BLOOD FORMING CELL SYSTEM

Cell Lineage, Stem Cells and Cell Determination
INSERM Symposium No. 10
Editor: N. Le Douarin
© *1979 Elsevier/North-Holland Biomedical Press*

POTENTIALITIES AND MIGRATIONS OF HEMOPOIETIC STEM CELLS OF YOLK SAC AND INTRA-EMBRYONIC ORIGINS, STUDIED IN AVIAN CHIMERAS OBTAINED BY BLASTODERM RECOMBINATION.

FRANCOISE DIETERLEN-LIEVRE, DENISE BEAUPAIN and CLAUDE MARTIN.
Institut d'Embryologie du CNRS et du Collège de France, 49bis, Avenue de la Belle-Gabrielle, 94130 Nogent-sur-Marne (France).

INTRODUCTION

Hemopoietic stem cells (HSC) arise early in ontogeny and invade the rudiments of the various blood forming organs. There they constitute a permanent self replicating reserve and undergo diverging differentiation pathways depending on their microenvironment. When, where and how they become segregated, how they are conveyed to their differentiation site and retained there are still points of investigation. One fact is well documented : they arise outside the hemo-poietic organ anlagen, as demonstrated in mammals[1,2], birds[1-8] and amphibians[9-11]. According to Moore and Owen's hypothesis[12] all HSC originate from the yolk sac blood islands and are conveyed through the circulation to the embryo. We have been able to demonstrate since the existence of intraembryonic stem cells [13,14]. Thus a unique origin of HSC from the yolk sac is no longer a tenable hypothesis. This demonstration was made possible by an original experimental approach devised in the avian embryo[15]. It consists in tracing cell lineages in chimeras obtained by exchanging equivalent areas between two blastodiscs at early organogenesis stages. The foreign area is grafted *in ovo*, the composite blastodisc is allowed to resume development. Substitutions are chosen so that areas presumably responsible for the formation of stem cells are associated with regions containing prospective hemopoietic organs. Stem cell origin, movements and fate can be traced after further development if donor and host blastoderms bear appropriate markers, such as the quail-chick nuclear marker[16]. The data obtained so far concern unfolding of erythropoiesis and colonization of hemo-poietic organs in some types of chimeras[13,14,17-19].

We will present here the picture of HSC potentialities and migrations, which emerges from these previous studies and from the analysis of other unpublished combinations.

I. Design of chimeras

The different chimeric models are schematized in plate 1. The substituted area is grafted by simultaneously clipping off with small scissors the margins of the recombined areas.

In the figure 1 pattern, the prospective body region of a quail is grafted on a chick host blastoderm. This results in a quail embryo developing with a chick yolk sac ("yolk sac chimeras"). Grafting is made before circulation is established, that is before any cells are seen in the blood vessels. Figures 2 and 3 patterns yield "partial chimeras" in which the head and neck of quail are associated with the remainder of the body of a chick or alternatively the head, neck and wings of quail with the abdomen and legs of a chick. In both patterns, the yolk sac is chick.

The last pattern (figure 4) is termed a "supernumerary chimera". The quail embryo is grafted side by side with the chick embryo on the chick yolk sac. Presumably due to antagonist heart beats and difficulties in the establishment of vascular patterns, this type of chimera has low viability. Two pairs only were obtained, but they yield informative data.

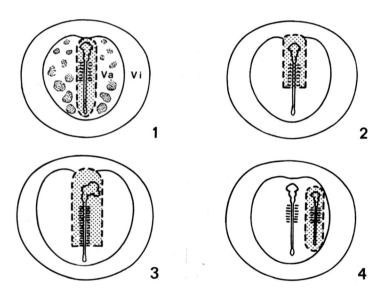

Figures 1 - 4 : Grafting schemes resulting in different types of chimeras. Quail areas (stippled) are grafted on chick blastoderms. Va : vascular area with blood islands ; Vi : vitelline area.
1. "Yolk sac chimera"
2. "Partial chimera". Grafted quail central area extends from head to somite 10.
3. "Partial chimera". Grafted quail area extends to somite 17.
4. "Supernumerary chimera".

II. <u>Demonstration of the existence of intraembryonic stem cells.</u>

The development of the hemopoietic system in the chick and quail embryos is fairly well known, having been the subject of abundant experimental research. Erythropoiesis has been described extensively in the chick, and the two species have often been used as models for the study of ontogeny of lymphopoietic organs. Moore and Owen were the first who showed a traffic of cells between the various hemopoietic compartments. Using the sex-chromosomal difference of the chick as a marker they found cell exchanges between hemopoietic organs of two partners parabiosed *in ovo* through vascular anastomosis[3]; they also demonstrated homing to the organs of cells of different origins injected into sublethally irradiated embryos[5]. They inferred that extrinsic HSC must seed the organ rudiments in order that they become hemopoietic. This was confirmed by experiments in the quail/chick system in which the timing of colonization of thymus and bursa of Fabricius was precisely assessed in the two species[6-8,20]. It was established by coelomic grafting of rudiments taken at different times of development that the thymus is colonized at a very early stage (5-6 days of incubation in the quail, 6-7 1/2 days in the chick) and that this first inflow is limited in time ; from 10 days onwards inflow of HSC is resumed at a slower rate. In the bursa, on the other hand, colonization begins around day 8 and is continuous, rather than sharply timed.

The bone marrow and spleen are also colonized by extrinsic stem cells, though the timing of colonization has been less precisely determined. This leaves the yolk sac as the only organ which possesses its own stem cells. The yolk sac is the earliest hemopoietic organ of amniote embryos and in birds it maintains that function for a major part of embryonic development. In the quail and chick, erythropoiesis begins there as early as the 2nd day of incubation. Hence the idea put forward by Moore and Owen that the yolk sac is the sole progenitor of all HSC.

This proposition was tested in quail-chick "yolk sac chimeras" (figure 1, 5 & 6). The origin and fate of cells were monitored in two different ways : the quail or chick nature of hemopoietic cells in different organs was analyzed by means of the nuclear marker ; the percentage of quail to chick erythrocytes in the blood was measured by an immunohemolysis technique. Briefly, mixed blood was hemolysed by rabbit antibodies directed against quail or chick erythrocytes. The ratio of released hemoglobin to hemoglobin liberated by total hemolysis is proportional to the ratio of red cells from the two species.

178

In the majority of these chimeras, composed of the body of a quail and the yolk sac of a chick, the thymus, bursa, and bone marrow were exclusively populated by quail hemopoietic cells. The spleen often harbored a mixture of chick and quail hemopoietic cells at 11-12 days of incubation ; at 13 days chick cells were usually absent. By virtue of the experimental design, the reticular framework of these different organs was always quail.

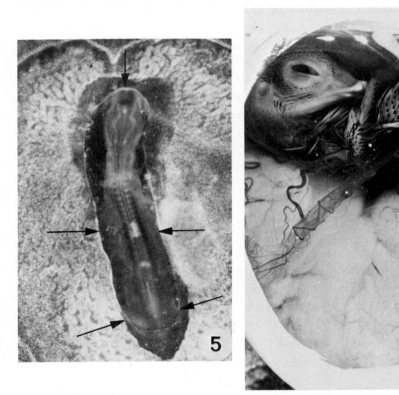

Figure 5 : A "yolk sac chimera" *in ovo* shortly after the operation. The white line (arrows) is the suture between quail and chick areas.(With permission of Cell Differentiation).

Figure 6 : After 11 more days of incubation, the graft (figure 5) has developed into a quail embryo (identified by its pigmented feathers) associated to a chick yolk sac. The chorio-allantois has been moved aside to allow full view of the embryo. The white shell of the chick egg is seen at the margin of the picture.

In the yolk sac on the contrary the endodermal and mesodermal cell framework was chick. Until 6 days of incubation, erythropoietic cells in the blood islands were chick also ; however from 7 days onwards, chick haemocytoblasts and erythroblasts were admixed or replaced by quail erythropoietic cells (figures 7-9). Thus in these heterospecific chimeras the embryonic body produced HSC which were capable of flooding the whole system. These intraembryonic HSC populated the intraembryonic organ rudiments in preference to HSC from the yolk sac and eventually migrated centrifugally to the yolk sac.

Data on the evolution of blood agree with these results (figure 10). Up to 6 days of incubation 95% or more of the erythrocytes were chick, i.e. they derived from yolk sac stem cells. From 7 days onwards the proportion of quail erythrocytes increased reaching a means of 42% at 13 days. It should be noted that the percentage of quail red cells was highly variable between chimeras. The reasons for these fluctuations will be considered in the next section. At the period of development studied, erythropoiesis is very active in the yolk sac, it begins in the spleen at 10-11 days and has not occurred yet in the bone marrow. Another probable erythropoietic site is the general mesoderm of the embryo, around the dorsal aorta, where hemopoietic foci have been described[21]. In all likeliness the quail erythrocytes found in the blood of the chimeras differentiated both in these intraembryonic foci and in the host yolk sac colonized by quail stem cells.

III. Respective potentialities of yolk sac and intraembryonic stem cells :
     Analysis of hemoglobins in erythrocytes of each derivation.

In the chimeric design used, red cells derived from yolk sac stem cells, i.e. chick, may be separated from red cells derived from intraembryonic stem cells, i.e. quail, by differential immune hemolysis (figures 11 & 12). Evolution of hemoglobin patterns was studied in these two populations. Normal ontogeny of chick erythrocytes has been studied many times (for a review see 22). In a first period (2-5 days of incubation) primitive erythrocytes are produced, characterized by two hemoglobin bands which may be separated by polyacrylamide gel electrophoresis, the so-called E and P + M in Ingram's terminology (cf. 22). After 5 days of incubation, the first definitive red cells formed have three new bands, A,D and H. The latter, a transitory Hb which disappears 1 month after hatching, co-migrates in this system with band E. Quail developmental patterns[19] have revealed very similar (figure 13). For the sake of comparison, the same terminology as that for chick bands has been used.

When the hemoglobins in the two red cell populations of chimeras were compared, they were found identical at 5 days (E and P + M bands) and 13 days (H, A and D bands) ; thus the small number of erythrocytes derived at 5 days from

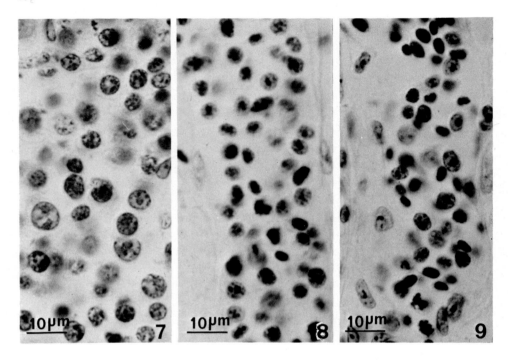

Figures 7 - 8 - 9 : Yolk sac blood islands. Feulgen-Rossenbeck staining.
7. Normal 7-day chick embryo. Large erythropoietic cell nuclei with faint heterochromatin masses.
8. Thirteen-day "yolk sac chimera". Erythropoietic cell nuclei are of quail type.(compare to nuclei in figures 7 and 9).
9. Normal 7-day quail. Small nuclei with heavy heterochromatin patches.

Figure 10 : Evolution of quail erythrocyte percentage with age of incubation in yolk sac chimeras.
%Q : number of quail red cells per 100 erythrocytes .
( ) : number of chimeras tested.
Bars; SE

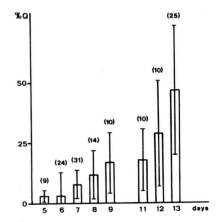

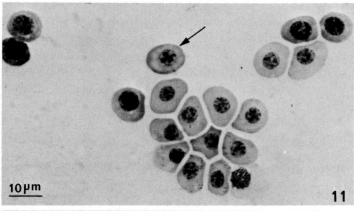

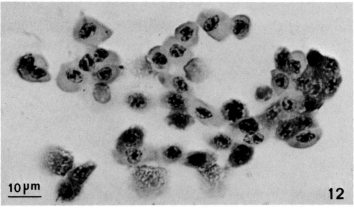

Figure 11 : Blood smear from a 6-day "yolk sac chimera".May-Grünwald-Giemsa staining. Most erythrocytes are chick. Arrow : one quail primitive erythrocyte. Figure 12 : Smear from the blood of the same embryo after immune hemolysis by anti-chick erythrocyte serum. Quail red cells are left, they are characterized by heavy chromatin patches. Some ghosts of chick erythrocytes are present. May-Grünwald-Giemsa staining.

intraembryonic stem cells (0-5 % of the total red cells), belonged to the primitive series ; the 3-band pattern found in the chick red cells at 13 days indicated further that yolk sac stem cells had given rise to some definitive erythrocytes, an occurrence demonstrated earlier by another experimental devise[23]. The quail 13-day pattern also reflected the presence of definitive erythrocytes.

By contrast at 7 days (figure 14), in the most frequent pattern, the two red cell populations appeared different : the chick erythrocytes (yolk sac stem cell derived) yielded 4 bands as in the control pattern, and thus comprised primitive and definitive red cells . The quail erythrocytes gave three bands only, A, D and presumably H. Thus early phase hemoglobins were no longer detectable, because the minute amount of primitive erythrocytes formed was negligible by comparison with the expanding definitive erythrocyte population.

These data lead to the following interpretation. Stem cells arise in the central part of the blastoderm, or presumptive embryonic body, as well as in

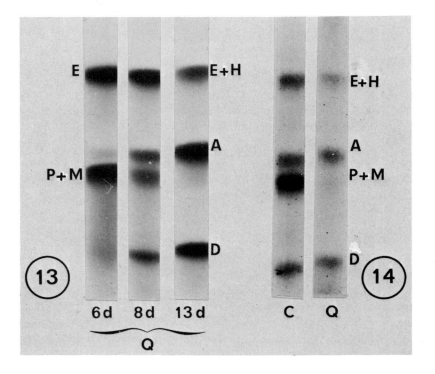

Figure 13 : Quail hemoglobin patterns during embryogenesis , analyzed by poly-acrylamide gel electrophoresis(Ref.19).For sake of comparison, the chick termi-nology has been used to designate the bands.

Fig. 14 : Comparison of hemoglobin patterns found in the quail (q) and chick (c) erythrocytes of a 7-day chimera.

the peripheral part, i.e. the presumptive yolk sac. Potentialities, as regards
erythropoiesis, are identical in the different regions,and commitment towards
the primitive or definitive red cell series appears to result from a time programme. However most primitive red cells are derived from peripheral (= yolk
sac) stem cells, whereas definitive cells derive mostly from central (= intraembryonic) stem cells. The distribution in the blastoderm of these two populations are schematized in figure 15. Whether all these stem cells become segregated from the mesoderm during a unique, early, event, or whether there are two
sequential waves of determination remains to be found. If the first instance
were true, commitment or dormancy of segregated stem cells in the different
regions of the blastoderm might result from the dissimilar nutritional conditions between yolk sac and embryo, at the beginning of development when vitelline nutrients are transferred through endodermal cells.

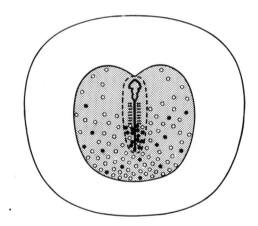

Figure 15 : Stem cell distribution
in the blastoderm. o : stem cells
which differentiate into primitive
erythrocytes; ● : stem cells which
differentiate into definitive
erytrocytes.

In figure 15 , no stem cells have been represented in the anterior most
region of the blastoderm, to take into account two facts. The first is that,in
the young blastoderm,blood islands occupy a posterior horse-shoe shaped area
and are absent in the anterior area. The second relates to the peculiar patterns
of thymic colonization found in partial chimeras (see section IV).
    One last point will be considered. In yolk sac chimeras, the replacement of
chick by quail erythrocytes is irregular. Since stem cells from central and

peripheral regions appear to have similar potentialities and since the total
quantity of red cells at a given stage of development must be regulated, it is
clear that small differences in timing of differentiation of the two components
of the graft may result in large fluctuations. Differences in growth potential
of the two species probably also bias the results, in a manner impossible to
foresee. The main conclusion from the yolk-sac chimera study is the existence
of intraembryonic stem cells and the prevalence of these over yolk sac stem cells
in the second phase of avian embryo hemopoiesis.

The analysis of chick-chick chimeras has confirmed quail-chick results. These
chimeras were constructed on the same model, an embryo being grafted on a foreign yolk-sac. The two components were from the same histocompatible chick line
and differed either by their genetic sex, or by their prospective immunoglobulin
G allotype. These embryos were able to hatch and could be raised until adulthood. The analysis of sex chromosome assortments after specific mitogen stimulation of T or B lymphocytes and the determination of the IgG allotype showed
that lymphoid cells were always descended from intraembryonic precursors[24-26].

IV. Regionalization of hemopoietic cell populations in "partial" chimeras.

In this pattern (figures 2, 3 & 16) only the anterior part of the area pellucida of a quail was grafted on a chick blastoderm. The constitution of the
thymus appeared strictly determined by the level of the suture. When the quail
contribution extended to the level of   somite 10, yielding embryos with
head and neck of quail on the thorax of chick, the thymus reticular cells were
quail and the lymphoid cells were chick (figure 17). When the quail also contributed the wings (suture at somite 17 level), the thymus was entirely quail
(figure 18). Thus some tissues at the wing level introduced stem cells, which
migrated cephalad towards the thymic epithelial rudiment. On the other hand,
in both combinations, the spleen and bursa,entirely located in chick regions,
had chick somatic and hemopoietic cells.

These partial chimeras thus possess several rather remarkable features :
- 1) no stem cells seem to be formed from the mesoderm of the head and neck
presumptive regions ; - 2)introducing the area pellucida between somites 10 and
17 results in changing the thymic lymphoid population - 3) some partial chimeras have different hemopoietic cell populations in their different organs.

Thus it appears that organ rudiments are colonized by stem cells arising
from neighbouring tissues. Closely similar patterns of colonization have been
observed in amphibian chimeras in which a diploid anterior half had been combined to a triploid posterior half[27]. In our opinion, these findings suggest that
stem cell colonization proceeds essentially through short range migrations,

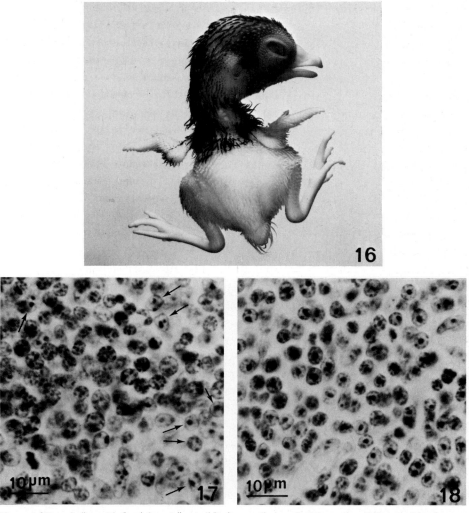

Figure 16 : A "partial chimera" at 13 days of incubation. In this particular specimen, quail feathers extend on the thorax below the wing level, but are scarce on the wings. Suture was made below the 12th somite.

Figure 17 : Thymus of a 13-day quail"head-neck chimera".Reticular cells are quail (arrows). Lymphoid cells are chick.

Figure 18 : Thymus of a 13-day quail"head-neck-wings chimera".All cells are quail.

either through an interstitial pathway or through strictly local vascular connections.

This does not exclude the possibility that dissemination of stem cells also occurs through the blood, especially at later stages of development. Indeed the last type of chimera which will be described here displays evidence for both migration routes.

V. Migrations of hemopoietic cells in "supernumerary" chimeras.

The quail partner in this model (figure 4) was reduced to the body of the embryo while the chick body and whole yolk sac were present. The scheme clearly reveals that the quail has a developmental advantage, due to which its hemopoietic cells invade the chick embryo. In the two pairs which were obtained and sacrificed at 10 days of incubation the hemopoietic organs in the quail embryo were entirely composed of quail cells. By contrast in the chick thymus, among a dominant chick prelymphoid population, there was a substantial minority of quail prelymphoid cells (figure 19).

Bursa and spleen were not chimeric. It should be stressed that only the thymus at that stage has already received a sizeable batch of stem cells while bursa and spleen are only partly colonized.

By virtue of the experimental scheme, the only connections between the two embryos were vascular ; any quail cells present in the chick could only have migrated in the blood and necessarily belonged to the hemopoietic system.

The different models of chimeras provide evidence for two possible routes of stem cell dissemination. One is the circulatory pathway followed in yolk sac chimeras by cells from the embryo settling in the yolk sac blood islands, or in supernumerary chimeras by cells from the quail invading the chick. The existence of this "blood-borne" traffic has been demonstrated earlier by Moore and Owen in parabiosed chick embryos[3]. The other is a strictly local migration pathway, operational in the case of partial chimeras. As a hypothesis we propose that it occurs through the general mesoderm or/and through lymphatic vessels.

In the supernumerary chimeras hemopoietic cells may actually be visualized in both situations. Quail cells were found in tightly packed groups in several small vessels in the neighbourhood of the bursa . In the vicinity of the thymus on the other hand clusters of quail cells were seen in the mesoderm, next to clusters of chick cells . Cells of the two species always appeared in separate groups, an observation suggesting that they may be clones.

We interpret these observations as meaning that the two pathways are possible and that their occurrence depends on the stage of development and timing of

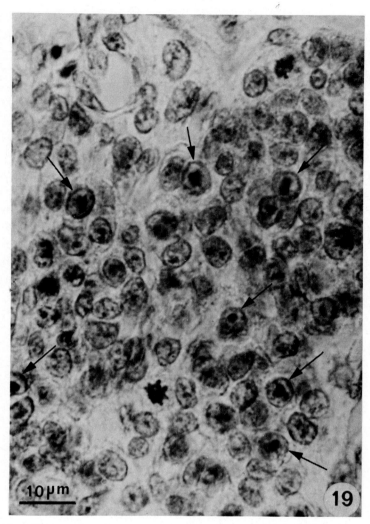

Figure 19 : Thymus of a 10-day chick embryo in a "supernumerary association".
Chimeric lymphoid population. Arrows : quail prelympoid cells. Feulgen-
Rossenbeck staining.

colonization of the rudiments. Indeed they may occur concomitantly, in which
case cells travel in the blood, then probably divide in the general mesoderm before they enter the organ rudiments.

CONCLUSION

The existence of hemopoietic stem cells arising within the embryo proper is demonstrated by several lines of evidence in different models of chimeras composed of complementary parts of chick and quail blastoderms. Despite the totipotency of yolk sac stem cells[17,28], intraembryonic stem cells colonize prevalently the organ rudiments. The results could be influenced by the differences in developmental rythm between the two species. However they have been confirmed in a chick-chick system. Migration of stem cells between the different hemopoietic compartments of the embryo is interpreted as occurring either through an interstitial or a circulatory pathway. The first is probably functional at the early stages of development of the hemopoietic system and becomes later associated with or replaced by the second. The developing hemopoietic system evinces considerable pliability. Several categories of stem cells with comparable potentialities can be found and several mechanisms of migration seem to exist. It is hoped that the events normally occurring during the ontogeny of the hemopoietic system will ultimately be understood through the analysis of monospecific chimeras distinguishable by appropriate markers.

REFERENCES

1. Moore, M.A.S. and Owen, J.J.T. (1967) J. exp. Med., 126, 715-725.
2. Owen, J.J.T. and Ritter, M.A. (1969) J. exp. Med., 129, 431-442.
3. Moore, M.A.S. and Owen, J.J.T. (1965) Nature, 208, 956-990.
4. Moore, M.A.S. and Owen, J.J.T. (1966) Dev. Biol., 14, 40-51.
5. Moore, M.A.S. and Owen, J.J.T. (1967) Nature, 215, 1081-1082.
6. Le Douarin, N. and Jotereau, F. (1973) Nature, N.B. 246, 25-27.
7. Le Douarin, N. and Jotereau, F. (1975) J. exp. Med., 142, 17-40.
8. Le Douarin, N., Houssaint, E., Jotereau,F. and Belo, M. (1975). Proc. Nat. Acad. Sc., 72, 2701-2705.
9. Hollyfield, J.G. (1966) Dev. Biol. 14, 461-480.
10. Deparis, P. et Jaylet, A. (1976). Am. Immunol. Inst. Pasteur, 127C, 827-831.
11. Tochinai, S. (1978). Dev. Comp. Immunol. 2, 627-636.
12. Moore, M.A.S. and Owen, J.J.T. (1967) Lancet II, 658-659.
13. Dieterlen-Lièvre, F. (1975). J. Embryol. exp. Morphol. 33, 607-619.
14. Dieterlen-Lièvre, F., Beaupain, D. and Martin, C. (1976). Ann. Immunol., 127C, 857-863.
15. Martin, C. (1972). C. R. Soc. Biol., 166, 283-285.
16. Le Douarin, N. (1969). Bull. Biol. Fr. Belg., 103, 435-452.
17. Martin, C., Beaupain, D. and Dieterlen-Lièvre, F. (1978). Cell Differentiation, 7, 115-130.
18. Dieterlen-Lièvre, F., Martin, C. and Beaupain, D. (1977). Folia biologica, 23, 373-375.
19. Beaupain, D., Martin, C. and Dieterlen-Lièvre, F. (1979). Blood, 53, 212-225.
20. Le Douarin, N. (1976) in Phylogeny of Thymus and Bone marrow- Bursa cells. R.K. Wright and E.L. Cooper, eds. Elsevier/North Holland Biomedical Press, Amsterdam, pp. 217-226.
21. Dantschakoff, V. (1908). Anat. Hefte, 37, 471-589.
22. Bruns, G.A.P. and Ingram, V. (1973). Philos. Trans. R. Soc. London B 266, 225-305.
23. Hagopian, H.K. and Ingram, V. (1971). J. Cell Biol., 51, 440-451.
24. Martin, C., Dieterlen-Lièvre, F., Lassila, O. and Toivanen, P. (1977) Folia biologica, 23, 371-372.
25. Lassila, O., Eskola, J., Toivanen, P., Martin, C. and Dieterlen-Lièvre, F. (1978). Nature, 272, 353-354.
26. Lassila, O., Martin, C., Dieterlen-Lièvre, F., Nurmi, T. E.I., Eskola, J. and Toivanen, P. (1979) Transpl. Proc. XI, 1085-1088.
27. Volpe, E.P. and Turpen, J.B. (1975). Science 190, 1101-1103.
28. Jotereau, F.V. and Houssaint, E. (1977) In Developmental Immunobiology. J.B. Solomon and J.D. Horton (Eds.) Amsterdam-New-York-Oxford, North-Holland Biomedical Press, pp. 123-130.

Cell Lineage, Stem Cells and Cell Determination
INSERM Symposium No. 10
Editor: N. Le Douarin
© 1979 Elsevier/North-Holland Biomedical Press

GRANULO-MONOCYTE COLONY FORMING CELLS FROM BONE MARROW, BLOOD, CORD
BLOOD AND FOETAL LIVER IN NORMAL MAN

CATHERINE DRESCH, ANNICK FAILLE
Institut de Recherches sur les Maladies du Sang, Formation INSERM
n° 4, Hôpital Saint-Louis, 75010 Paris (France)

INTRODUCTION

The distribution of granulo-monocytic colony-forming cells
(C.F.C.) differs in adult and foetus as differs the distribution
of hemopoietic tissue. However these C.F.C are also in different
kinetic states and seem different in their self replicating possibilities.

MATERIALS AND METHODS

Culture conditions. All cultures were done in semi solid agar.
Mononuclear cells were separated on lymphoprep (D = 1.077 g/cm^3)
and were cultured in Mac Coy's medium with 15 % Fetal Calf Serum
in 0.3 % agar. Colony formation was stimulated by either the use
of 0.5 % agar underlayers containing 10^6 peripheral blood cells
from normal donors or the addition of 10 % PHA-stimulated leukocyte conditioned medium (C.M.). Cultures were incubated at 37°C
in 100 % relative humidity in an atmosphere of 7.5 % CO_2 in air.

Counting of colonies and clusters. Colonies were counted with
a dissecting microscope. Aggregates of more than 50 cells were
scored as colonies, 5 to 50 cells were termed clusters.

Specimens. Normal adult bone marrow was taken out of bone
fragments from hematologically normal patients undergoing ortho-
pedic surgery. Cord blood was taken immediately after the accou-
chemant from the placenta cord. 13 to 22 weeks foetuses were
results of spontaneous abortion. Liver was sliced finely and
ground ; cells were filtered through a gauze tissue and mononuclear cells were separated on lymphoprep.

RESULTS

The concentration of C.F.C for 2.10^5 mononuclear cells in 14
days cultures is shown in Table 1 with the percentage of cells

out of S phase as estimated by Hydroxyurea suicide (ratio of hydroxyurea treated specimen colonies on control specimen colonies).

Specimen		C.F.C.	S / T
Adult bone	colonies	64 + 41	.60 + 0.21
marrow	col + cl	222 + 111	.78 + 0.16
Adult blood	colonies	8 + 12	.92
	col + cl	17 + 18	.85
	colonies	25 + 14	0.35 + 0.24
Cord blood	col + cl	41 + 25	0 .49 + 0.25
	colonies	236	0.56
Foetal liver	col + cl	261	0.56

From these data, two facts are dominant on a kinetic point of vue. First a
large number of clusters are found in adult bone marrow culture and nearly no
cluster forming cells are found in foetal liver, adult and cord blood cultures
giving an intermediate picture. Second a high rate of suicide is found in
C.F.C from adult bone marrow, cord blood and foetal liver, but most adult
blood C.F.C are not in S phase.

However the suicide level of C.F.C varied with the date of the development
of the colonies and the cytological type of the colonies, as already known for
adult bone marrow (1). In cord blood, as shown in fig. 1 and 2, early developing C.F.C giving rise to neutrophil colonies were more in S phase than late
developing C.F.C which gave rise to eosinophil and macrophage colonies. On the
other hand suicide level remained in the same range in three weeks cultures of
foetal liver cells.

There was no correlation between the number of mixed G.M. colonies and the
suicide rate ; mixed colonies were very seldom seen in adult bone marrow, and
represented 4 % of colonies in adult blood with a maximum in 21 days cultures.
They were much more numerous in cord blood and foetus liver. 16 % of colonies
were mixed in cord blood (neutrophils and macrophages in 12 % and / or eosinophils in 4 %), and 18 % in foetus liver (neutrophils and macrophages) in 10
and 14 days cultures.

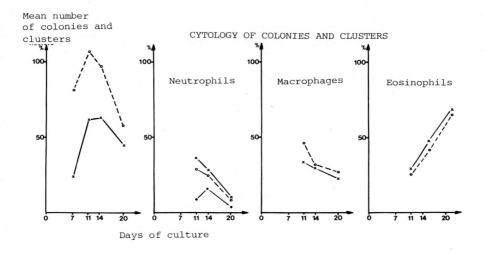

Fig. 1. Evolution of colonies and clusters in cord blood cultures (same symbols as in Fig. 2)

The repartition of C.F.C in hematopoïetic organs from 15 to 22 weeks foe-tures is shown in table II.

TABLE II

MEAN NUMBER OF C.F.C FOR 2.10^5 MONONUCLEAR CELLS SEEDED

Foetus age (number studied)	Liver			Spleen			Bone marrow		
	col.		clusters	col.		clusters	col.		clusters
3 months (2)	270	–	50	5	–	35	150	–	70
4 months (1)	620	–	200	3	–	45	124	–	300
5 months (1)	300	–	150	25	–	24	180	–	90

these preliminary studies seem to show a peak of C.F.C in liver between 16 and 18 weeks, and an earlier hematopoïesis than usually thought in bone mar-row. No colonies were found in the thymus, in our culture conditions.

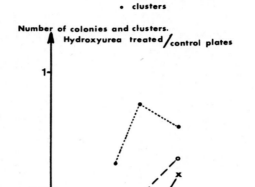

Fig. 2. Evolution of suicide rate in cord blood cultures

<u>Heterogeneity of G.M.-C.F.C.</u> We have already shown with others the hetero-
geneity of G.M - C.F.C in adult human bone marrow (2). At least two subpopulations of C.F.C can be separated by velocity sedimentation (Fig. 2): large cells
(sedimenting between 7 and 12 mm/hr), with a high suicide rate, develop small
granulocyte and monocyte colonies during the first week of culture; smaller
cells (sedimenting between 3 and 6 mm/hr), with a low suicide rate, develop larger colonies of granulocytes, monocytes and eosinophils between two and three
weeks of culture.

Adult blood cell velocity sedimentation (Fig. 3) shows two peaks of C.F.C,
a major one in the fraction sedimenting at 4-5 mm/hr and a minor one in the
fractions sedimenting between 7-8 mm/hr.

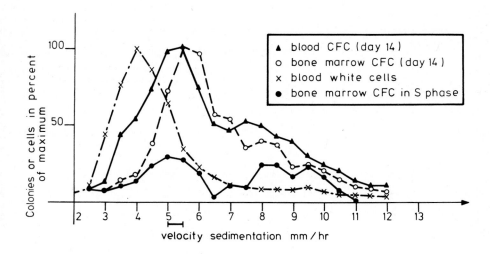

Fig. 3. Velocity sedimentation of adult blood and bone marrow C.F.C

These two peaks correspond approximatively to the cells in G 1 of the two peaks of adult bone marrow C.F.C (3)

Cord blood mononuclear cells sedimentation shows only one peak of C.F.C. between 5 and 6 mm/hr. Foetal liver mononuclear cells sedimentation shows a more complex distribution of C.F.C., according to cell size: In 4 and 5 month old foetuses two studies showed two peaks of C.F.C. at 4 mm/hr and 9-10 mm/hr; in a 3 month old foetus the maximum of C.F.C. was found in the fraction of cells sedimenting at 12 mm/hr, but a high level of colony formation was found in all the fractions of cells sedimenting between 5 and 11 mm/hr. Fig. 4 shows the results of these three studies compared with the profile of cord blood C.F.C.

Multiple colonies (like bursts in the erythropoïetic line) were found in a high proportion (between 30 and 60 % of all colonies) in 3 month old foetus liver, in cultures of cell fractions sedimenting between 4 and 6 mm/hr. Few burst erythroïd colonies were found in 14 days cultures with erythropoïetin in these same fractions, but none in cultures without erythropoïetin.

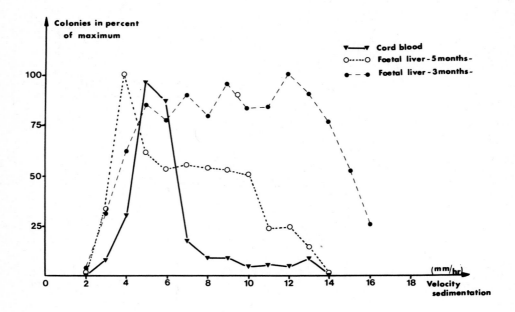

Fig. 4. Velocity sedimentation profile of cord blood, 4-5 months and 3 month old foetus liver C.F.C.

DISCUSSION

Hematopoïesis in human foetus has been studied essentially by anatomical and cytological techniques. Liver hematopoïesis is said to begin at 7-8 weeks (4 - 5 - 6) even for some 4-5 weeks after ovulation (7). Most authors insist on the predominance of erythropoïesis in liver hematopoïesis (4 - 6 - 8), with granulopoïesis essentially in spleen and bone marrow from 12 weeks onwards. Thomas and Yoffey even consider that haemopoïesis in the liver of human foetus is exclusively erythropoïetic (5 - 9). The distribution of G.M.-C.F.C. seems to be at variance with these facts. We found a high concentration of G.M. - C.F.C in liver from 3 month onwards with a maximum at 4 month, very few C.F.C in spleen and a high percentage in bone marrow. But liver volume in 3 and 4 month foetus is much more important than that of bone marrow and the repartition of C.F.C. seems to be predominantly in liver before 5

month of gestation. This discrepancy could suggest that liver environmental
conditions "in vivo" promote erythropoïetic differentiation and that our conditions "in vitro" promote granulopoïetic differentiation, although erythropoïetin adjunction to the agar culture or methyl-cellulose culture produced
some erythropoïesis but never predominant. This raises the problem of a common progenitor cell for erythropoïesis and myelopoïesis in human foetus, the
differentiation of which is controled by different stimulus or environmental
conditions, as suggested by Fukuda (7) or the existence of two different progenitor cells in liver and bone marrow as suggested by Thomas (9).

We found a mean concentration of G.M. - C.F.C. in cord blood much lower
than that found by others (10 - 11), different probably because of conditions
of collections and culture. However all authors found a very large range of
results. No data have been published about the suicide rate of cord blood
C.F.C., which seems to be comparable to that of adult bone marrow. Our data
on the number of circulating C.F.C. and suicide rate in adult blood are in
agreement with those of Tebbi (12).

Velocity sedimentation of G.M. - C.F.C. In different hemopoïetic organs
shows three major peaks of cell size. The more interesting one is at 4 - 6
mm/hr. It is the only peak of cord blood C.F.C., the major one for adult
blood and late developing C.F.C of adult bone marrow, the major one for 4 - 5
month liver C.F.C. These cells, either in cycle or out of cycle, have a high
multiplication potential (giving rise to multiple (G.M. colonies in liver or
large colonies in blood and bone marrow). Their sedimentation rate corresponds
to cells $\leqslant$ 10 μm in diameter and to the peak of mixed erythroïd-granulocytic
colonies found by Fauser in adult blood (13). These C.F.C. could be either
pluripotential progenitors the differentiation of which depends on different
stimulus or environmental conditions, and/or the committed daugters of this
cell, which remains hypothetical in man. Our data and those of Fauser (13)
seem to imply that both pluripotent and committed progenitors are found in
this cell population. During the haemopoïesis development these cells are
highly proliferative in foetal liver, and cord blood. In adult their proliferative rate decreases in bone marrow and only out of cycle or G 1 phase cells
circulate from bone marrow to blood.

The second peak of G.M. - C.F.C., sedimenting between 7 and 11 mm/hr is not
found in cord blood and is of minor importance in adult blood. It is the
major peak for early developing C.F.C. in adult bone marrow and an important
part of the total C.F.C. in foetal liver. These cells have a high suicide
rate, but lower self replicating possibilities than the first peak cells.

The third peak of very large C.F.C., sedimenting between 11 and 16 mm/hr, characterizes very early granulopoïesis and is found only in 2 to 3 month foetal liver cells.

The study of the characteristics of foetal granulopoïesis seems to indicate some research openings in pathological granulopoïesis. For exemple it is interesting to note that C.F.C. of myelomonocytic leukemia have the same sedimentation profile and the same suicide rate as cord blood.

REFERENCES

1. Dresch, C. et al. (1979) Expl. Hematol., to be published

2. Johnson, .G.R. et al. (1977) Blood, 50, 823-832

3. Dresch, C. and Faille A. (1978) Expl. Hematol., 6, suppl. 3, 80

4. Wintrobe, M.M. (1967) Clinical Hematology, Lea and Febiger, Philadelphia
   pp 2-5

5. Thomas, D.B. and Yoffey, J.M. (1964) Brit. J. Haemat., 10, 193-201

6. Enzan, H. and Kawakami, M. (1978) Acta Haem. Jap., 41, 1214-1230

7. Fukuda, T. (1978) Acta Haem. Jap., 41, 1204-1213

8. Oguro, M. et al. (1978) Acta Haem. Jap., 41, 1231-1241

9. Thomas, D.B. et al. (1960) Nature, 187, 876-877

10.Knudtzon, S. (1974) Blood, 43, 357-361

11.Prindull, G. et al. (1978) Acta Paediatr. Scand., 67, 413-416

12.Tebbi, K. et al. (1976) Blood, 48, 235-243

13.Fauser, A.A. and Messner, H.A. (1978) Blood, 52, 1243-1248

Cell Lineage, Stem Cells and Cell Determination
INSERM Symposium No. 10
Editor: N. Le Douarin
© *1979 Elsevier/North-Holland Biomedical Press*

THE COMMITMENT OF MULTIPOTENTIAL HEMOPOIETIC STEM CELLS: STUDIES IN VIVO AND
IN VITRO

G. R. JOHNSON AND D. METCALF
Cancer Research Unit, Walter and Eliza Hall Institute of Medical Research,
P.O. Royal Melbourne Hospital, 3050, Victoria, Australia.

INTRODUCTION

The hemopoietic system in mammals is a clonal system. Thus in mice and
humans, where the most extensive analyses have been performed, it is generally
accepted that all of the morphologically-recognizable cells can ultimately be
derived from a single multipotential stem cell. Most of the mature hemopoietic cells can be recognized morphologically and their relative position in the
differentiation sequence can be visualized directly. The detection of immature hemopoietic cells has depended on the development of clonal assays which
allow normal hemopoietic differentiation and maturation to occur. Multipotential hemopoietic stem cells (HSC) are detected by their ability to give rise to
clones of mature progeny in pre-irradiated spleens (the HSC that initiates the
spleen colony being defined as a CFU-S, colony-forming unit spleen)[1]. A second class of hemopoietic cells can be detected by their ability to produce
clones of mature hemopoietic cells in vitro. Since these in vitro clones
usually contain differentiated cells of a single hemopoietic lineage, the cells
giving rise to these clones are believed to be already committed to one line of
hemopoietic differentiation. The proliferation and differentiation of these
committed hemopoietic cells (progenitor cells) and their progeny are dependent
on specific regulatory hormones, several of which have been purified and their
mode of action extensively characterized[2,3,4].

Although the control of progenitor cells is beginning to be understood, the
factors controlling the differentiation of HSC into committed progenitor cells
remain unknown. Two theories have been proposed for the differentiation of
HSC into single lines of hemopoietic development based upon observation of the
growth and differentiation of CFU-S-derived spleen colonies. When it was
observed that colonies differed greatly from each other in their content of
differentiated cells and of new CFU-S, it seemed logical to conclude that the
single cell of origin was a pluripotent stem cell and that a variable proportion of its progeny differentiated early and randomly into each of several

hemopoietic cell lines[5,6]. This "stochastic" theory of hemopoiesis has produced a model in which HSC differentiation to erythroid or granulocytic cell lines is a random event, the model fitting published experimental results[7].

The second major theory on the commitment of CFU-S to determined progeny is based upon the observation that the majority of spleen colonies contain differentiated erythroid cells during the early growth phase and later acquire cells of a second line of differentiation, usually at the periphery. Although morphologically "pure" erythroid colonies are in the majority at the earliest time after hemopoietic cell transplantation, a smaller but fixed proportion of CFU-S-derived splenic colonies are morphologically defined as "pure" granulocytic. Because of the distinctive and different distributions in the spleen of these two colony types, it has been proposed that these differences occur due to the presence of distinct hemopoietic inductive microenvironments (HIM)[8,9]. The commitment of CFU-S that lodge in these microenvironments is then due to the inductive influence of radioresistant non-hemopoietic microenvironmental cells[9].

The HIM theory was developed from observations on morphologically-recognizable cells within spleen colonies although these cells are not the immediate progeny of the multipotential stem cell. The validity of assuming that only a single line of differentiation is occurring within a CFU-S-derived spleen colony, based upon morphological criteria, has been seriously challenged by in vitro progenitor cell assays of morphologically "pure" erythroid spleen colonies[10,11,12]. These studies have shown that committed progenitor cells of the granulocyte-macrophage lineage (GM-CFC) can be present in such erythroid colonies. Analysis of individual spleen colonies, although unable to resolve the problem of what controls the commitment of CFU-S to a single line of hemopoietic differentiation, has provided information on the relationships between CFU-S and the various progenitor cells[13,14].

The present communication describes the results of experiments designed to test the microenvironmental theory of hemopoietic commitment using in vivo and in vitro assays that detect the clonal progeny of HSC. The in vivo data has been obtained from the analysis of individual spleen colonies. The in vitro analysis has been performed with a recently described clonal assay for members of the hemopoietic multipotential stem cell compartment[15,16,17]. In the presence of media conditioned by pokeweed mitogen-stimulated spleen cell conditioned media it is possible to stimulate the formation of colonies containing differentiated erythroid, neutrophilic, eosinophilic, macrophage and megakaryocytic cells[15,16]. In addition to differentiated progeny these mixed-erythroid colonies also contain CFU-S and committed progenitor cells[17].

MATERIALS AND METHODS

Analysis of Individual Spleen Colonies.   C57BL/6J mice maintained under
conventional conditions in this Institute were irradiated with X-rays (total
750 rads, with a Phillips RT 250 Unit operating at 250 kV 15 mA: HVL was 0.8
mm^{Cu} at a focal distance of 50 cm with full back scatter conditions used at a
dose rate of 127 rads/min).   Within 2 hours of irradiation individual mice
were transplanted with 75,000 syngeneic bone marrow cells by intravenous injection.   Twelve days later mice were killed by cervical dislocation and their
spleens removed and placed in Eisen's balanced salt solution.   All spleen colonies visible at X 20 magnifications with indirect lighting and an Olympus (SZ)
dissection microscope were dissected free of surrounding splenic tissue using
cataract knives, 10 - 12 individual colonies being obtained from each spleen.
Dispersed cell suspensions of individual colonies were produced by aspiration
through needles of decreasing bore size.   The total and viable cell content
of each colony was determined by hemocytometer counts and eosin dye exclusion.
Where possible, four replicate cultures each of 5×10^4 cells were established
to determine the number of granulocyte-macrophage colony-forming cells (GM-CFC)
present in each suspension.   The remaining cells were spun in a cytocentrifuge
(Shandon Cytospin) air-dried, stained with May-Grunewald Giemsa, and differential cell counts determined at X 1200 magnifications on 500 cells.   Correlation coefficients on total cells, total erythroid cells, total granulocytic
cells and total GM-CFC per spleen colony were calculated using a Hewlett-Packard
HP-25 calculator using the program outlined in the Applications Programs booklet
supplied.   Tests for significance were performed using the Students t test.

In Vitro Cultures for GM-CFC and Multipotential Cells (Mixed Erythroid
Colony-Forming Cells).   The isolation and culture of hemopoietic cells has been
described extensively previously[2,15,16].   Briefly, cells to be assayed were
cultured in 35 mm petri dishes to which was added an equal part mixture of 0.6%
agar and double strength Dulbecco's Modified Eagle's Medium containing either
40% fetal calf serum or human plasma (1 ml), which after gelling, was placed in
a fully humidified 37°C incubator containing 10% CO_2 in air.   Cultures were
scored after seven days.   Stimulation of granulocyte-macrophage colony-forming
cells (GM-CFC) was provided by the addition of 0.1 ml of partially purified
(Stage II) GM-CSF from mouse lung conditioned medium[3] to each 1 ml culture.
Stimulation of multipotential colony formation was obtained by the addition of
0.2 ml of pokeweed mitogen-stimulated spleen cell conditioned medium (SCM) to
each culture[18].

Buoyant Density Separation.   Separation of fetal CBA peripheral blood cells into 20 fractions on the basis of buoyant density was accomplished by centrifugation of the cells to equilibrium (4000g; 30 minutes; 4^0) in a continuous gradient of bovine serum albumin (BSA), pH 5.1, isosmotic with mouse serum. Density measurements were made on each fraction using the method described by Shortman[19].   All distribution profiles were expressed as cells per density increment, plotted against fraction density, to provide a true density distribution profile, and to correct for any small deviations of the gradient from linearity.

Density Cut Separation.   Cells were suspended in 1 ml BSA, (pH 5.1, density 1.064 g/cm^3, isosmotic with normal mouse serum) then layered over 1 ml of albumin of the same density.   One ml of phosphate buffered saline was added above the albumin and the interfaces mixed.   The tube was then centrifuged at 3500 g for 15 minutes.   Cells of density equal to or lighter than 1.064 g/cm^3 remained in suspension and denser cells formed a pellet.   Supernatant and pelleted cells were harvested separately, washed and viable cell counts performed. These cells were then cultured, differential cell counts were determined on May-Grunewald Giemsa stained smears of the remaining cells.

RESULTS

Analysis of Different Cell Parameters in Spleen Colonies.   Individual 12 day spleen colonies were dissected out and the total cellularity (N), total morphologically-recognizable erythroid (E) and neutrophilic (G) cells, and total GM-CFC content of each colony were determined.   In total, 81 colonies were analysed.   As reported by others, extreme variability was noted for all the parameters measured.   Mean colony size was found to be 5.83 x 10^6 with the range in colony size varying from 0.12 x 10^6 to 34.2 x 10^6.   Nine of the 81 colonies contained more than 90% erythroid cells; no colonies were found with more than 90% neutrophils and only 2 of the 81 had more than 80% morphologically-recognizable neutrophilic cells.   GM-CFC were detected in 58 of the colonies and within positive colonies the calculated total number of GM-CFC per colony varied from 20 to 13,653 with a mean of 1998.   Correlation coefficients were determined upon the numbers of each cell type assayed.   These values for pairs of parameters are shown in Table 1.

TABLE 1

CORRELATION COEFFICIENTS BETWEEN PAIRS OF DIFFERENT CELL TYPES FOUND IN SPLEEN
COLONIES

Pair No.	Cell Parameters[+]	Correlation Coefficient (r)	Significance* P> 0.95	P>0.99
1	GM-CFC:N	0.28	Yes	Yes
2	GM-CFC:G	0.37	Yes	Yes
3	GM-CFC:E	0.23	Yes	No
4	G:N	0.58	Yes	Yes
5	E:N	0.99	Yes	Yes
6	G:E	-0.003	No	No

* Calculated assuming data represent a normal distribution.
+ GM-CFC, total number of granulocyte-macrophage colony-forming cells per
  spleen colony; N, total number of cells per spleen colony; G, total number of neutrophils per spleen colony; E, total number of erythroid cells
  per spleen colony.

As expected, the strongest correlation existed between pair number 5, i.e. the
total number of cells and the total number of erythroid cells per colony. The
weakest correlation occurred between pair number 6, i.e. total number of neutrophils per colony with total number of erythroid cells per colony. This
latter result is also expected as these two cell types do not share any common
pathway as assessed by morphology. Five of the six pairs of parameters showed
significant correlations at the 0.95 level, the only non-significant pair being
pair 6 (total neutrophils per colony with total erythroid cells per colony).
The weakest correlation that was significant at this level was that between
GM-CFC and total erythroid cells per colony (pair No. 3, Table 1), the correlation coefficient (r) being only slightly above the value (0.22) required for
significance at this level (P>0.95). This was probably due to the fact that
most of the colonies were predominantly erythroid (as seen with the strong
correlation between E:N, pair 5). Pair 3 (GM-CFC:E) lost its significance when
the level of significance was raised to P values greater than 0.99 (r > 0.28)
(Table 1).

It has been suggested that the reason why spleen colonies develop a second
line of hemopoietic differentiation is that outgrowth of colony cells occurs
from one HIM to an adjacent different HIM[20]. If this were the case, then as
a pure erythroid colony becomes larger it should ultimately impinge upon a

neutrophilic inductive microenvironment and the HSC's persisting in the colony should begin to produce neutrophils. The earliest detectable change in such a colony should be the appearance of committed progenitor cells for the neutrophilic differentiation pathway (GM-CFC). One might expect therefore to find a strong correlation between the increase in cellularity of "pure" erythroid colonies and the appearance of GM-CFC. Such an analysis has been performed and the results are shown in Table 2. Nine colonies were found to contain more than 90% recognizable erythroid cells, however the correlation coefficient calculated for the total number of cells in these nine colonies and their individual content of GM-CFC was not significant (Table 2). Since this sample was small, a second calculation was performed taking as "pure" erythroid colonies, those that contained more than 80% recognizable erythroid cells. When the total number of cells in each of the 37 colonies was compared with the total number of GM-CFC in each, no significant correlation was observed (Table 2).

TABLE 2

CORRELATION COEFFICIENTS BETWEEN GM-CFC AND TOTAL CELLULARITY IN "PURE" ERYTHROID COLONIES

Percent Erythroid Cells	No. of Examples	Correlation Coefficients	Level of Significance*
>90	9	-0.04	$P < 0.1$
>80	37	0.11	$P < 0.5$

* Calculated assuming data represents a normal distribution.

In Vitro Studies on the Clonal Differentiation of Multipotential Hemopoietic Stem Cells. It has previously been demonstrated that when single cells are placed individually into semisolid cultures containing SCM, growth and differentiation along several distinct hemopoietic lineages can occur[15]. The present experiments were performed to analyse the stage of commitment of the earliest cells produced by the division of multipotential cells obtained from CBA fetal peripheral blood. The use of fetal peripheral blood cells has several advantages over those obtained from fetal liver. Since fetal peripheral blood is already a single cell suspension, this overcomes the problem of viability loss due to mechanical separation of cells. More importantly, every hemopoietic colony generated in vitro by peripheral blood has almost certainly arisen from a single cell. Thirdly, fetal peripheral blood contains 3 uniform cell populations - yolk sac erythroblasts, macrophages and large blast cells.

Since the proportion of yolk sac erythroblasts greatly exceeds the number of other cell types, separation procedures can produce fractions enriched for blast cells (the colony-forming cell population).

Density Separation of Fetal Peripheral Blood. Peripheral blood cells from 12 day old CBA fetuses were separated on a continuous BSA gradient. The distribution of yolk sac erythroblasts was determined from hemocytometer counts and served as an internal control. In all experiments, yolk sac erythroblasts were found to segregate as a single peak with a buoyant density of 1.073 - 1.074 g/cm^3 (Fig. 1). The yolk sac erythroblasts were segregated from the blast cells and macrophages which segregated between 1.056 and 1.068 g/cm^3. Although comprising only 3% of the total unfractionated population (Table 3), the blast cell and macrophage populations displayed a slight peak in fractions segregating between 1.061 and 1.063 g/cm^3 (Fig. 1). However these two cell types were not separated significantly from each other in any of the fractions.

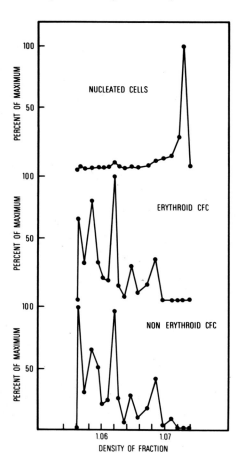

Fig. 1. Segregation of 12-day CBA fetal peripheral blood cells following equilibrium density centrifugation in a continuous gradient of bovine serum albumin. All data are plotted as percentages of the fraction with peak activity expressed as cells per density increment. The erythroid colony profile includes both pure and mixed erythroid colonies.

The erythroid mixed-erythroid and non-erythroid colony-forming cells were found to separate into a heterogeneous distribution pattern and no segregation between the various colony types was observed. The majority of colony-forming cells segregated with a relatively light buoyant density between 1.056 - 1.069 g/cm^3 (Fig. 1). Identical results were obtained with 11 day CBA fetal peripheral blood.

Due to the almost complete separation of yolk sac erythroblasts (the major population) from the blast cell and macrophage population and the correlation between the distribution of these latter cells and the in vitro colony-forming cells, further experiments were conducted with the simpler density cut procedure using BSA at a density of 1.064 g/cm^3. Unfractionated 11 or 12 day CBA fetal peripheral blood contained approximately equal proportions of macrophages and blast cells which comprised 3% or less of the total cell population (Table 3). When cells equal to or lighter than 1.064 g/cm^3 were taken, the proportion of macrophages and blast cells increased significantly (Table 3). From 5 separate experiments with 11 day fetal peripheral blood the mean proportion of non-erythroblast cells was found to be 17% (range 8 - 31) and with 12 day peripheral blood the mean proportion of these cells was found to be 46% (range 14 - 76) from 9 separate experiments. Two experiments are shown in Table 3.

TABLE 3

FREQUENCY OF COLONY-FORMING CELLS IN FRACTIONATED AND UNFRACTIONATED CBA FETAL PERIPHERAL BLOOD

Age of Fetal Donor	Density of Fraction Cultured (g/cm^3)	Differential* Cell Count of Sample Cultured (%)			Colony-Forming Cells[+] per 10^5 Cells	
		YS	Macro.	Blast	Eryth.	Non-Eryth.
11 D	Unfraction.	98	1	1	85	98
	$\leq$ 1.064	76	3	21	452	1847
12 D	Unfraction.	97	2	1	6	21
	$\leq$ 1.064	37	22	41	1340	4660

* YS = Yolk-sac erythroblasts, Macro = Macrophages.

+ Eryth. = Erythroid and mixed erythroid colony-forming cells, Non-Eryth. = Non-erythroid colony-forming cells (predominantly macrophage). Differential cell counts determined from counts of 500 May-Grunewald Giemsa stained cell smears.

It is also evident from this table that a significant enrichment for colony-forming cells occurred (up to 220-fold) although no segregation of erythroid or mixed erythroid colony-forming cells from the non-erythroid (predominantly macrophage) colony-forming cells occurred. If one assumes that the blast cells are the colony-forming cells then with the 12 day data presented in Table 3, 23% of blast cells were capable of producing a colony (>50 cells) or a cluster (<50 cells) (with the experiment shown in Table 3 there were 53 colonies and clusters per 10^5 unfractionated cells and 9400 per 10^5 light density cells).

Single Cell Transfer Experiments. Since it is now possible to obtain clonal growth and differentiation of at least five separate hemopoietic lineages in vitro, analysis of these developing clones should give new insight into the cellular events occurring from the initial multipotential cell to the committed progeny that it produces. With this aim the following experiments were performed as diagramatically represented in Figure 2. Light density fractions

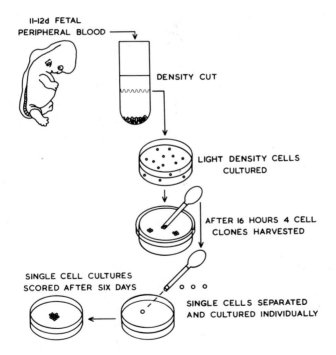

Figure 2.   Diagramatic representation of the experimental procedure used for reimplantation of single cells derived from primary hemopoietic clones.

(<1.064 g/cm^3) of CBA fetal peripheral blood cells were cultured in the presence of SCM. As low numbers of peripheral blood cells were used no aggregates were observed immediately after preparation of the agar cultures. After 16 - 18 hours' incubation, developing clones containing between 3 and 8 cells were individually removed from the primary cultures. The individual clones were then gently pipetted to yield single cells. In some instances, cells were tightly bound to each other so that only one or two single cells were obtained along with cell doublets or triplets. The isolated cells from a single primary clone were then implanted into marked areas of a second culture containing gelled agar-medium and SCM. The secondary cultures were then incubated for a further six days, at which time all cell aggregates were counted and stained with benzidine and aceto-orcein for assessment of total cellularity and state of differentiation. In this manner, a total of 47 primary clones were analysed. Following cell dispersion, 107 single cells, 30 doublets and six triplets were obtained and successfully transplanted into secondary cultures. Of the 143 transplanted single cells or doublets and triplets, 85 produced clusters (<50 cells) and 21 produced colonies (>50 cells), an overall reculturing efficiency of 74%. The largest colony obtained contained 2,800 cells and when the 21 colonies were examined morphologically, 6 were composed of neutrophils and macrophages, 3 macrophages, 7 erythroid cells and 5 mixtures of erythroid, megakaryocyte, neutrophil-macrophage and blast cells. Four of these latter mixed-erythroid colonies were derived from the transfer of single cells and thus represent the proliferation of multipotential cells.

The results obtained from the dispersion and reculture of the cells from three primary 4-cell clones are shown in Table 4. Since each clone generated cells of multiple hemopoietic lineages, the single cell initiating each primary clone must have been a multipotential cell. In each of the three examples shown the primary clones consisted of 4 cells, and 2 single cells and one doublet was recultured from each of these primary clones. In each of the 3 examples a secondary colony was obtained which displayed multiple hemopoietic differentiation (i.e. erythroid cells with other hemopoietic cells) and of these, two were obtained from single cells (from primary clone numbers 19 and 38, Table 4). This indicates that it is possible after 2 or 3 divisions from a multipotential cell, to obtain at least one cell retaining multipotentiality. The remaining cells obtained from the primary clones displayed a single line of commitment. This is most clearly seen in the secondary colonies obtained from primary clone number 38 (Table 4).

In this example, apart from the multipotential clone obtained from one cell, the other single cell gave rise to a colony of erythroid cells, suggesting that the starting cell was a committed erythroid progenitor.   The remaining two cells were not separated but nevertheless gave rise only to neutrophils and macrophages.   Since these latter differentiated cells are known to arise from a common committed progenitor[2], it can be concluded that one or both of the transfered cells were GM-CFC.   With the secondary colonies obtained from primary clones numbers 3 and 19 apart from those expressing multiple differentiation, it is not possible to determine accurately the stage of commitment of the transfered cells, since variable numbers of morphologically-unrecognizable blast cells were present in addition to the differentiated cells.

TABLE 4

SINGLE CELL TRANSFER OF DEVELOPING MIXED HEMOPOIETIC CLONES

Primary Clone Number	Number of Cells Transfered	Number of Cells Derived from Transfer				
		Eryth-roid	Neutro-phil	Macro-phage	Mega-karyocyte	Blast
	2	121	0	8	4	33
3	1	0	0	30	0	4
	1	0	458	53	0	56
	2	14	0	0	0	40
19	1	27	0	0	0	19
	1	63	17	0	0	56
	1	181	0	0	0	0
38	1	29	207	39	0	62
	2	0	217	8	0	0

Cells transfered 16 - 18 hours after initiation of primary culture, secondary cultures scored 6 days later.   All primary clones contained 4 cells at time of dispersion and transfer.

During the mechanical procedure of transfer, dispersion and reimplantation, unidentified factors may alter the commitment and subsequent differentiation of the cells transfered.   To explore this possibility, the total number of cells and their pattern of differentiation was ascertained from all the secondary transfers obtained from each of the 47 primary clones.   When considered this way, cells from 20 of the 47 primary clones gave rise to colonies (the largest

number of cells obtained from a dispersed primary clone being 4800) and 26
gave rise to clusters.   Of the colonies, 5 were neutrophil-macrophage (13%),
7 macrophage (67%), 3 erythroid (7%) and 5 mixed-erythroid (13%).   All of the
26 clusters obtained from dispersed primary clones were macrophage.   These
data agree closely with data obtained from analysis of replicate primary cultures that were established from the same cell suspension used to generate
the transfered clones, but which were not subjected to manipulation.   In these
control cultures, 51% of clones produced after seven days' incubation were colonies and of these 4% were neutrophil-macrophage, 57% macrophage, 22% erythroid
and 17% mixed-erythroid.   Thus, the procedure of dispersion and retransplanta-
tion does not appear to alter the patterns of differentiation obtained from
primary clones.

DISCUSSION

   The nature of the factor/s controlling the commitment of multipotential hemopoietic cells to committed progenitor cells remains the most fundamental question in experimental hematology.   A related problem is the manner in which self-
replication by multipotential cells is regulated, if indeed genuine self-repli-
cation does occur.

   As outlined in the introduction, two major theories have been proposed.   The
problem with both is that they are based upon data obtained from the growth of
spleen colonies and therefore can never be tested directly, since by the time
that a spleen colony is recognizable and capable of being manipulated, the
events leading to commitment have already occurred.   Moreover in vivo studies
abound with difficulties when one attempts to isolate the molecular events
occurring during such complex commitment events.

   Nevertheless, the theories developed from the studies of spleen colony development provide information which may ultimately be tested in other ways.   Correlation analysis has revealed some of the relationships between the various
stages of hemopoietic differentiation[10,13,14,21].   While these studies can
never demonstrate the factors causing the effects that they measure, they can
however test models of hemopoiesis based upon the microenvironmental theory[8,9,20].
One basic premise of this theory is that multiple lines of hemopoietic differentiation arise by expansion of the primary clone into microenvironments capable
of inducing the second line of differentiation.   On this basis, one would expect that as an erythroid colony enlarges there should be a correlation between
total cellularity of these "pure" erythroid colonies and the appearance of
GM-CFC.   Analysis of these parameters (Table 2) revealed a very low correlation

coefficient that was not statistically significant. Although based upon statistical evidence, this failure to document one of the predictions of the microenvironmental theory highlights a major deficiency in the experimental data on which this theory was based. The original microenvironmental inductive theory was developed from observations on morphologically-recognizable progeny in spleen colonies. The morphologically-identifiable cells are the progeny of committed progenitor cells which themselves are the progeny of multipotential cells. The primary event in the microenvironmental model would therefore be the induction of committed progenitor cells, but it is physically impossible to isolate and subsequently culture such cells from the earliest stages of development of an individual spleen colony.

The "stochastic" theory of hemopoietic commitment and differentiation similarly suffers from the same problems of direct testing. Unless it becomes possible to manipulate multipotential stem cells to differentiate in a particular desired fashion, the questions of whether or not the self-renewal or commitment decisions are random will remain inconclusive.

The recent development of a method for cloning multipotential hemopoietic stem cells in vitro[15,16,17], provides another means to answer some of the questions relating to the commitment and differentiation of these cells. The ability to place a single cell in a culture dish and obtain a clone expressing multiple hemopoietic differentiation states[15] (Table 4) argues strongly against the necessity for induction via cell-cell contact between non-hemopoietic microenvironmental inductive cells and HSC. The results shown in Table 4 also demonstrate that in vitro cloning of HSC can provide information about self-renewal or commitment of HSC. The data presented were obtained from primary clones containing four cells which might have been produced by two symmetrical divisions or three asymmetrical divisions. From the patterns of differentiation obtained from the transplanted cells it can be stated that, at least under in vitro conditions, within the first three divisions of an HSC and its progeny, at least one cell with pluripotentiality can be produced and at least two committed hemopoietic progeny can arise from the two or three divisions. A larger series of experiments utilising the techniques described should make it possible to build a "family tree" of the early cellular events leading to multiple hemopoietic differentiation. Such an analysis may also determine the "randomness" or otherwise of these early hemopoietic events.

The study of many individual mixed-erythroid clones obtained from 7 day cultures suggests that the commitment of HSC to particular cell lineages may not be random, but is rather a predetermined event. More than 400 individual colonies have been isolated from cultures stimulated by SCM followed by smearing, staining and differential cell counting. In all cases multiple differentiation, within mixed colonies always included erythroid differentiation[15,17]. Mixed colonies of neutrophils, macrophages, eosinophils and megakaryocytes, without erythroid cells have never been observed. These observations suggest that at least under the culture conditions used, commitment and differentiation of cells from HSC involves, as an obligatory step, the development of erythroid progeny, a result not predicted by a truly random model.

The data presented give some indication of the role in vitro cloning of HSC can play in studying the differentiation of these cells and hopefully will allow the HIM (Hemopoietic Inductive Microenvironment) versus HER (Hemopoiesis Engendered at Random) controversy to be settled[22].

ACKNOWLEDGEMENTS

This work was supported by the Carden Fellowship Fund of the Anti-Cancer Council of Victoria, The National Health and Medical Research Council, Canberra and the National Cancer Institute, Bethesda, Contract No. NOI-CB-74148.

REFERENCES

1. Till, J.E. and McCulloch, E.A. (1961) Radiat.Res., 14, 213.

2. Metcalf, D. (1977) Hemopoietic Colonies. Springer-Verlag, Heidelberg, New York.

3. Burgess, A.W., Camakaris, J. and Metcalf, D. (1977) J.Biol.Chem., 252, 1998.

4. Miyake, T., Kung, C.K.H. and Goldwasser, E. (1977) J.Biol.Chem. 252, 5558.

5. Siminovitch, L., McCulloch, E.A. and Till, J.E. (1963) J.Cell.Comp.Physiol. 62, 327.

6. Till, J.E., McCulloch, E.A. and Siminovitch, L. (1964) Proc.Nat.Acad.Sci., 51, 29.

7. Korn, A.P., Henkelman, R.M., Ottensmeyer, F.P. and Till, J.E. (1973) Exp.Hemat., 1, 362.

8. Curry, J.L. and Trentin, J.J. (1967) Develop.Biol.15,395.

9. Trentin, J.J. (1970) Regulation of Hematopoiesis. Ed. A.S. Gordon, Appleton-Century-Crofts, New York, p.161-186.

10. Metcalf, D. and Moore, M.A.S. (1971) Haemopoietic Cells. North-Holland. Amsterdam.

11. Johnson, G.R. and Metcalf, D. (unpublished observations).

12. Wu, A.M., Siminovitch, L., Till, J.E. and McCulloch, E.A. (1968) Proc.Nat.Acad.Sci. (U.S.A.) 59, 1209.

13. Gregory, C.J., McCulloch, E.A. and Till, J.E. (1973) J.Cell.Physiol., 81, 411.

14. Gregory, C.J. and Henkelman, R.M. (1977) Experimental Hematology Today, Ed. S.J. Baum and G.D. Ledney. Springer-Verlag, New York,p.93-101.

15. Johnson, G.R. and Metcalf, D. (1977) Proc.Natl.Acad.Sci. (U.S.A.) 74, 3879.

16. Johnson, G.R. and Metcalf, D. (1978) J.Cell.Physiol., 94, 243.

17. Metcalf, D., Johnson, G.R. and Mandel, T. (1978) J.Cell.Physiol., 98, 401.

18. Metcalf, D. and Johnson, G.R. (1978) J.Cell.Physiol., 96, 31.

19. Shortman, K. (1968) Aust.J.Exp.Biol.Sci., 46, 375.

20. Trentin, J.J. (1976) Stem Cells of Renewing Cell Populations. Eds. A.B. Cairnie, P.K. Lala and D. G. Osmond. Academic Press, New York, p.255-264.

21. Fowler, J.H., Wu, A.M., Till, J.E. and McCulloch, E.A. (1967) J.Cell.Physiol. 69, 75.

22. Till, J.E. (1976) Stem Cells of Renewing Cell Populations. Eds. A. B. Cairnie, P.K. Lala and D.G. Osmond. Academic Press, New York, p.269.

Cell Lineage, Stem Cells and Cell Determination
INSERM Symposium No. 10
Editor: N. Le Douarin
© *1979 Elsevier/North-Holland Biomedical Press*

DIFFERENTIATION AND MATURATION IN VITRO OF HUMAN MEGAKARYOCYTES
FROM BLOOD AND BONE MARROW PRECURSORS.

William VAINCHENKER and Janine BRETON-GORIUS.
Unité de Recherches sur les Anémies. INSERM U.91
Hôpital Henri Mondor. 94010 CRETEIL   FRANCE.

INTRODUCTION

The regulation of megakaryocytopoiesis is difficult to
study in vivo, particularly in man, and many problems remain to
be solved. In vitro culture systems may provide a new method by
which to analyse this regulation.

Murine megakaryocyte (MK) colonies have been grown in vitro,
using several semi-solid media and stimulating factors (1-5).
Recently, we were able to culture human MK colonies from the
precursors of fetus, newborn and adult blood, by the plasma clot
technique using erythropoietin (Epo) preparations as the stimulating factor (6, 7). In the present study, we have investigated
the role of Epo in the differentiation and maturation of MK
in vitro. For this purpose, cultures of blood and marrow cells
were seeded in the absence or presence of different sources and
various concentrations of Epo.

MATERIAL AND METHODS

 - Cell culture technique

Samples of human blood or bone marrow cells were collected
on 10 units/ml of heparin (preservative free). Light density cells
were separated by Ficoll metrizoate centrifugation. The plasma
clot technique (3) was used with slight modification (7) ; the
culture dishes were subsequently incubated for up to 14 days in
a fully humidified atmosphere of 3% CO_2 in air.

 - Epo preparations

Four different sources of Epo were used. Three of them were
either unpurified, i.e. a crude serum from anemic mice (8) or were
poorly purified, i.e. step III preparation from sheep plasma

(12 units/mg of protein, Connaugh Laboratories, Toronto, Canada),
and a human urinary Epo (9 u/mg of protein, Los Angeles pool M15
TaLSL). Another human urinary Epo was highly purified (70 000 u/mg
of protein (9)) and a gift from Dr. GOLDWASSER. The Epo was added
at day O, from 0 to 3 u/ml

- ## Light microscopic staining procedure

The cultures were directly stained in petri dishes. The
erythroblasts colonies were scored by revelation of the pseudo-
peroxidatic activity of hemoglobin as described by Mac LEOD et
al. (10). MK were identified by cytological examination using
Harris hematoxylin counterstained. Some cultures were observed
using an inverted microscope.

- ## Electron microscopic (EM) procedure

Cultures which had been grown either in the absence or in
the presence of Epo were prepared for ultrastructural studies.
The fibrin network was lyzed with a solution of Pronase (1°/oo).
The free cells were first washed once in Hank's medium with 10%
fetal calf serum, and then twice in Hanks medium. Platelet peroxidase was revealed as previously described (11) in the pellet
which was subsequently treated for electron microscopic examination.

RESULTS

- ## Evolution of MK colonies

The MK were identified in culture by their morphology, i.e.
large size, multilobulated nucleus and presence of blebs. The
first recognizable MK (Fig. 1) were observed at day 7 or 8 in
cultures derived from the bone marrow as well as in those from the
blood cells (7). Each colony consisted of 2 to 30 typical MK. The
colonies were spread over an area as large as an erythrocytic
burst. The number of colonies increased till day 10. After day 12,
their number fell as a result of the lysis of the MK. In the cultures, typical MK (Fig. 1) and some atypical smaller cells (Fig. 2)
were present. The megakaryocytic nature of small cells was sus-
pected by the presence of cytoplasmic blebs and of typical MK in
their close proximity.

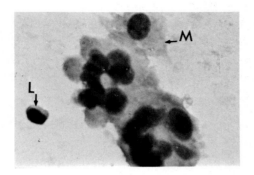

Fig. I . Two megakaryocytes showing multilobulated nuclei and
cytoplasmic blebs.A macrophage (M) and a lymphocyte-
like cell (L) are indicative of the size of megakaryo-
cytes.Culture from bone marrow cells,at day 12.

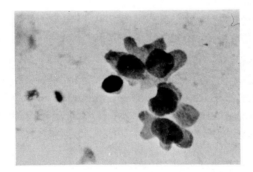

Fig. 2. Four cells have a size approximatively twice that of a
lymphocyte-like cell.The single nucleus is atypical of
megakaryocytes but cytoplasmic blebs are highly suggestive of such cells.Culture from bone marrow cells,at
day 12.

- Effect of Epo on MK colony formation

In the absence of added Epo, spontaneous colonies could be observed. They represented about 1/5 of the maximum plating efficiency either in the blood or the bone marrow cell cultures. Under these conditions, no colonies of mature erythroblasts could be observed.

With added Epo, the number of MK quickly increased, and reached a plateau at 1.5 u/ml of Epo. At doses higher than 3 u/ml, the number of MK colonies was reduced. Two types of colonies were observed : pure MK colonies which represented 75% of the MK, and mixed colonies usually containing erythroblasts and MK. Granulocytes could be rarely observed in these colonies. The average plating efficiency for 10 different normal adults was $19/10^5$ cells for the bone marrow, and $3/10^5$ cells for the blood samples, but with high individual variations.

- Effect of Epo on the size of the colonies and of MK

No major difference was observed in the size of the colonies, and of the megakaryocytes cultured in the presence or absence of Epo. In both cases atypical MK were present.

- Influence of the origin or purification of Epo

No difference was observed with the 4 different Epo, at the same concentration. Use of the highly purified Epo permitted us to obtain a similar number of MK colonies to those seen in the other Epo preparations.

- Influence of the number of plated cells

A critical number of plated cells was necessary for the growth MK colonies.

In the bone marrow cultures, no MK colony formation was observed for less than 1×10^5 plated cells while erythroid bursts were still in evidence. For a number of plated cells ranging from 4×10^5 to 7×10^5, a linear relationship was found. For blood cells, 5×10^5 plated cells were usually necessary for the identification of MK colonies.

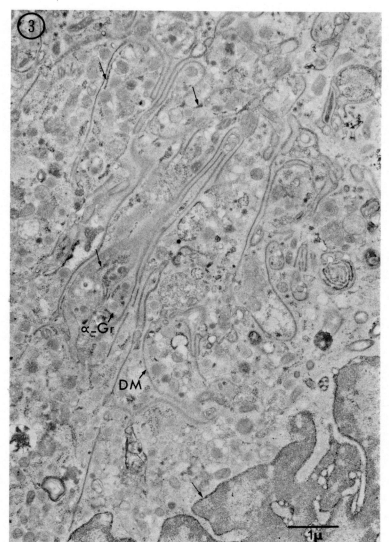

<u>Fig.3.</u> Portion of a large megakaryocyte examined by EM,after per-
oxidase staining.Culture in the presence of Epo from bone
marrow cells,at day 12.
The nuclear envelope of the multilobulated nucleus and the
ER contain weak reaction product due to the platelet peroxidase (arrows).Demarcation membranes (DM) divide the
cytoplasm into platelet territories containing α-granules
(α-Gr) and small mitochondria.

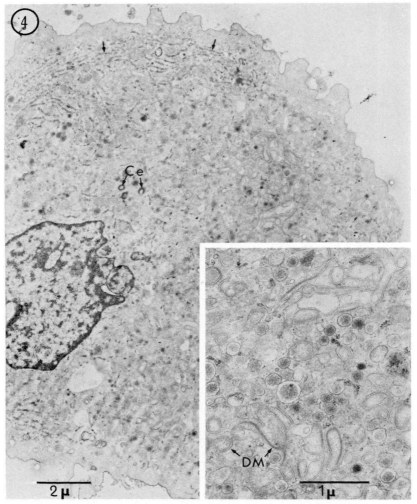

Fig.4. A large megakaryocyte treated as in Fig.3.Culture without
Epo from blood cells,at day 12.
The ER identified by the black staining of the platelet
peroxidase is principally localized at the cell periphery
(arrows).Four centrioles (Ce) indicate the polyploid
pattern.

Inset:Enlargement of an area showing the demarcation
membrane system (DM) and numerous granules.

- <u>Maturation of MK in culture</u>

    At the EM level, most of the large MK exhibited an essen-
tially normal maturation. No major differences could be observed between
the MK grown from the blood or bone marrow cultures with
(Fig. 3) or without added Epo (Fig. 4).

    α-granules, glycogen, the demarcation membrane system and
platelet peroxidase were produced as in vivo (Fig. 3, 4).

    As the platelet peroxidase is restricted to the MK lineage,
its presence has permitted to identify the atypical MK (Fig. 5).

<u>Fig. 5 and 6</u>. Culture in presence of Epo from bone marrow cells,
            at day 12

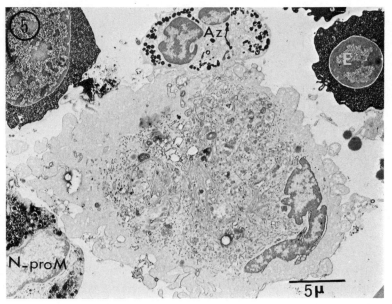

<u>Fig. 5</u>. Small megakaryocyte treated as in the Fig. 3.
         An erythroblast (E), well hemoglobinized, as indicated
         by the density of the cytoplasm due to pseudoperoxidatic
         activity is located near a megakaryocyte. Some concentric
         ER saccules exhibit platelet peroxidase staining. The
         other organelles are poorly produced with the exception
         glycogen (Gly) particules which are aggregated in cyto-
         plasmic blebs.

Demarcation membranes were sometimes regularly distributed and
divided the cytoplasm into platelet territories (Fig. 3). As a
consequence, naked nuclei and platelet shedding could be observed
either in bone marrow or blood cell cultures. In other MK, the
demarcation membranes remained located at one place.

Small MK exhibited a poor cytoplasmic maturation (Fig. 5)
as compared to that of large MK (Fig. 6). In consequence, platelet shedding from the small MK could not be observed.

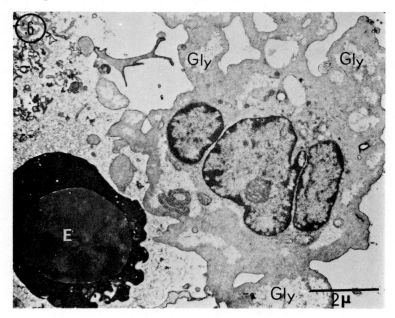

Fig. 6. A megakaryocyte, large in size, is compared to that of
well hemoglobinized erythroblasts (E), neutrophil pro-
myelocytes synthesizing myeloperoxidase (N-proM) and a
mature neutrophil with numerous reactive azurophils (Az).
The excentric nucleus of the megakaryocyte is surrounded
by a cisterna stained by the peroxidase reaction. The
cytoplasm shows an essentially normal density of typical
organelles (demarcation membranes and non reactive granules).

DISCUSSION

With Epo, two types of colonies could be grown ; the first included only MK while the second involved both MK and erythroblasts. In cultures from adult bone marrow cells, as well as from blood cells (7) most of the MK colonies were pure while in fetal and newborn cultures, most of them were mixed (6, 7). These data suggest that two different types of MK precursors can be cloned although no definitive proof of the clonal origin of the mixed colonies has been obtained. The first type would be a multipotential stem cell, frequent in newborn and fetal hemato-poietic cells, while the second would be committed only to the MK line. It should be pointed out that mixed colonies are also detected in murine cultures (3, 12, 13).

In the mouse, several stimulating factors can induce a differentiation towards megakaryocytopoiesis, but till now, none is specific. Conditioned medium derived from pokeweed stimulated spleen cells has been used (1, 2). In such conditioned medium, it has been suggested than four different colony stimulating factors were present and that these were for eosinophils, erythroblasts, granulocytes/monocytes and MK respectively. (14).

WILLIAMS et al. (4) have grown murine MK colonies, in their culture (agar), two factors seemed necessary. The first was a conditioned medium prepared from a murine myelo-monocytic leukemia WEHI-3, the second a conditioned medium from long term bone marrow cultures. It appeared that the first factor acted on the differentiation of the precursor while the second was impli-cated in the maturation of MK. However, it remains undetermined as to whether these in vitro stimulating factors have a physio-logical relevance, and whether they are related to the humoral factor, thrombopoietin, responsible for controlling platelet pro-duction (see in recent review (15)). WEHI-3 was able to stimu-late platelet production in irradiated, bone marrow reconstituted mice (16) but had no effect on the rebound thrombocytosis assay (17). Thrombopoietin derived from supernatants of a human embryo-nic kidney cell line could itself induce murine MK colony forma-tion in plasma clots (18) ; in contrast, in agar, it has no acti-vity of its own but was able to potentialize the activity of WEHI-3 in a similar manner to the bone marrow-conditioned medium (17).

Under these conditions, the exact role of Epo in MK colony formation must be clarified. In vivo, there is evidence that erythropoietic and thrombopoietic activities are different ; particularly, a chronic hypoxia does not stimulate thrombopoiesis (19). For murine MK colonies cultured by the plasma clot technique, Mac LEOD et al. (3) have shown that Epo induced MK colony formation with maturation of MK reaching platelet shedding. MK colony formation has also been obtained in agar with Epo (AXELRAD, personnal communication). In contrast, ERSLEV et al. (20) could grown murine megakaryocytic colonies without the addition of a specific conditioned medium by the plasma clot technique. In the present study, spontaneous human MK colony formation has been obtained, although the addition of Epo increased plating efficiency. The role of a contaminant present in the Epo preparations which could enhance MK colony formation has been ruled out since similar results were obtained for the same concentration with four different Epo, particularly with the highly purified one. Similar results have been obtained in the mouse (AXELRAD, personnal communication). For erythroblast differentiation, ISCOVE (21) has clearly shown that the early erythroid precursor (BFU-E) is regulated by factor other than Epo and termed burst promoting activity ; Epo apparently acts later in the differentiation process of erythroblasts and mainly at the level of the late precursor (CFU-E).

We have particularly studied the possibility that Epo was acting mostly on the late stages of the differentiation of MK. No major differences could be observed in the size of the colonies and of the MK grown with and without added Epo. Furthermore, in the absence of Epo, large mature MK exhibited a normal maturation ruling out a direct role of Epo in the maturation of MK . It seems probable that the minute amount of Epo present in the serum is unable to stimulate MK maturation, since in this condition no erythroid colonies are present.

In our culture technique, a critical factor was the number of plated cells. At a low cell density, no MK colony formation was observed in the presence or absence of Epo. A high cell density favoured the growth of MK by a mechanism distinct from the burst promoting activity, since in contrast to MK, erythroid bursts could be grown in the presence of a low number of cells.

Thus, it can be suggested that either bone marrow or blood cells are able to synthesize an MK colony-stimulating factor. However it remains to be determined whether in the plasma clot technique at least 2 factors are required for maximum plating efficiency, one of cellular origin and Epo itself, or alternatively whether Epo is acting indirectly to increase the level of the MK colony stimulating factor by stimulation of the cell population responsible for its secretion

REFERENCES

1. METCALF, D., Mac DONALD, H.R., ODARTCHENKO, N., SORDAT, B. (1975) Proc. Nat. Acad. Sci. USA, 72, 1744-1748.

2. NAKEFF, A. and DANIELS-Mc QUEEN, S. (1976) Proc. Soc. Exp. Biol. Med. 151, 587-590.

3. Mac LEOD, D.L., SHREEVE, M.M., AXELRAD, A.A. (1976) Nature, 261, 492-494.

4. WILLIAMS, N., JACKSON, H., SHERIDAN, A.P.C., MURPHY, M.J., ELSTE, A., MOORE, M.A.S. (1978) Blood, 51, 245-255.

5. PENINGTON, D.G. (1979) Blood Cells, 5, 13-23.

6. VAINCHENKER, W., GUICHARD, J., BRETON-GORIUS, J. (1978) C.R. Acad. Sci. Paris, 287, 177-179.

7. VAINCHENKER, W., GUICHARD, J., BRETON-GORIUS, J. (1979) Blood Cells, 5, 25-42.

8. TAMBOURIN, P.E., WENDLING, F., GALLIEN-LARTIGUE, O., HUAULME, D. (1973) Biomedicine, 19, 112-116.

9. MIYAKE, T., KUNG, C.K.H., GOLDWASSER, E. (1977) J. Biol. Chem. 252, 5558-5564.

10. Mac LEOD, D.L., SHREEVE, M.M., AXELRAD, A.A. (1974) Blood, 44, 517-534.

11. BRETON-GORIUS, J., REYES, F., DUHAMEL, G., NAJMAN, A., GORIN, N.C. (1978) Blood, 51, 45-60.

12. JOHNSON, G.R., METCALF, D. (1977) Proc. Nat. Acad. Sci. USA, 74, 3879-3882.

13. HARA, H., OGAWA, M. (1978) Am. J. Hemat. 4, 23-34.

14. BURGESS, A.W., METCALF, D., NICOLA, N.A., RUSSELL, S.H.M. (1978) Hematopoietic cell differentiation. New York, Academic Press, pp 399-416.

15. LEVIN, J. EVATT, B.L. (1979) Blood Cells, 5, 105-121.

16. KRIZSA, F., DEXTER, T.M., LAJTHA, L.G. (1978) Biomedicine, 29, 162-163.

17. WILLIAMS, N., Mc DONALD, T.P., RABELLINO, E.M. (1979) Blood Cells, 5, 43-55.

18. FREEDMAN, M.H., Mc DONALD, T.P., SAUNDERS, E.F. (1977) Blood, 50, suppl. 1, 146.

19. LANGDON, J.R. ,   Mc DONALD, T.P. (1977) Exp. Hematol. 5, 191-198.

20. ERSLEV, A., SILVER, R., CARO, J., PAIST, S., COBBS, E. (1978) In vitro aspects of erythropoiesis, Ed. Murphy, Springer Verlag, New York, pp 58-63.

21. ISCOVE, N.N. (1977) Cell Tissue Kinet. 10, 323-334.

Cell Lineage, Stem Cells and Cell Determination
INSERM Symposium No. 10
Editor: N. Le Douarin
© *1979 Elsevier/North-Holland Biomedical Press*

REGULATION OF BONE MARROW STEM CELL KINETICS.

EMILIA FRINDEL

Institut de Radiobiologie Clinique INSERM U-66 - Institut Gustave-Roussy,
94 Villejuif, France.

INTRODUCTION

It is well known that pluripotent bone marrow stem cells are quiescent in
normal mice[1]. These cells (CFU-S) have the capacity of self renewal and differentiation towards all the hematological cell lineages. The first step of
differentiation leads to the progenitor cells which maintain a certain degree
of self renewal capacities but which can only differentiate into one determined
pathway.

The mechanisms controlling self replication of the pluripotent stem cells
are not entirely elucidated but there is now some data indicating that in the
steady state, humoral modulators are involved[2].

It has been shown that various types of aggressions such as drugs, irradiation, antigens, bleeding, etc... can recruit quiescent stem cells into cycle[3].
However, the mechanism of the stimulation is controversial and short range
microenvironmental factors are usually evoked[4]. We have recently demonstrated
that long range humoral factors play an important role in the stimulation and
the inhibition of CFU-S proliferation[5-6-7].

The last few years have made it clear that the committed progenitor cells
are sensitive to regulatory mechanisms which are specific for each one of the
cell lineages considered[8-9]. However, very little is known about the regulation
of CFU-S differentiation towards the progenitor cells. Random differentiation[10]
and the importance of the microenvironment[11] have been suggested. We now have
preliminary data which evoke the possibility that long range humoral factors
may determine the direction of CFU-S differentiation pathways[12].

In this paper, experiments on CFU-S proliferation and inhibition, the effect
of the thymus and the thymic factor on CFU-S proliferation, and preliminary
studies on CFU-S differentiation will be reported. The mechanisms of these phenomena and the eventual role of CFU-S membrane receptors will be discussed. The
biochemical studies of the humoral factors themselves will not be mentioned as
they are as yet too preliminary to arrive at any conclusions.

MATERIALS AND METHODS

Mice. All mice used in these experiments were male or female CBA/OLA aged 2-3
months and housed in specific pathogen free conditions.

Assessment of stem cell kinetics. The technique of TILL et al.[13] and BECKER[1] et al. were used throughout to determine the CFU-S kinetics of donor mice in vivo and of the responder cells in the in vitro method[5].

In vivo experiments. At various times after treatment, bone marrow cells were harvested from at least three donor mice per point by flushing the cells from the bones with tissue culture medium. Cells were pooled within each group and counted. Two vials were prepared : one contained 200 µCi of tritiated thymidine ([3]HTdR) (s.a. 25 Ci/mM) in 2 ml of 199 medium containing buffer. The second vial was prepared as above but without [3]HTdR. To each vial 2.5 x 10[6] bone marrow cells were added. Both vials were incubated at 37°C for 20 minutes. 8 ml 199 medium were then added to each vial and 5 x 10[4] cells were injected intraveinously to recipient mice (fig. 1). The proportion of CFU-S in DNA synthesis is calculated by the following formula :

$$\% \, S = \frac{(No. \ nodules \ without \ ^3H) - (No. \ nodules \ with \ ^3H)}{(No. \ nodules \ without \ ^3H)} \times 100$$

In vitro experiments. The secretion of a stimulating factor was tested by the method of FRINDEL et al.[5] reported previously. The system was composed of two cellular compartments separated by a millipore filter which permits the diffusion of molecules but isolates the two cell populations from direct contact. The impermeability of the filters to cell passage was tested by labelling the treated cells. No labelled cells were present in the responder cell population. Bone marrow from Ara-C treated (Cytosine arabinoside 20 mg i.p. per mouse) antigen treated (oxazolone or allografts) or irradiated mice was placed in the form of plugs on each filter which floated on the surface of tissue culture medium containing the responder cells (normal bone marrow) at the bottom of the Petri dish. The system was incubated for 24 hours at 37°C in a continuous flow incubator (95 % air and 5 % CO_2). The responder cells and the treated cells were always of the same strain. In some experiments bone marrow was fractionated using a Ficoll-Isopaque continuous linear gradient. In this case, the marrow was deposited on the filter in the form of clots containing either a CFU-S enriched population or a population poor in CFU-S. After incubation, the responder bone marrow cells were harvested and pooled in order to assess the proliferation kinetics of their CFU-S (Fig. 1).

Inhibition of CFU-S proliferation.

In vivo. Bone marrow extracts were prepared from a pool of fetal calf bone marrow taken from animals immediately after death and frozen. The bone marrow was rapidly homogenized and centrifuged at 50000 g for 60 minutes at 4° C. The pellet was discarded, the supernatant was dialyzed overnight against demineralized water at 4° C and the dialyzate was lyophilized. The protein content of the dialyzate was measured by the Lowry's micromethod[14]. Bone marrow extract (BME) was injected i.p. at a dose corresponding to 2 mg of protein, to mice having received 150 rads irradiation in order to stimulate CFU-S proliferation 22 and 24 hours previously. One hour after the last injection, the mice were killed for CFU-S studies.

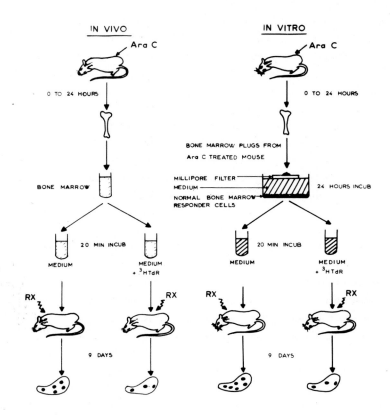

RESPONSE OF CFU TO Ara C TREATMENT IN SITU   SECRETION OF FACTOR BY Ara C TREATED BONE MARROW : EFFECT ON NORMAL RESPONDER CELLS

Fig. 1

In vitro. The technique of FRINDEL et al.[5] was used for these experiments. The bone marrow extract (170-330/μg per ml) was added to Petri dishes at the beginning of the incubation. The treated bone marrow plugs were harvested from mice 2 hours after 20 mg Ara-C treatment or 15 minutes after 500 rad whole body irradiation. In some experiments the BME was injected simultaneously with Ara-C. Differentiation.

In vivo. Five donor mice were used for each point at various times after 3 x 10 mg Ara-C injections given at 24 hour intervals. The bone marrow of these mice was injected I.V. into 8 irradiated recipient mice which were killed 9 days

later. The spleens were fixed in BOUIN'S and 4 μ histological sections were
prepared. Each spleen was analysed at 100 μ intervals. In one of the experiments the treated bone marrow (16 hours after 20 mg Ara-C) was incubated in
vitro for 20 hours and then injected into the recipient mice.

In vitro : The secretion of a stimulating factor was tested by the method
reported above. After 20 hours of incubation, the responder bone marrow cells
from three Petri dishes per group were harvested, pooled and injected into 8
lethally irradiated recipient mice and the spleens of these mice were processed
as above. The E/G ratio of the spleen colonies was determined by scoring the
various types of colonies and relating the number of erythroid to granulocyte
spleen nodules. In some cases, the responder cells were tested for the progenitors of the granulocytic series (CFC) by the method of WHORTON et al[15].

Thymic factor studies (FTS).

Eight-week-old mice were thymectomized under anesthesia by an aspiration
technique ; these animals were used as donors of bone marrow 10-15 days later.
Normal and thymectomized mice were treated with FTS as described by Bach et al.
at a dose of 5 ng protein/dose (natural FTS) or 0.1 ng/dose (synthetic FTS)
mixed with CMC (carboxy methyl cellulose). The treatment was repeated every day
for 5 days. Control mice were treated according to the same protocol, either
with CMC alone or with a nonsense peptide (a synthetic peptide in which the
amino acid sequence is completely different from that of FTS) mixed with 15 mg
CMC. FTS treatment began on day 0 and bone marrow was tested on day 7. AKR
spleen cells (2×10^7) previously washed and diluted in medium 199, were injected I.V. into donor mice on the fourth day of FTS treatment. Mice grafted with
syngeneic CBA spleen cells served as controls. Bone marrow was tested 4 days
after the antigenic challenge. Oxazolone (4 ethoxy methylene-2-phenyl oxazolone)
was painted on each shaved shoulder and one drop deposited on each foreleg of
the mice on the third day of FTS treatment. Bone marrow was tested 5 days after
antigenic challenge. Both types of antigenic stimulants have been shown to stimulate CFU-S into cycle in normal mice but not in Tx mice.

RESULTS.

CFU-S Proliferation Kinetics.

The peak of secretion of stimulating factors is reached 2 hr after the injection of Ara-C[6] (Fig. 2). Whereas the proportion of CFU-S in DNA synthesis is
about 7 % when control bone marrow is floated on the millipore filter, it is
about 45 % when bone marrow is harvested two hours after Ara-C treatment. In
vivo, the peak of 36 % occurs at 12 hours after the injection. TABLE I shows

the results with inhibitors[7]. It can be seen that the triggered CFU-S population have about 44 % in DNA synthesis but after BME this proportion falls to 3 %. When BME was added in vitro, the % CFU-S was nil whereas it was 30 % after Ara-C treatment without BME[16] (TABLE II).

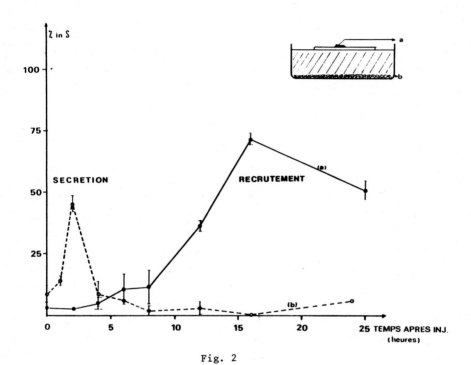

Fig. 2

TABLE I

Estimation of CBA bone marrow susceptibility to tritium suicide : effect of fetal calf bone marrow and other tissue extracts.

	Number of experiments	Number of splenic nodes/10^6 cells Mean $\pm$ S.E.		% in S Mean $\pm$ S.E.
		Without H^3	With H^3	
Control mice	5	125 $\pm$ 14	119 $\pm$ 12	5 $\pm$ 6
Irradiated mice	9	34 $\pm$ 5	19 $\pm$ 5	44 $\pm$ 5
Irradiated mice treated with				
. bone marrow extract	6	38 $\pm$ 6	37 $\pm$ 6	3 $\pm$ 12
. thymic extract	3	40 $\pm$ 14	27 $\pm$ 10	33 $\pm$ 1
. liver extract	1	35	15	58

TABLE II

	Number of experiments	Number of nodes 10^6 cells - Mean $\pm$ SE		Percentage of CFU-S in S
		Without H^3-TdR	With H^3-TdR	
Controls	6	8 $\pm$ 1.5	7.4 $\pm$ 1.2	8 $\pm$ 1.4
Irradiation	3	9 $\pm$ 1.6	6.5 $\pm$ 1.1	28 $\pm$ 4.3
BME added in vitro	4	5.6 $\pm$ 0.8	6.5 $\pm$ 0.9	0
Ara C	12	6.2 $\pm$ 0.7	4.4 $\pm$ 0.6	30 $\pm$ 1.7
BME added in vitro	11	6.3 $\pm$ 0.6	6.8 $\pm$ 0.5	0
BME injected with Ara C	4	4.8 $\pm$ 0.8	5.4 $\pm$ 0.7	0
BME injected to donors of				
receptors cells	1	7.3	7.3	3

Role of thymic factor

in vivo. In normal mice 30 % of the CFU-S were in S phase after allografting and 37 % after oxazolone painting. In thymectomized mice, 13 % of the CFU-S were in DNA synthesis after allografts and 9 % after oxazolone. The percent CFU-S in DNA synthesis was 5 $\pm$ 7 and 11 $\pm$ 4 in normal mice, and 5 $\pm$ 6 and 12 $\pm$ 5 in Tx mice, with and without FTS, respectively. After injection of iso-genic cells into normal or thymectomized (Tx) mice, treated or not with FTS, the percentage of CFU-S susceptible to ^{3}H suicide remained as low as 1 $\pm$ 8 and 8 $\pm$ 3 in normal and Tx non treated mice respectively and 10 $\pm$ 8 and 2 $\pm$ 8 in normal and Tx treated mice, respectively. CFU-S of normal mice were stimulated to enter into DNA synthesis after allograft (30 % in S phase). This stimulation was unchanged by FTS treatment (35 %). In contrast, while only about 13 % of CFU-S were killed by ^{3}H-TdR in Tx mice, 35 % of the CFU-S in the bone marrow of Tx mice were susceptible to ^{3}H suicide following FTS treatment. Results obtained with oxazolone painting were similar to those described above for the allogeneic grafts. In normal mice the percentage of CFU-S in S-phase was 37 % and 26 % with or without FTS treatment, respectively. In Tx mice only 9 % of CFU-S were in S phase, while after FTS injection the percentage of CFU-S in DNA synthesis rose to 28 %.[17]

in vitro. When bone marrow or spleen of antigen treated mice were placed on the filters, the percent of responder cells of normal marrow was about 29 %. However, in thymectomized responder bone marrow, the percent of CFU-S in S phase was about 7.5 %. In one experiment, Ara-C stimulated bone marrow was floated on the filter and in this case the CFU-S response was identical in normal and thymectomized responder cells[18].

TABLE III

Percent CFU-S in DNA synthesis							
BONE MARROW				SPLEEN			
Normal		Thymectomized		Normal		Thymectomized	
Controls	Oxaz.	Controls	Oxaz.	Controls	Oxaz.	Controls	Oxaz.
3.4	28.8	7.5	7.4	9	28.5	13.7	7.5

Différentiation

in vivo.

Normal bone marrow E/G ration is 1.9 for CBA mice. 24 hours after 3 x 10 mg Ara-C injections at 24 hours intervals, the E/G ratio of the recipient spleen colonies produced by the treated bone marrow CFU-S was 8.8. It was 3.0 and 2.0 when bone marrow was taken from mice treated 2 and 7 days previously (table IV).

TABLE IV

EXPERIMENT	No. COLONIES ANALYSED	No. SPLEENS	% TOTAL				RATIO
			ERYTH.	GRANUL.	UNDIFF.	MEGA	E/G
NORMAL CBA BONE MARROW	240	18	48.6	25.3	28.0	5.3	1.9
NORMAL BALB/C BONE MARROW	52	5	40.3	23.0	28.8	7.6	1.8
3 x 10 mg ARA-C (24hr. intervals) CBA : TIME AFTER LAST INJECTION :							
. 24 HRS	81	4	65.4	7.4	27.1	1.2	8.8
. 48 HRS	198	7	61.1	20.7	8.0	10.1	3.0
. 7 DAYS	76	7	51.3	26.3	18.4	3.9	2.0

in vitro.

When normal bone marrow plugs were floated on the millipore filters, the responder cell population CFU-S produced colonies having an E/G ratio of 1.7 when plugs of bone marrow were harvested 2 hours after Ara-C treatment of mice (one injection of 20 mg), the responder CFU-S produced colonies having an E/G ratio of 6.3 in experiments where the filter with the plugs was left for one hour and the incubation continued for a total of 20 hours. The same plugs on the same filter transferred to a fresh responder population induced the latter to produce colonies with an E/G ratio of 5.2. When the plug-bearing filters were left for 5 hours the CFU-S gave rise to colonies having an E/G ratio of 7.9 and an E/G ratio of 3.2 when the same filter was transferred to a fresh responder population. In the experiments using fractionated bone marrow, the total population (540 CFU-S) in the form of a clot induced the same response as did the bone marrow plugs (E/G = 5.4). When the CFU-S enriched population (about 1410 CFU-S) was placed on the filter, the responder cell population CFU-S gave rise to colonies having an E/G ratio of 11.7 and the "poor" fraction (390 CFU-S), an E/G ratio of 1.4. None of these fractions influenced the responder population if the latter was taken from Ara-C treated mice in which the bone marrow CFU-S gave rise to spleen colonies with an E/G ratio of 6.5. The number of CFC from the responder cell population decreased to about 70 % of the controls when Ara-C treated bone marrow was tested for the secretion of factors (Table V).

DISCUSSION

The aim of this work was to try and understand the mechanism underlying bone marrow stem cell regulation in response to various types of aggressions. The two parameters we study are CFU-S proliferation and CFU-S differentiation. We have shown[3], as have others[19], that phase-specific drugs recruit bone marrow stem cells into DNA synthesis. Partial body irradiation studies[20] have also shown that as early as 4 hours after irradiation, CFU-S of the protected areas are stimulated into DNA synthesis. These results suggest that soluble factors capable of triggering the quiescent undamaged cells into mitotic cycle may be released by other undamaged cells. Feedback mechanisms controlling these phenomena may be different for the various aggressions envisaged.

Data reported recently suggest that humoral factors affecting stem cell kinetics are released by cells after different treatments but the influence of these factors have been difficult to study in vivo. We have therefore elaborated a technique permitting us to study the cells that secrete the regulatory modulators, the cells that respond to these factors and the characterization of the factors themselves. The present data seem to suggest a number of points concerning the regulation of bone marrow stem cells. There is a temporal correlation between the secretion of factors followed by entry of CFU-S into cycle and not vice versa. This suggests that the factor is responsible for cell recruitment and that it is the quiescent cell population that secretes these factors. They are secreted very rapidly after treatment and cease to be secreted after a short time. They are secreted by live cells and are not unspecific products of dead or dying cells. This is evidenced by the fact that bled or antigen treated mouse

TABLE V

	No. COLONIES ANALYSED	No. SPLEENS	ERYTH.	% TOTAL GRANUL.	UNDIFF.	MEGA	RATIO E/G
EXPERIMENT	No. COLONIES ANALYSED	No. SPLEENS	ERYTH.	GRANUL.	UNDIFF.	MEGA	E/G
(A) NORMAL BONE MARROW PLUGS ON							
a) NORMAL RESPONDER CELLS	189	13	48.0	28.0	18.5	5.0	1.7
b) STIMULATED RESPONDER CELLS	122	5	73.7	11.4	9.0	5.7	6.5
(B) PLUGS FROM ARA-C TREATED MICE (2 hrs AFTER TREATMENT)							
1 hr	107	7	64.4	10.2	21.5	3.7	6.3
1 hr T	69	5	68.1	13.0	13.0	5.7	5.2
5 hr	104	6	75.9	9.6	6.7	7.6	7.9
5 hr T	122	8	62.3	19.6	17.2	0.8	3.2
20 hrs	133	7	63.9	9.7	20.3	6.0	6.6
(C) FRACTIONATED BONE MARROW							
1. NORMAL							
TOTAL	280	7	54.6	25	10	10	2.1
P.F.	177	6	49	30	13	7	1.6
R.F.	142	6	51.4	30.9	10.5	7	1.7
2. ARA-C TREATMENT							
a) NORMAL RESPONDER CELLS							
TOTAL	79	4	62.0	11.4	26.5	0	5.4
P.F.	72	5	37.5	26.3	34.7	5.5	1.4
R.F.	69	3	66.6	5.7	24.6	4.3	11.7
b) STIMULATED RESPONDER CELLS							
TOTAL	163	7	76.6	14.1	4.2	3.0	5.4
P.F.	71	3	67.6	11.3	16.9	4.3	6.0

bone marrow can secrete the factors as well as the protected bone marrow in a partially irradiated mouse. A fetal calf bone marrow extract can inhibit CFU-S entry into cycle when it is injected in vivo into mice previously stimulated by irradiation or drugs. The in vitro experimental system used allows the study of interactions between stimulating factors and inhibitors that control the regulation of CFU-S kinetics. In those experiments where the BME was added for the entire extent of the incubation suggest that the BME can prevent the action on CFU-S of stimulating factors liberated after drug treatment or irradiation. However, a purely chemical interaction between both factors cannot be ruled out. The results observed when BME is given at the same time as Ara-C may indicate either that the stimulating factor is not liberated in this case or that the kinetics of its liberation are changed. A physiologic purified regulator, the FTS, in itself has no effect on CFU-S kinetics in normal and thymectomized mice. However, when injected into thymectomized mice, which do not respond by CFU-S entry into DNA synthesis after antigen treatment, FTS restores the capacity of CFU-S to initiate DNA synthesis. A control non-sense peptide was not capable of restoring the response, thus implying a specific mechanism of restoration. The mode of action of FTS in this system is not clear but preliminary experiments seem to indicate that it may act on CFU-s membrane receptors. Indeed, responder CFU-S of bone marrow harvested from thymectomized mice do not respond to factors secreted by antigen stimulated mice. They seem to respond to factors secreted by drug stimulated mice. It thus seems that CFU-S have specific receptors for each type of regulatory factor.

The results reported in this paper seem to indicate that CFU-S differentiation as well as CFU-S proliferation is under the influence of humoral factors. If these factors exist in the steady state, the opposing regulators (stimulators-inhibitors, inducers of the different hematological lineages) balance their effect. When this equilibrium is disrupted by various aggressions some of the factors become predominant either because they are secreted in abnormally increased quantities or because the amount of the opposing factors decrease.

Several studies have indicated that CFU-S differentiation in vivo is modified by irradiation and that granulocytic differentiation is favored at the expense of erythropoiesis[21]. Partial body irradiation[22] showed modified differentiation patterns in the protected areas and this suggested the possibility of humoral factors affecting differentiation. Factors, capable of triggering quiescent CFU-S into cycle were previously shown to be secreted 15 min. after irradiation. GIDALI et al.[21] analyzed spleen colonies in recipient mice following injection of irradiated bone marrow. They found a decrease in the E/G ratio but did not give a clear explanation for the phenomena.

Most of the studies concerning differentiation of stem cells reported in the litterature concern the already committed stem cells and the factors influencing their maturation. CFU-S differentiation has been thought to be under the influence of microenvironments. The elegant studies of WOLF and al.[23] have shown that E/G ratios are different in the spleen and in the bone marrow. It is also known that in polycythymic recipients, erythroid colonies do not appear. They are, however, potentially present and mature under the influence of ery-thropoietin. These studies seem to indicate that the microenvironment is impor-tant for the expression of differentiation but not for its determination, whe-reas our preliminary results suggest that long range humoral factors play a role in the determination of CFU-S differentiation.

Some authors[24] suggest that leukocyte progenitor units and erythroid proge-nitor units with a limited differentiation can give rise to colonies in the spleen. This would make it possible to imagine that irradiation or drug treat-ment would kill preferentially one or the other type of unit. However, the dif-ferential sensitivity of these hypothetical units cannot explain the in vitro results in which the responder cells are not killed but respond to a diffusible factor. Moreover, we have found that when normal bone marrow was incubated for 20 hours with the conditioned medium taken from Ara-C treated bone marrow, the number of CFC (unipotent granulocyte oriented stem cells) decreased to about 70 % of the control values (unpublished data). This agrees with the increased E/G we found in the spleen colonies.

When responder bone marrow was tested for CFC content after incubation with an irradiated bone marrow on the floating filter, an important increase of CFC was demonstrated[25]. This is in agreement with the decrease of E/G spleen colony values when irradiated bone marrow was injected.

The "transfer" experiments seem to indicate that one hour of secretion is sufficient to induce the preferential differentiation and that after 5 hours, the secretion of the factor is exhausted.

When fractionated bone marrow was placed on the filters, only the total and the enriched fraction secreted a factor capable of modifying the CFU-S diffe-rentiation of the receptor cells. The fact that the difference in the CFU-S concentration of the total population (540 CFU/clot) and the poor fractions (390/clot) was very slight while the difference in the effect was considerable, suggests that CFU-S are not the cells responsible for the secretion of the fac-tor. The candidate may be the "regulator" cell of the bone marrow population[26].

In conclusion, the existence of humoral regulators of CFU-S proliferation and differentiation have been demonstrated after various treatments. They are capa-ble of inducing the pluripotent stem cells to proliferate and to differentiate along a specific pathway. This induction is most probably effective via the cell membrane receptors and explains the "dilution" of the effect as the time

238

between treatment and the assays is increased. The cells responsible for the secretion of this factor are found in the CFU-S enriched fraction of the bone marrow.

REFERENCES

1. Becker, A.J., Mc Culloch, E.A., Siminovitch, L., Till, J.E. (1965). The effect of differing demands for blood cell production on DNA synthesis by haemopoietic colony forming cells of mice. Blood, 26, 296-308.

2. Lord, B.I., Mori, K.J., Wright, E.G., Lajtha, L.G. (1976). An inhibitor of stem cell proliferation in normal bone marrow. Brit. J. Haemat., 34, 441-450.

3. Vassort, F., Winterholer, M., Frindel, E., Tubiana, M. (1973). Kinetic parameters of bone marrow stem cells using in vivo suicide by tritiated thymidine or by hydroxyurea. Blood, 41, 789-796.

4. Mc Culloch, E.A., Till, J.E. (1970). Cellular interaction in the control of hemopoiesis. Hemopoietic cellular proliferation. Edit. by Stohlman Jr., New-York, Grune & Strattonlne, 15-25.

5. Frindel, E., Croizat, H., Vassort, F. (1976). Stimulating factors liberated by treated bone marrow. In vitro effect on CFU kinetics. Exp. Haematol., 4, 56-61.

6. Frindel, E., Guigon, M., Dumenil, D., Fache, M.P. (1978). Stimulating factors and cell recruitment in murine bone marrow stem cells and EMT_6 tumours. Cell. Tis. Kinet., 11, 393-403.

7. Frindel, E., Guigon, M. (1977). Inhibition of CFU entry into cycle by a bone marrow extract. Exp. Haematol., 5, 74-76.

8. Krantz, S.B. and Jacobson, L.O. "Erythropoietin and the regulation of Erythropoiesis". University of Chicago Press, Chicago.

9. Bradley, T.R. and Metcalf, D. The growth of mouse bone marrow cells in vitro. Aust. J. Exp. Biol. Med. Sci., 1966, 44, 297.

10. Till, J.E., Mc Culloch, E.A. and Siminovitch, L. (1964). A stochastic model of stem cell proliferation, based on the growth of spleen colony-forming cells. Proc. Nat. Acad. Sci., 51, 29.

11. Trentin, J.J., Rauchwerger, J.M. and Gallagher, M.T. (1974). In "control of proliferation in animal cells" (B. Clarkson and R. Baserga, eds), 927-932. Cold spring harbor laboratory, cold spring harbor, N.Y.

12. Frindel, E. Humoral regulation of pluripotent stem cell differentiation (submitted to Biom.).

13. Till, J.E. and Mc Culloch, E.A. (1961). A direct measurement of the radiation sensitivity of normal mouse bone marrow cells. Radiat. Res., 14, 213.

14. Lowry, O.H., Rosenbrough, N.J., Farr, A.L. and Randall, R.J. (1951). Protein measurement with the folin phenol reagent. J. Biol. Chem., 193, 265.

15. Worton, R., Till, J.E., Mc Culloch, E.A. (1969). Physical separation of hemopoietic stem cells from cells forming colonies in culture. J. Cell. Physiol., 74, 171.

16. Guigon, M., Frindel, E. (1978). Inhibition of CFU-S entry into cell cycle after irradiation and drug treatment. Biomed., 29, 176.

17. Lepault, F., Dardenne, M., Frindel, E. Restoration by serum thymic factor of colony forming unit (CFU-S) entry into DNA synthesis in thymectomized mice after T-dependent antigen treatment. Europ. J. Immunol. (in press).

18. Lepault, F., Frindel, E. Effect of thymectomy on CFU-S response to stimula-

ting factors in vitro (in preparation).

19. Van Putten, L.M. (1973). Recrutement, une arme à double tranchant dans la chimiothérapie du cancer. Bull. Cancer, 60, 131.

20. Croizat, H., Frindel, E. et Tubiana, M. (1970). Proliferative activity of the stem cell in the bone marrow of mice after single and multiple irradiation. Int. J. Radiat. Biol., 18, 347.

21. Gidali, J., Feher, I., Varteresz, V. (1972). Differences in the growth and differentiation of the CFU fraction surviving sublethal irradiation. Radiat. Res., 52, 499.

22. Croizat, H., Frindel, E. and Tubiana, M. (1976). Abscopal effect of irradiation on haemopoietic stem cells of shielded bone marrow-role of migration. Int. J. Radiat. Biol., 30, 347.

23. Wolf, N.S. and Trentin, J.J. (1968). Hemopoietic colony studies : I. Effect of hemopoietic organ stroma on differentiation of pluripotent stem cells. J. Exp. Med., 125, 205.

24. Bennett, M. and Cudkowicz, G. (1968). Hemopoietic progenitor cells with limited potential for differentiation : erythropoietic function of mouse marrow "lymphocytes". J. Cell. Physiol., 72, 129.

25. Croizat, H., and Frindel, E. CFU-S differentiation after total body irradiation (in preparation).

26. Mc Culloch, E.A., Gregory, C.J. and Till, J.E. (1973). Cellular communication early in hematopoietic differentiation. In : Haematopoietic stem cells. Ciba foundation Symposium, 13, 183.

Cell Lineage, Stem Cells and Cell Determination
INSERM Symposium No. 10
Editor: N. Le Douarin
© *1979 Elsevier/North-Holland Biomedical Press*

ALLOGRAFT REACTION: ATAVISM OR IMMUNOLOGICAL <u>TOUR DE FORCE</u>?

JAN KLEIN

Max-Planck Institut für Biologie, Abteilung Immungenetik, Correns-
straße 42, 7400 Tübingen, Federal Republic of Germany

An allograft transplanted from one individual to another is
destroyed (rejected) whenever the two individuals differ in certain of their genes (the so called histocompatibility or <u>H</u> genes).
The allograft reaction is a complex immunological process involving many cellular and humoral components of the host's defense
system. The most puzzling aspect of the allograft reaction is
that in many living forms -- particularly the most advanced ones
in which grafting is purely an experimental situation -- it
appears to be totally useless. Since in nature, a bird or a
mammal almost never encounters a tissue graft from another bird
or mammal, why do they then maintain the potential to reject such
a graft?

There are two possible ways of answering this question: Either,
the allograft reaction is an atavism, a function which was once
needed in the normal life of the ancestors of present-day animals,
but which is not needed or used anymore, and is in the process
of regression. Or, the allograft-reaction machinery is very much
used even by the most advanced present day forms, though not
normally for rejection of tissues of other individuals but for
some other purpose. In the latter case, the allograft reaction
would be an incidental and for the organism totally inconsequen-
tial, sideeffect of cells that normally function in syngeneic
interactions.

The strongest argument against the former alternative is the
strength of the allograft reaction in animals of the different
phyla. Were the allograft reaction an atavism, one would expect
it to be most strongly developed in the less advanced forms
living in conditions that provide an opportunity for an allogeneic
body contact, and to be receding in the upper branches of the
phylogenetic tree. In reality, however, just the opposite occurs[1].
The ability to reject allografts is only poorly developed (and

sometimes absent) in invertebrates, improves with the evolution of lower vertebrates, and is most strongly expressed in birds, and particularly in mammals. In fact, in mammals, the allograft reaction is the most vigorous immune response these animals can mount. A variety of experiments indicate that, in preparation for allograft rejection, a mammal mobilizes some one to ten percent of all the lymphocytes available for defense [2-4]. These figures are 100 to 1000 times higher than those for any other (nonhistocompatibility) antigen tested[5].

If the allograft reaction is not an atavism, what then is the true function of the machinery underlying it? Before we attempt to answer this question, let us first pose another one, namely: What makes the allograft reaction so vigorous? Several possible answers to this question have been proposed. Some investigators have suggested that an allograft reaction, expecially as measured in vitro, represents an anamnestic response of lymphocytes activated by natural (crossreactive) stimuli, and thus a response of clones already expanded. Others have argued that, during allograft reaction, rapid nonspecific expansion of the activated clones occurs by soluble, diffusible products. Still others, explain the high frequency of responding lymphocytes by low specificity (and crossreactivity) of the lymphocyte receptors recognizing H antigens.

Although at least some of these factors may contribute to the vigorousness of the immune response during the allograft reaction, the main reason so many lymphocytes are activated by an allograft probably lies in the activating stimulus, that is in the histo-compatibility antigen itself.

Numerous experiments spanning almost half a century have demonstrated that although antigens encoded by many H loci can elicit the allograft reaction, by far the most potent stimulus for this reaction comes from the major histocompatibility complex (MHC) of the species[6]. Also, in the phylogeny, the development of strong allograft reaction correlates with the development of the MHC (although this statement is somewhat of a tautology, because rapid graft rejection is one of the criteria used for establishing the presence of the MHC in a given phylogenetic group[1]).

Why then do MHC antigens stimulate such a vigorous immune response? Again, there could be many answers to this question, but

here I shall mention only the one that I favor. In my view, the
reason for the potency of the MHC in eliciting the allograft
reaction is the complexity of the MHC antigens. In the murine
MHC -- the H-2 complex -- some 15 loci are now recognized as
members of this family of loci[7]. Of these, eight have been impli-
cated in allograft rejection. Since the effect of individual
H-2 loci is a cumulative one (two loci together provide a stronger
stimulus than each one singly[8]), a partial reason for the strong
effect of the MHC, is in the number of H loci it contains.
However, we have demonstrated that even when dealing with disparity at a single H-2 locus, the allograft reaction is still
stronger than that induced by any single non-H-2 histocompatibility locus[8]. There appears to be, therefore, something special
about the MHC molecule in terms of its immunogenicity. There are
probably two aspects to this high MHC immunogenicity, one pertaining to the MHC molecules themselves, and the other pertaining
to the receptors on T lymphocytes recognizing the molecules during
the allograft reaction.

The products of MHC loci are glycoprotein molecules, in which
antigenicity resides in the protein moiety. The MHC molecules
possess a feature not known in any other genetic system in mammals,
namely an extreme polymorphism. Our studies on wild mice indicate
that a single MHC locus may exist in a natural population in more
than 200 alternative forms (alleles[9]). At the same time, biochemical studies suggest that two MHC molecules controlled by alleles
at a single locus may differ by some 40 amino acid substitutions[10].
This enormous variability of MHC molecules probably leads to their
extreme antigenic complexity, creating an intricate mosaic of
antigenic determinants. These determinants, however, would not be
recognized were there not a system of receptors finely tuned
for the detection of minor antigenic differences. All indications
are that T-cell receptors represent such a system. Furthermore,
it appears that the receptors are tuned specifically for the
recognition of MHC molecules.

It is a common experience with all non-MHC systems that the
closer the immunizing molecule to the corresponding molecule
carried by the recipient, the more difficult it is to elicit an
immune response. With the MHC, however, just the opposite occurs.

Here, it is more difficult to obtain allograft reaction (or at
least some of its in vitro forms) when the graft comes from a
donor that is phylogenetically very distant to the recipient,
than in situations where the donor and the recipient are more
closely related[11]. In fact, the strongest allograft reaction (in
quantitative and relative terms) occurs between two most closely
related individuals. The evidence for these assertions derives
from the study of H-2 mutations[12].

When one exchanges skin grafts among genetically homogeneous
individuals (members of an inbred strain or F_1 hybrids between
two inbred strains), one occasionally finds individuals that
reject such grafts. Genetic tests performed with such aberrant
individuals then reveal the presence of H mutations, some of them
occuring in the MHC loci. Several of the available H-2 mutant
strains have been shown to differ from their corresponding
standard strains in a single amino acid substitution in the
glycoprotein molecule controlled by one of the H-2 loci. In
addition to graft rejecion, the mutants react to their corresponding standard strains in a variety of in vitro assays, presumably
measuring different phases and forms of the allograft reaction.
One of these assays, the cell-mediated lymphocytotoxicity (CML)
test, allows dissection of the target antigen into individual
determinants -- a dissection that would be difficult to carry out
using the in vivo assay. The principle, on which this dissection
is based is this.

Several mutations affecting the same gene, say $H-2K^b$, are
obtained, the mutant and standard strains, are arranged into as
many responder-stimulator combinations as theoretically possible,
effector cells are produced in each combination, and each combination is tested against all the mutant and standard strains. The
distribution of positive reactions in the different strains
indicates the strain-distribution pattern of the determinant or
a combination of determinants detected by a given responder -
stimulator combination. To distinguish whether one determinant
or a combination of determinants are dealt with, inhibition of
CML with target cells of a third strain is done or the effector
cells are adsorbed on a third-strain monolayer and then the
reactivity of the nonadherent cells is tested on the panel of
strains.

Using this approach and a collection of five K^b mutants, some
25 different determinants could be identified (Table 1). A single
mutant (standard) allele was shown to differ from another mutant
(standard) allele in at least 14 determinants. Adsorptions on
monolayers have demonstrated that the removal of T lymphocytes
reacting with one determinant (or one group of determinants) still
left T cells reacting with another determinant (or another group
of determinants), and thus indicated the existence of separate
clones of T lymphocytes reacting with individual determinants[13].
A single amino acid substitution thus produces an alteration
(probably configurational) in the MHC molecule, of which different
parts are recognized by different T-cell clones. The recognition
of these different parts then results in the stimulation and activation of such clones. How many different T-cell clones can recognize such a simple change in the MHC molecule remains to be
determined, but the number will clearly be large. Since two
unrelated MHC molecules differ not in one but in multiple amino
acid substitutions, the number of determinants differentiating
two molecules may run into several hundreds or thousands.
The number of determinants differentiating two unrelated haplotypes is probably higher by an order of magnitude because of the
number of genes composing the MHC complex.

Complexity of MHC determinants is also indicated by yet another
experiment (Table 2). We have choosen five responder-stimulator
strain combinations in the H-2 mutant system, produced effector
cells in these combinations, and tested the cells against a
panel of 30 unrelated H-2 haplotypes. Except for the stimulating
haplotype, none of the unrelated haplotypes reacted with any
of the effector cells. This result can be interpreted in one
of two ways: Either the effector cells were directed against
a single determinant which was absent in all 30 strains tested;
or they were directed against a composite of determinants and
it was this composite that was missing in the unrelated haplotypes.

In view of the preceding discussion, the latter interpretation
seems to be the more likely of the two. According to this view,
some of the determinants present in the composite might have
occurred in the strains tested, but the reactivity of a single

TABLE 1

H-2K antigenic determinants defined by cell-mediated lymphocytotoxicity (CML)

H-2K allele	*Determinant																								
	1	2	3	4	5	6	7	8	9	10	11	12	13	14	15	16	17	18	19	20	21	22	23	24	25
b	1	2	-	-	5	+	+	8	9	+	+	12	13	14	+	+	-	-	-	-	-	-	-	-	-
bm1	-	+	3	+	-	-	+	+	+	10	+	-	-	-	-	-	+	+	-	-	!	-	-	-	-
bm4	1	+	-	4	-	+	7	+	-	-	-	-	13	+	+	+	17	+	+	-	-	-	-	-	-
bm5	1	2	-	4	.	+	-	-	9	+	+	+	13	-	-	-	17	-	+	-	-	-	-	-	-
bm8	+	-	-	+	.	-	+	+	+	+	11	12	-	14	15	-	+	18	19	20	-	-	-	-	-
bm9	1	2	-	+	5	+	-	-	9	+	.	.	13	-	.	-	17	-	+	.	-	-	-	-	-
bm11	+	2	+	4	+	+	7	+	-	-	.	.	13	+	.	+	+	+	+	.	-	-	-	-	-
f	-	-	-	-	-	.	.	.	.	.	.	.	.	.	.	.	.	.	.	.	-	-	-	24	-
fm1	-	-	-	-	.	.	.	.	.	.	.	.	.	.	.	.	.	.	.	.	-	-	-	-	25
k	-	-	-	-	.	.	.	.	.	.	.	.	.	.	.	.	.	.	.	.	21	-	23	-	-
km1	-	-	-	-	-	.	.	.	.	.	.	.	.	.	.	.	.	.	.	.	-	22	23	-	-

*1,2,3, etc. indicates strongly positive CML against a given determinant; + indicates weakly positive CML; -= absence of CML reactivity; . = not tested.

Determinants 1 through 5 were defined by Klein and Forman[18], Geib et al.[13], and Melief et al.[19]; determinants 6 through 20 were defined by Melief et al.[19]; and determinants 21 through 25 by J. Klein (unpublished data). The allelic combinations defining individual determinants were as follows: 1, bm1 anti-b; 2, bm8 anti-bm5; 3, b anti-bm1; 4, b anti-bm4; 5, bm1 anti-bm4; 6, bm8 anti-bm1; 7, bm5 anti-b; 8, bm5 anti-b; 9, bm4 anti-b; 1o, bm4 anti-bm1; 11, bm4 anti-bm8; 12, bm1 anti-bm8; 13, bm1 anti-b; 14, bm1/bm8 anti-b; 15, bm8 anti-bm5; 16,bm5/bm8 anti-b; 17, b anti-bm8; 18, b anti-bm5; 19, b/bm1 anti-bm8; 2o, b/bm5 anti-bm8; 21, km1 anti-k; 22, anti-k; 23, o2 anti-k; 24, f anti-fm1; 25, fm1 anti-f.

T-cell clone in the mixture of effector cells was probably far below the level of detection of the assay used. Only in a situation where several of the determinants had occurred in the same combination as in the stimulating strain, would crossreactivity have been detected.

TABLE 2

Distribution of H-2K antigenic determinants among 34 H-2K alleles

H-2K allele	Determinant									
	1	2	3	4	5	21	22	23	24	25
b	1	2	–	–	5	–	–	–	–	–
bm1	–	2	3	–	–	–	–	–	–	–
bm4	1	2	–	4	–	–	–	–	–	–
d	–	–	–	–	–	–	–	–	–	–
f	–	–	–	–	–	–	–	–	24	–
fm1	–	–	–	–	–	–	–	–	–	25
j	–	–	–	–	–	–	–	–	–	–
k	–	–	–	–	–	21	–	23	–	–
km1	–	–	–	–	–	–	22	23	–	–
p	–	–	–	–	–	–	–	–	–	–
q	–	–	–	–	–	–	–	–	–	–
r	–	–	–	–	–	–	–	–	–	–
s	–	–	–	–	–	–	–	–	–	–
u	–	–	–	–	–	–	–	–	–	–
v	–	–	–	–	–	–	–	–	–	–
w1 through w19	–	–	–	–	–	–	–	–	–	–

Since such a combination, apparently did not occur in the tested strains, there must be large number of MHC determinants that have the ability to stimulate separate clones of T lymphocytes.

The fact that so many T-cell clones recognize and are activated by MHC determinants, suggests that the T-cell receptors might, indeed, be directed primarily against MHC molecules, and that recognition of MHC molecules is part of the physiological function of a T lymphocyte. This suggestion is in line with a

large body of data on the so-called MHC restriction of T lymphocyte function[14]. The data indicate that T lymphocytes always
recognize all nonself entities (foreign antigens) in the context
of self, where self is represented by MHC molecules. The specificity of a T lymphocyte is thus restricted by MHC molecules:
When the lymphocyte encounters an antigen without an MHC molecule
or in the presence of an MHC molecule different from that in which
it was trained to recognize an antigen, recognition (with all its
consequences) fails to occur.

We thus come to the conclusion that the vigorousness of the
allograft reaction results from a combined effect of

- the number of loci in the MHC;
- antigenic complexity of individual MHC molecules, with each
  molecule representing a mosaic of several thousands of
  determinants, each of which is capable of stimulating a
  separate T-cell clone;
- tuning of T lymphocytes to recognize fine differences in
  MHC molecules.

By combining the two sets of information -- one concerning the
vigorousness of the allograft reaction, and the other concerning
MHC restriction -- one reaches the conclusion that the allograft
reaction is not an atavism but an expression of an important
physiological function. This function requires complexity of
MHC determinants and a repertoire of T-cell receptors directed
against these determinants. Normally, under physiological conditions, the function works in such a way that a foreign antigen
(let us refer to it as nominal, indicating any non-MHC molecule)
is recognized by a T lymphocyte in the context of the individual's
own MHC molecules. But during the allograft reaction, the
complex of a nominal antigen and self MHC is replaced by an
MHC alloantigen and the T cells respond to this antigen as they
would normally respond to the complex. One can propose several
models of how this "fooling" of T lymphocytes during the allograft
reaction can occur[15]. The one I favor is based on two assumptions:
First, during T-lymphocyte differentiation, a selection of cells
carrying receptors for minor variants of the individual's own
MHC molecules occurs. And second, to a T lymphocyte, the complex
of a nominal antigen and the individual's own MHC molecule looks like

a minor variant of this molecule. An allograft reaction is, therefore, equivalent to immunization of an individual with a mixture of several thousand nominal antigens. Hence the vigorousness of the response. Details of this hypothesis have been discussed elsewhere[16,17]. However, at this stage of investigation, it is not important whether we do or not not have the correct hypothesis explaining the allograft reaction (to this date, we do not possess enough experimental data to choose among the various hypothesis proposed). All that matters is that we _can_ propose hypothesis which are not complete flights into a fantasy-land. This state of affairs is a great progression from where things stood not so long ago.

ACKNOWLEDGMENTS

I thank Ms. Chin-Lee Chiang for technical assistance in the experiments referred to in this communication, and to Ms. Rosemary Franklin, Roswitha Lange, Erika Schmidt, and Birgit Köhler for editorial and secretarial help.

REFERENCES

1. Klein, J. (1977) In D. Götze (ed.) The Major Histocompatibility System in Man and Animals, Springer-Verlag, New York, pp. 369-378.

2. Dutton, R.W. (1965) J. Exp. Med., 122, 759.

3. Nisbet, N.W., Simonsen, M., and Zaleski, M. (1969) J. Exp. Med., 129, 459.

4. Lindahl, K.F. and Wilson, D.B. (1977) J. Exp. Med. 145, 5o8.

5. Marrack, P., Kappler, J.W., and Kettman, J.R. (1974) J. Immunol. 113, 83o.

6. Klein, J. (1975) The Biology of the Mouse Histocompatiblity-2 Complex. Springer-Verlag, New York.

7. Klein, J. (1979) Science, 2o3, 516.

8. Klein, J. (1972) Tissue Antigens, 2, 262.

9. Duncan, W.R., Wakeland, E.K., and Klein, J. (1979) Immuno-genetics, in press.

1o.Vitetta, E.S. and Capra, J.D. (1978) Adv. Immunol., 26, 147.

11.Asantila, T., Vahala, J.,and Toivanen, P. (1974) Immunogene-tics, 1, 272.

12.Klein, J. (1978) Adv. Immunol., 26, 55.

13.Geib, R., Chiang, C., and Klein, J. (1978) J. Immunol.,12o,34o.

14. Zinkernagel, R.M. and Doherty, P.C. (1979) Adv. Immunol., in press.

15. Dutton, R.W., Panfili, P.R., and Swain, S.L. (1978) Immunol. Rev., 42, 2o.

16. Zaleski, M. and Klein, J.(1978) Immunol. Rev., 38, 12o.

17. Klein, J. (1979) In Ciba Foundation Symposium on Enzyme Defects and Immune Dysfunction, in press.

18. Klein, J. and Forman, J.(1976) In V.P. Eijsvoogel, D. Roos, and W.P. Zeylemaker (eds.) Leukocyte Membrane Determinants Regulating Immune Reactivity, Acad. Press, New York,pp.443-452.

19. Melief, C.J.M., van der Meulen, M., and Postma P. (1977) Immunogenetics, 5, 43.

Cell Lineage, Stem Cells and Cell Determination
INSERM Symposium No. 10
Editor: N. Le Douarin
© *1979 Elsevier/North-Holland Biomedical Press*

TWO STAGES OF H-2 DEPENDENT T CELL MATURATION

ROLF M. ZINKERNAGEL,[1] ALANA ALTHAGE,[1] ELIZABETH WATERFIELD,[1] PIERRE PINCETL,[1]
GERRY CALLAHAN,[1] AND JAN KLEIN[2]
[1]Departments of Immunopathology and of Molecular Immunology, Scripps Clinic and
Research Foundation, La Jolla, California 92037.
[2]Institute for Immunogenetics, Max Planck Institute, Tubingen, German Federal
Republic

INTRODUCTION

The thymus is crucially involved in the differentiation of some lymphocytes;
they are the T lymphocytes that are processed in or derived from the thymus and
are the principal effector cells of cell-mediated immunity[(Reviewed in 1, 2)].
Recently, it has become clear that T cells of mice express dual specificity for
a foreign antigenic determinant (e.g., viral antigen) and for a self-cell surface determinant coded by the major histocompatibility gene complex (MHC; H-2
in mice)[(Reviewed in 3, 4)]. Cytotoxic T cells are generally restricted to the
H-$2K$ or D structures which code for serologically defined major transplantation
antigens, whereas most nonlytic (e.g., helper) T cells are restricted to H-$2I$
determinants. Some connections between the thymus' role in T cell maturation
and T cell restriction have emerged from recent experiments with lymphohemopoietic chimeras formed by reconstituting lethally irradiated mice with stem
cells or by reconstituting mice lacking a thymus with thymus tissue. They
established the following points: First, T cells are intrinsically biased toward recognizing self-H-2 as expressed by the radioresistant portion of the
thymus; thus selection of the restriction specificity for self-H-2 occurs in
the thymus before T cells encounter antigen[5-17]. Second, the H-2 type of cells
from the lymphoreticular systems (e.g., macrophages) seems to determine the
effector T cell specificities but only within the spectrum dictated by the
thymus[8, 9]. Third, irradiation chimeras formed with histoincompatible or H-$2I$
incompatible stem cells do not generate a measurable primary cytotoxic T cell
immune response against virus *in vivo*[6, 9, 12]; however, upon repeated stimulation cytotoxic T cells against minor transplantation antigens have been received from allogeneic chimeras[16]. This need for H-$2I$ compatibility may indicate that I restricted T helper cells are necessary to induce the cytotoxic T
cell response or that the thymus selects *self-recognition,* but does *not promote
full maturation* of T cells. The question is then: Are T cell differentiation

and maturation dependent upon thymic selection *alone*, or is there an additional mechanism necessary involving nonthymic cells? The results presented here suggest that T cells mature in at least two MHC-dependent steps: The thymus selects the restriction specificity, after which maturation of T cells is promoted by lymphohemopoietic cells that must be histocompatible with the thymus.

MATERIALS AND METHODS

Mice. C57BL (H-2^b), BALB/c (H-2^d), C3H (H-2^k) and the respective F$_1$ hybrids were bred at Scripps. Genetically thymus deficient nude mice on a C57BL (H-2^b) CBA (H-2^k), BALB/c (H-2^d) and (C57BL x BALB/c)F$_1$ background were obtained from breeding colonies maintained by Drs. W. O. Weigle, E. Parks, M. B. A. Oldstone, G. Sato, J. Watson and S. Hedrick at Scripps and at the University of California, San Diego and at Irvine. The nude mice did not respond to ConA or PHA and failed to generate virus-specific cytotoxic T cells.

Chimeras. Reconstitution of nude mice with fetal thymuses was performed as described by Miller and Osoba[1]. Two to three thymus lobes were transplanted under the kidney capsule; thymus chimeras were tested 6-10 weeks after reconstitution. Irradiation bone marrow chimeras were made and tested according to published methods[4, 6, 9].

Virus, Immunization and Cytotoxicity Test. Mice were infected with about 2-5 plaque forming units (PFU) of vaccinia virus WR (a gift from Dr. W. Joklik, Duke University, Durham, N.C.). Six days later the spleen cells of these mice were tested for cytotoxicity as described elsewhere[5-9]. The target cells used were established transformed fibroblast tissue culture cell lines MC57G (H-2^b), D2 (H-2^d), L929 (H-2^k)[4, 6, 9]. The results are corrected for spontaneous ^{51}Cr release and are compared by using Student's *t* test.

RESULTS AND DISCUSSION

To investigate the role of lymphohemopoietic cells in T cell maturation, we used homozygous C57BL *H-2*^{b} nude mice, which lack both thymus and functional T cells as measured by their inability to generate virus-specific cytotoxic T cells. These animals became thymically chimeric by virtue of reconstitution with semi-allogeneic thymus grafts from newborn (C57BL x BALB/c) (*H-2*^{b} *x H-2*^{d})F$_1$ mice. If thymic selection alone was sufficient for full T cell maturation, we expected that T cells of both restriction specificities should be generated. If, however, only the nude host's *H-2*^{b} restriction specificity was found, the results would indicate that, besides the thymus, lymphohemopoietic host cells must be involved in full T cell maturation.

Four to seven months after reconstitution, these thymus chimeras were injected with vaccinia virus. Six days later the virus-specific cytotoxic spleen cells taken from the chimeras effectively lysed infected H-2^b targets, but left infected H-2^d targets unharmed (Table 1, Group 1). The kidneys of these chimeras contained histologically normal thymus grafts; their lymphocytes were of recipient H-2^b type alone as determined by H-2 typing. Therefore, these nude mice were thymically reconstituted and had functional T cells. However, since the chimeras contained antigen-presenting lymphoreticular cells of H-2^b but not of H-2^d type, the results were as expected; effector T cells had been generated solely against infected H-2^b targets.

Now that these C57BL (H-2^b) nude mice possessed functional thymus grafts of (H-2^b x H-2^d)F$_1$ origin, did they contain precursor effector T cells that were restricted to H-2^d and could these cells be triggered? Spleen cells from these mice were sensitized against vaccinia infected H-2^b and H-2^d antigen-presenting stimulator cells in lethally irradiated and infected (C57BL/6 x BALB/c)F$_1$ mice. Six days later, the adoptively sensitized chimeric spleen cells lysed infected H-2^b but not infected H-2^d target cells (Table 1, Group 2). Thus, the transplanted F$_1$ thymuses were functional and selected T cells to express a restriction specificity for recipient H-2^b. The thymic chimeras were also tolerant to the thymic H-2^d haplotype, since they did not react against H-2^d targets after this adoptive sensitization. However, the hosts had not developed mature T cells restricted to the allogeneic tolerated H-2^d that could later become effector T cells. Mixing experiments (Compare Groups 3 and 4, Table 1) indicate that normal (C57BL x BALB/c)F$_1$ spleen cells mixed or not with an equal number of chimeric lymphocytes vaccinia infected H-2^d targets to comparable extent. Therefore, the failure of the nude mice reconstituted with an F$_1$ thymus to lyse H-2^d targets cannot be explained readily by suppression directed against H-2^d restricted T cells. The result that parental stem cells differentiating in an F$_1$ thymus do not express immunocompetence and restriction for the second parental H-2 type is not unique to nude mice. As shown in Table 1, Group 5, the same result was obtained with adult thymectomized lethally irradiated and bone marrow reconstituted (ATXBM) mice that were transplanted with an F$_1$ thymus. That the thymic MHC selects the restriction specificity of maturing T cells in nude mice is documented in Table 1, Group 6 in which F$_1$ nude mice were reconstituted (as previously shown for ATXBM) with parental thymus grafts. Nude F$_1$ (BALB/c x C57BL) (H-2^d x H-2^b) hybrid mice were reconstituted with 19 day old fetal thymus grafts from C57BL (H-2^b) mice. The reconstituted recipients generated virus-specific cytotoxic T cells specific for infected H-2^b

TABLE 1

F₁ - THYMUS TRANSPLANTS RECONSTITUTING PARENTAL NUDE MICE: EFFECTOR T CELLS ARE RESTRICTED TO RECIPIENT NUDE H-2

Group	RECIPIENT MICE LACKING THYMUS AND T CELLS[a]	THYMUS GRAFT[b]	INFECTED SENSITIZING RECIPIENT (925r)[c]	RATIO OF SPLEEN CELLS TO TARGET CELLS	% SPECIFIC RELEASE[d] FROM VACCINIA TARGET (MC57G) H-2[b]	(D2) H-2[d]	(L929) H-2[d]
Experiment A1							
1	C57BL nu/nu (H-2^b)	C57BL/6 x BALB/c (H-2^b x H-2^d) Newborn		40:1 / 13:1 / 4:1	90 / 50 / 23	0 / 0 / 0	N.T
Controls:	BALB/c (H-2^d)			40:1 / 13:1	6 / 9	57 / 22	N.T
	C57BL/6 (H-2^b)			40:1 / 13:1	100 / 100	0 / 0	N.T
Experiment A2 - Adoptive Secondary Sensitization of Cells from Group 1 in Expt. 1.							
2	[C57BL nu/nu (C57BL/6 x BALB/c)] (H-2^b) (H-2^b x H-2^d)	→	(C57BL/6 x BALB/c)F₁ (H-2^b x H-2^d)	13:1 / 4:1	90 / 62	0 / 0	N.T
3	[Chimeric lymphocytes + normal C57BL/6 x BALB/c]	→	(C57BL/6 x BALB/c)F₁	13:1 / 4:1	100 / 73	60 / 21	N.T
4	Normal C57BL/6 x BALB/c	→	(C57BL/6 x BALB/c)F₁	13:1 / 4:1	95 / 58	64 / 27	
Experiment B							
5	C57BL/10 ATXBM	(C3H x C57BL)F₁	(C3H x C57BL)F₁	40:1 / 13:1 / 4:1	70 / 57 / 32	N.T	0 / 0 / 0
	Control B10.BR (H-2^k)			40:1 / 13:1 / 4:1	0 / 0 / 0	N.T	46 / 30 / 10
Experiment C1							
6	(BALB/c x C57BL)F₁ nu/nu C57BL			40:1 / 13:1 / 4:1	55 / 22 / 8	1 / 0 / 0	
	Control (BALB/c x C57BL)F₁			40:1 / 13:1 / 4:1	103 / 91 / 40	76 / 53 / 18	
Experiment C2 - Adoptive Secondary Sensitization of Cells of Group 6 in Expt. C1.							
7	(BALB/c x C57BL)F₁ nu/nu C57BL		(BALB/c x C57BL)F₁	40:1 / 13:1 / 4:1	113 / 58 / 31	0 / 0 / 0	
	Control (BALB/c x C57BL)F₁			40:1 / 13:1	100 / 58 / 17	80 / 61 / 32	

[a] The experimental protocol is similar to that pictured on the left in Figure 1.

[b] Chimeras were formed by transplanting < 19 day fetal thymus grafts under the kidney capsule of 6-24 week old nude mice (C57BL nu/nu mice were from Dr. W. Weigle and E. Parks). Mice were infected 6-12 weeks after reconstitution. 6 days later mice were killed and the lymphocytes tested for cytotoxicity. Thymus grafts were examined histologically and lymphocytes were typed for H-2 (> 90-95% of recipient nu type).

[c] Chimeric lymphocytes were transferred alone or mixed with normal F₁ cells into irradiated (950r) and virus-infected recipients; 5 days later these recipients were killed and their stem cells tested for cytotoxic activity.

[d] ^{51}Cr release assay conditions were as follows: Expt. A1:Duration 16 h; Spontaneous release D2: 29%; MC57G:21%; Expt. B:Duration 6 h; Spontaneous release MC57G:26%; L929:13%; Expt. C1:Duration 6 h; Spontaneous release D2:21%; MC57G:13%; Expt. C2:Duration 16 h; Spontaneous release D2:32%; MC57G:19%. These results are representative for 6 similar experiments. Results that are statistically significantly greater than negative or H-2 incompatible controls are boxed (p < 0.05).

targets only. Therefore, nude mice given thymic tissue do not seem to differ generally from chimeras formed by reconstituting lethally irradiated homozygous parental mice with F_1 bone marrow stem cells, or from adult F_1 ATXBM hybrids then grafted with a parental type thymus. In all examples, whenever the variety of MHC determinants expressed by the thymus is smaller than that expressed by lymphohemopoietic cells, the thymic MHC is the limiting factor in determining the expressed restriction specificity of mature T cells that can be triggered to become effector cells. These contrasting results from Table 1 suggest that thymic selection of T cells' restriction specificity for thymic *H-2* is a *necessary* requirement but not sufficient for T cell maturation.

Researchers in various laboratories have found that zygote fusion chimeras between $H-2^k$ and $H-2^d$ mice[15], or irradiation bone marrow chimeras made by reconstituting lethally irradiated F_1 ($H-2^k$ x $H-2^d$) hybrid mice with bone marrow stem cells from both parents, generate T cells of $H-2^k$ and $H-2^d$ [18, 19] types and both types are restricted in response to $H-2^k$ or $H-2^d$ targets. The difference between these chimeras and parental homozygous nude mice receiving F_1 thymus grafts is that in the latter lymphohemopoietic cells are of one parental MHC type only, whereas in the former both MHC haplotypes are presented on lymphohemopoietic cells as well as in thymuses. These combined results suggest then, that lymphohemopoietic cells carrying the same MHC haplotype as the thymus are instrumental in promoting full T cell maturation, probably after thymic selection has occurred.

This possibility was tested in the following experiment (Fig. 1). CBA nu/nu mice were grafted with (BALB/c x C3H) ($H-2^k$ x $H-2^d$) fetal thymus grafts under the kidney capsule. Some mice of this group were "thymectomized" 5 weeks later by nephrectomy, at a time when immunocompetence and $H-2^k$ restricted effector T cells were detected. These nude mice possessing thymus-processed lymphocytes were then injected with spleen cells from unmanipulated BALB/c nu/nu donor mice as a source of lymphohemopoietic cells of $H-2^d$ origin that themselves contained no functional T cells. When CBA nu/nu mice with intact (BALB/c x C3H)F_1 thymus grafts were infected with vaccinia virus, the mice generated virus-specific $H-2^k$ restricted but not $H-2^d$ restricted T cells (Table 2, Group 1); again upon adoptive sensitization only a very minor $H-2^d$ restricted response was measurable, contrasting with the substantial $H-2^k$ restricted response (data not shown). However, CBA ($H-2^k$) nude mice that had been deprived of the transplanted ($H-2^d$ x $H-2^k$) thymus and had been given $H-2^d$ lymphohemopoietic cells 3 weeks earlier, expressed a high level of $H-2^k$ as well as $H-2^d$ restricted effector T cell activity (Table 2, Group 2). Effector activity was by host CBA ($H-2^k$) T

TABLE 2

LYMPHOHEMOPOIETIC CELLS PROMOTE MATURATION OF THYMICALLY PROCESSED LYMPHOCYTES[†]

GROUP	RECIPIENT[a]	THYMUS GRAFT[b]	ANTISERUM + C TREATMENT	RATIO OF LYMPHOCYTES TO TARGET CELLS	% SPECIFIC ^{51}CR RELEASE FROM INFECTED TARGET CELLS[c] H-2^k (L929)	H-2^d (D2)	H-2^b (MC57G)
1	No addition of H-2^d lymphohemopoietic cells						
	CBA nu/nu	(BALB/c x C3H)F$_1$	None	40	52[d]	6	N.T[*]
	(H-2^k)	(H-2^d x H-2^k)		13	21	0	
				4	6	2	
2	Thymectomy plus injection of H-2^d lympho-hemopoietic cells[§]						
	CBA nu/nu	(BALB/c x C3H)F$_1$	C alone	40	41	93	N.T
	(H-2^k)	(H-2^d x H-2^k)		13	11	33	
				4	4	11	
3			anti-H-2$^{d\,o}$ + C	40	37	82	N.T
				13	14	35	
				4	5	15	
4	Control: C57BL			40	0	10	100
				13	0	5	52
				4	0	6	21
5	BALB/c + C3H mixture		C alone	40	66	90	N.T
				13	34	55	
				4	12	13	
			anti-H-2^d	40	60	10	N.T
				13	29	8	
				4	8	4	

[†]The experimental protocol is summarized in Figure 1.

[a]Female CBA nu/nu mice of 6-24 weeks of age were used. (These mice are derived from stock obtained from the Walter and Eliza Hall Institute, Melbourne, and were obtained from Drs. M.B.A. Oldstone and M. Dutko). The thymus graft recipients were tested 8-9 weeks after reconstitution.

[b]Thymus grafts were obtained from 15-18 d old fetuses; thymus lobes were transplanted under the kidney capsule of one kidney.

[c]Immune spleen cells were tested at the indicated ratios for 16 h at 37°C. Spontaneous release from L929:23%; D2:30%; MC57G:31%.

[d]Results were compared with ^{51}Cr release by H-2 incompatible immune control lymphocytes; statistically significant results ($p < 0.05$) are boxed.

[*]N.T. - not tested.

[§]Thymus transplanted nude mice were nephrectomized to eliminate the thymus grafts 3-5 weeks after reconstitution. These mice received spleen cells from BALB/c/nu mice on the same day. Three weeks later they were infected with vaccinia virus and their lymphocytes tested 6 d later. Serological typing of these spleen cells determined: 70% H-2^k, 30% H-2^d.

[o]Cells were tested with anti-H-2^d (B10 anti-B10.D2, 100 µl per 10^7 cells) for 30 min. 4°C and rabbit Complement (C) (diluted 1:15, 1 ml per 10^7 cells) 30 min. 37°C. The treated cells were tested at the concentrations of live effector to target cells of 40, 13 and 4:1.

TWO STAGES OF T CELL DIFFERENTION

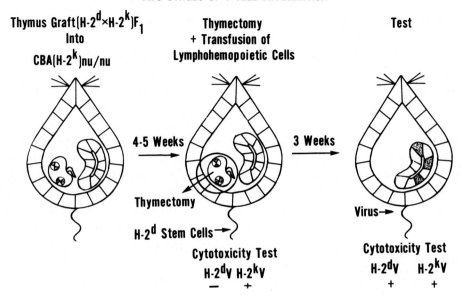

Fig. 1. Experimental protocols: CBA/nu/nu (H-2^k) mice were reconstituted with fetal thymus grafts from (BALB/c x C3H) (H-2^d x H-2^k)F$_1$ donors. When infected with virus 6 weeks later directly (or when sensitized in an infected and irradiated (H-2^d x H-2^k)F$_1$ recipients), these chimeric spleen cells lysed only infected H-2^k type targets, histocompatible with the recipient chimeric nude CBA.

Some thymus chimeras were thymectomized by nephrectomy 4-5 weeks after reconstitution and injected with 6-10 x 10^7 lymphohemopoietic cells from BALB/c nu/nu (H-2^d) donor mice. These chimeras were infected with virus three weeks later and their lymphocytes tested for cytotoxic activity at 6 days.

cells since 1) thymectomy prevented the added H-2^d lymphohemopoietic cells from differentiating into T cells and 2) anti-H-2^d plus complement treatment did not abrogate activity (Table 2, Group 3), whereas the activity of a mixture between BALB/c (H-2^d) plus CBA (H-2^k) was abrogated on H-2^d infected targets (Table 2, Group 5). Apparently addition of lymphohemopoietic cells promoted differentiation of H-2^d restricted effector cells in thymus chimeras whose effector cells of this type did not mature otherwise. Since the effector cells were not treated with anti-H-2^k plus C to make sure that the H-2^d restricted effector cells were of H-2^k origin, the present result may still be caused by some sort of factor mediated maturation of the transferred nude H-2^d cells. One can also argue that the results obtained here may be caused by some form of suppression preventing the differentiation of an otherwise expected restriction specificity and that thymectomy has removed this suppression. Experiments to assess the influence of thymectomy alone in nude mice reconstituted with thymus grafts or in irradiation bone marrow chimeras are in progress.

Nevertheless, the foregoing results seem to agree with the postulate of Stutman[20] that after thymic processing, T cells must undergo post-thymic differentiation before becoming fully mature, immunocompetent and triggerable. These and earlier results with histoincompatible irradiation bone marrow chimeras extend the experiments by Kindred and Loor[21] who showed that nude mice reconstituted with allogeneic thymuses were not fully immunocompetent. In light of the present experiments, immunoincompetence of allogeneic or H-$2I$ incompatible irradiation bone marrow or thymus chimeras may be best explained as a *block* of full T cell maturation, possibly combined with the lack of functional T cell help as proposed earlier[9]. Thus, in allogeneic or H-$2I$ incompatible chimeras, the thymic self-H-2 and the H-2 type of the cells that help induce full maturation of T cells are not compatible. Therefore, despite thymic selection, these T cells may not undergo further maturation.

The presented results may also explain some differing data obtained when differing protocols were used to construct chimeras[6, 17-19]. For example, we previously used irradiated (C3H x C57BL) (H-2^k x H-2^b)F_1 that had been reconstituted with stem cells of H-2^k origin and infected them 6-12 weeks after reconstitution[9]. Upon *in vivo* infection, these 900r irradiated and infected F_1 hosts were able to generate and express cytotoxic effector T cells of H-2^k type restricted to infected H-2^k but also, to a smaller extent, to infected H-2^b target cells[22]. If a higher irradiation dose of 950r was used, primary infection of these chimeras revealed T cell activity for the shared parental haplotype. However, upon adoptive sensitization, activity restricted to the second parental haplotype was found[9]. When the doses of irradiation were higher (up to 1050r, or split dose irradiation using 650r and 10-14 days later 850r), the preferential restriction to the H-2 compatible haplotype was much more pronounced even upon sensitization in appropriate F_1 hosts (Table 3). Sometimes no T cells expressed significant restriction specificity for the second incompatible haplotype. Similar data were obtained in a model of T cell-macrophage interactions to induce helper cells[17]. The apparently small but constant percentage of contaminating F_1 lymphohemopoietic cells that survive incomplete irradiation in such chimeras seems quite sufficient to induce post-thymic maturation of parental T cells restricted to the incompatible H-2 type; occasionally high doses of irradiation may eliminate these few surviving host cells

TABLE 3

P → F₁ IRRADIATION BONE MARROW CHIMERA

GROUP	CHIMERA: BONE MARROW DONOR	LETHALLY IRRADIATED CHIMERIC RECIPIENT	SENSITIZING RECIPIENT	% SPECIFIC RELEASE FROM TARGET CELLS			
				H-2^k (L929)		H-2^b (MC57G)	
				Vacc.	Nor.	Vacc.	Nor.
1	[C3H . (H-2^k)	→ (C3H x C57BL/6)F₁ (H-2^k x H-2^b)	→ C3H x C57BL/6 (H-2^k x H-2^b)	100 [b] 85 63	0 2 0	12 [b] 8 5	0 0 2
2			→ C57BL/6 (H-2^b)	N.T		0 0 0	-2 0 1
	Control Mice:						
3	C3H (H-2^k) [a]		→ C3H (H-2^k)	100 102 60	0 2 -	5 3 2	0 - -
4	C57BL/6 (H-2^b) [a]		→ C57BL/6 (H-2^b)	0 1 0	0 - -	93 61 35	0 - -

[a] Chimeras were formed by irradiating (C3H x C57BL/6)F₁ mice with 1025r and reconstituting them with 2 x 10^7 twice with anti-θ plus C bone marrow cells from C3H donors. Four months later, mice were infected with about 5 x 10^6 plaque forming units of vaccinia WR virus; 6 d later immune spleen cells were typed for H-2 and found to be > 98% H-2^k. The immune spleen cells were transferred to acutely irradiated and infected sensitizing recipients. 6 d later cytotoxic activity was tested on infected and normal target cells.

[b] Means of triplicate determination; values which are statistically significantly different from negative controls are boxed (p < 0.05). Spontaneous release from L929:20%, MC57G:18%. Test duration 12 h.

and allow creation of "clean" Parent → F₁ chimeras.

In summary, the results indicate that full maturation of T cell immunocompetence takes place in two stages: 1) T cells' specificity for self-H-2 is selected during thymic maturation; 2) post-thymic maturation of T cells involves lymphohemopoietic cells which must share MHC antigens present in the thymus.

It is unclear whether this second stage reflects a need for some for of I dependent maturation mechanism during T cell differentiation or that cells of lymphohemopoietic origin are involved in driving generation of, or select, diversity of the T cell receptor repertoire.

ACKNOWLEDGEMENTS

We thank Drs. E. Park, M. B. A. Oldstone, M. Dutko, S. Hedrick, G. Sato and D. Mackensen for the nude mice, Dr. F. J. Dixon for support, and Ms. A. Parson and P. Minick for expert help in the preparation of this manuscript. This work was supported by USPHS grants A1-07007, A1-13779, A1-00248, CA-19108 and CA-13384. This is publication number 1546 from the Immunology Departments of Scripps Clinic and Research Foundation, La Jolla, California 93027.

REFERENCES

1. Miller, J. F. A. B. and Osoba, D. (1967) Phys. Rev. 47, 437-520.

2. Davies, A. J. S. (1969) Transplant. Rev. 1, 43-91.

3. Benacerraf, B. and Paul, W. (1977) Science, 195, 1293-1303.

4. Zinkernagel, R. M. and Doherty, P. C. (1979) Adv. Immunol. In press.

5. Bevan, M. J. (1977) Nature, 269, 417-419.

6. Zinkernagel, R. M., Callahan, G. N., Althage, A., Cooper, S., Klein, P. A., and Klein, J. (1978) J. Exp. Med. 147, 882-896.

7. Sprent, J. (1978) J. Exp. Med. 147, 1838-1842.

8. Bevan, M. J. and Fink, P. J. (1978) Immunol. Rev. 42, 4-19.

9. Zinkernagel, R. M. (1978) Immunol. Rev. 42, 224.

10. Katz, D. H., Skidmore, B. J., Katz, L. R. and Bogowitz, C. A. (1978) J. Exp. Med. 148, 727-745.

11. von Boehmer, H., Haas, W. and Jerne, N. K. (1978) Proc. Natl. Acad. Sci. U. S. A. 75, 2439-2442.

12. Miller, J. F. A. P., Gamble, J., Mottram, P. and Smith, F. I. (1979) Scand. J. Immunol. 9, In press.

13. Waldmann, H., Pope, H., Bettles, C. and Davies, A. J. S. (1979) Nature 277, 137.

14. Kappler, J. W. and Marrack, P. (1978) J. Exp. Med. 148, 1510-1522.

15. Matsunaga, T. and Simpson, E. (1978) Proc. Natl. Acad. Sci. U.S.A. 74, 6207-6210.

16. Matzinger, P. and Mirkwood, G. (1978) J. Exp. Med. 148, 84.

17. Erb, P., Meier, B., Matsunaga, T., and Feldman, M. (1979) J. Exp. Med. 149, 86-701.

18. von Boehmer, H. and Sprent, J. (1976) Transplant. Rev. 29, 3-23.

19. Waldmann, H. (1977) Immunol. Rev. 35, 121-145.

20. Stutman, O. (1977) Contemp. Topics in Immunobiology, 7, 1-46.

21. Kindred, B. and Loor, F. (1974) J. Exp. Med. 139, 1215-1227.

22. Zinkernagel, R. M. (1976) J. Exp. Med. 144, 933-945.

Cell Lineage, Stem Cells and Cell Determination
INSERM Symposium No. 10
Editor: N. Le Douarin
© 1979 Elsevier/North-Holland Biomedical Press

THE TARGET CELL OF THYMIC HORMONES

Jean-François BACH, Marie-Anne BACH, Mireille DARDENNE and Jean-Marie PLEAU
I.N.S.E.R.M.U 25 - Hôpital Necker - 161, rue de Sèvres - 75015 Paris -
France

INTRODUCTION

The existence of thymic hormones and their intervention in T cell differentiation are now well established (reviewed in Ref.1 and 2), even if there
remains much incertainty on the number and physicochemical characteristics of
the molecule(s) responsible for the humoral function of the thymus. In fact,
the main question is now to determine the precise site of action of thymic
hormones in the course of T cell differentiation. Do they act on lymphoid
stem cells or on more mature T cells already engaged along the T cell differentiation pathway ? If they act selectively on a minority of T cells, what is
the nature of their target cell in terms of its differentiation alloantigens
and its functions ? What is the nature of the signal given to the target cell,
in particular can one relate the effect on markers to functional changes ?
Lastly, do thymic hormones essentially act within the thymus or do they also
operate in the periphery at distance from the thymus ? Before approaching these
various questions we shall first review data obtained with the thymic factor
under study in our laboratory, the "facteur thymique sérique"(FTS), since it
is apparent that some of these data are directly relevant to the questions
listed above.

MAIN FEATURES OF FTS

We demonstrated in 1971 that thymic extracts induce the expression of cell
markers in immature bone marrow rosette forming cells (RFC)[3]. Thus, the theta
antigen is induced after 60 min incubation at 37°C with less than 0.1 µg/ml
thymosin Fraction 5. This assay was used to characterize a serum factor showing
the same activity as thymic extracts in the theta rosette assay. This serum
thymic factor (called Facteur Thymique Sérique, FTS) is absent in the serum
of nude or thymectomized (Tx) mice and reappears after thymus grafting. Chemical analysis[4] showed that it involved a peptide of low molecular weight. The
sequence of the amino acids of porcine FTS was obtained in collaboration with
J. ROSA[5] :   Glu-Ala-Lys-Ser-Gln-Gly-Gly-Ser-Asn

Synthesis of this factor was done by several laboratories, notably that of
E. BRICAS at Orsay. Recently, the latter synthesized a series of analogues which
made it possible to identify the biologically active site and the antigenic
site of the molecule [6].

We have compared synthetic FTS and natural FTS (extracted from pig serum)
in many biological and biochemical tests, without being able to detect the
least difference between the two products. The biological activities of synthetic FTS and natural FTS are likewise identical in all the biological tests
in which we compared them : in particular the rosette test, the autologous
rosette test, the induction of cytotoxic T cells and the rejection of sarcomas
induced by the MSV virus [7].

The presence of FTS in the thymus has been demonstrated by different
approaches. Firstly, fractionation of a thymic extract on Sephadex G-25 gel
reveals the presence of molecules with a molecular weight close to that of FTS,
that are fully biologically active in the rosette assay. The relationship
between such molecule(s) and FTS is supported further by its (their) removal
after passage on a specific anti-FTS immunoadsorbent. Second, by direct use
of this immunoadsorbent (prepared by coupling to Sepharose an antiserum obtained from a rabbit immunized to a conjugate of synthetic FTS and BSA), we
could remove molecules which proved to be, after elution, considerably more
active in the rosette assay, and had a molecular weight close to that of FTS.
We cannot exclude that the material thus extracted from the thymus is a slightly
larger molecule thatn FTS, and might be, for example, a precursor. In any case,
this material is closely related to FTS since in addition to very similar
molecular weight, it shares with it antigenicity and biological activity [7].
Note also that the level of FTS found in the thymus in the second experiment
is about 10 times higher than that found in serum, which excludes a mere conta-
mination of the thymus by serum. Lastly, we have recently shown that the anti-
FTS serum mentioned above raised against synthetic FTS, binds to epithelial
cells of rat and mouse thymus by immunofluorescence.

BIOLOGICAL ACTIVITIES OF THYMIC FACTORS

It is apparent that thymic factors do not act identically on various lymphocyte subsets. The analysis and the discussion of the functions that are the
most readily affected by the various available thymic factors should prove
useful for the understanding of the role of thymic factors in T cell differentiation.

Indirect evidence, essentially based on STUTMAN's work, indicates that thymic factors probably act at the level of so-called "post-thymic cells" as found in neonatal spleen[8]. Such a post-thymic cell has already encountered the thymic influence, probably by direct contact with the epithelium, where, in addition to the acquisition of its maturational features, it has gained its anti-H-2 receptors that will be needed for the various T cell cognitive functions.

Data obtained with purified or synthetic thymic factors are generally compatible with this hypothesis. There are some reports according to which thymic factors might act in nude mice or totally T cell-deprived mice (Tx, irradiated, reconstituted with antitheta serum-treated bone marrow cells) but these publications either deal with T cell markers, and do not have totally convincing implications for T cell differentiation, or relate to T cell functions, but have not been confirmed. Most data, either obtained in vitro or in vivo, derive from studies in normal, adult Tx, partially T cell-deprived, NZB or aged mice, that may show some degree of T cell deficiency, but that share the property of possessing post-thymic cells.

Marker studies indicate that the various types of T cell differentiation antigens may be induced in precursor cells that are devoid of such markers. This was initially shown by us for the theta antigen, using various thymic extracts[3], and has now been confirmed and extended for Ly 1, 2 and 3 antigens, TL antigens, and xenogeneic antigens. In particular, FTS induces the theta and Ly antigens in the mouse and xenogeneic T cell antigens in the human[7,9].

Other T cell markers are induced by thymic factors. In particular, terminal deoxynucleotidyl transferase (TdT) expression is modified by incubation of immature lymphoid cells with FTS. Interestingly, the effects differ according to the cell type considered. TdT is increased by thymosin in nude mouse spleen cells[10] and decreased in normal bone marrow cells by synthetic FTS in BSA gradient-separated human bone marrow cells[9]. Human E rosettes are seemingly increased in vitro and in vivo by all available factors[9].

Most T cell functions have been reported to be induced or enhanced by thymic factors (provided the adequate recipient is selected, as discussed above). It is not the place here to review all the biological activities of the various factors. We shall limit ourselves to considering the most striking properties of the well-defined peptide FTS (see Ref.5).

FTS is active on most T cell fucntions (Table 1). Most strikingly, it enhances T cell—mediated cytotoxicity in Tx mice. This effect is particularly clear in adult Tx mice using the BRUNNER assay[11]. It is not known whether FTS directly stimulates the generation of the cytotoxic cells or enhances the function of a regulatory cell that could be the Ly 123^{+} spleen cell. Similarly, FTS also acts on T cells involved in delayed—type hypersensitivity induced by DNFB[12]. It restores a normal response in adult Tx mice. Its effect on helper T cells as studied on anti-SRBC antibody production is much less clear (we have not obtained major effects in a reproducible manner), perhaps due to a simultaneous action on suppressor T cells.

In fact, FTS has recently proven to be remarkably active on suppressor T cells in various in vitro and in vivo systems. Given in vivo to normal mice, FTS suppresses the generation of alloantigen reactive T cells[11] or DNFB-sensitive T cells[12]. Given at 10-100 ng it may prolong skin allograft survival[7] or enhance the growth of MSV-sarcoma in T cell—deprived mice (while at lower doses it stimulates its rejection). Lastly, in vitro, FTS reconstitutes, in a very significant way, the depressed capacity of most lupus patients to generate suppressor T cells after Con A activation, assessed on PWM—driven immunoglobulin synthesis (R. KRAKAUER, in preparation).

This new effect of FTS probably has its counterpart for other thymic factors. It complicates the interpretation of the biological data observed in various functions, but widens the potential therapeutic applications. It appears, as far as FTS is concerned, that the suppressor effect is essentially observed at high "pharmacological" FTS dose, while other effects are seen at lower, presumably physiological doses. Whether this difference in dose is related to a difference in cellular receptors of suppressor T cells compared to helper T cells or other T cells, it not known. Whether this effect is related to a pharmacological stimulation of mature suppressor cells or to an induction or maturation of suppressor T cell precursors is similarly not determined. Note, however, that a non specific inhibitory effect on immune responses is made unlikely by the prevention of the effect by pretreatment of recipient mice by low doses of cyclophosphamide, known to selectively inhibit suppressor T cells in various systems.

It is interesting to note that this effect of FTS on suppressor cells probably explains most of its preventive effects observed in NZB autoimmune mice (decrease in anti-PVP antibody production, prevention of SJÖGREN syndrome[13])). A simultaneous effect on helper T cells probably explains the accelerated production of IgG anti-DNA antibodies also observed in these mice.

TABLE 1

BIOLOGICAL ACTIVITIES OF FTS[7,9,11,12,13]

	In vitro $(10^{-7}-10^{-5}$ µg/ml)	In vivo (0.1-1 ng per mouse)
- Induction of T lymphocyte markers		
Theta antigen	+	+
Heterospecific T cell antigen	+	
A-RFC (adult Tx and normal mice)	+	+
Antigen-binding receptors (thymus)	+	+
E-rosettes (T cell depleted humans)	+	
PHA and Con A responsiveness	−	+
Reduction in TdT	+	
- Effect on T cell-mediated cytotoxicity		
Generation of anti-H-2 cytotoxic T cells (adult Tx mice)		+
CML ("B" mice)	−	+
MSV sarcoma rejection ("B" mice)		+
- Stimulation of helper T cells		
Anti-SRBC antibody (PFC) ("B" mice)	−	$\overset{-}{+}$
+ effects on autoimmunity (anti-DNA antibodies)		+
- Enhancement of T cell-mediated suppression or less likely depression of amplifier T cells		
Decrease in PVP antibody production (NZB mice)		+
Depression of DNFB contact sensitivity (normal mice)		+
Depression of anti-H-2 cytotoxic T cells (normal mice)		+
Retardation of skin allograft rejection (normal mice)		+
+ effects on autoimmunity (Sjögren syndrome)		+
Stimulation of Con A-induced T-cell suppression (humans)	+	

Finally, thymic factors show a large variety of effects on T cell functions especially in relatively mature cells, including suppressor T cells. In addition to their effect on T cell maturation they seem to have a pharmacological effect on mature T cells, and particularly suppressor cells that would still possess receptors for them. A similar situation exists for corticosteroids, which reconstitute the various effects of adrenal insufficiency at low doses and show dramatic and varied biological effects at higher, supraphysiological doses. In any case, the multiplicity of well-defined and well-controlled biological effects of purified or synthetic thymic peptides argues in favor of their important role in T cell differentiation, at least in its late stages. Their action on the initial step could be also considered if one hypothesized that at this stage they only act locally at high concentrations on cells in direct contact with the thymic epithelium.

SPECIFIC FTS RECEPTORS ON T CELLS[14]

The binding to specific receptors on its target cell is the first step in the action of a polypeptide hormone. It is thus of utmost importance for the understanding of the cellular mode of action of FTS to search for and characterize FTS receptors on lymphoid cells. To do this, we have applied the methodology now well established for polypeptide hormones. This effort was significantly helped by the finding of two lymphoblastoid cell lines (derived from cell cultures of patients with acute lymphoblastoid leukemia) that showed high levels of FTS binding. FTS was labelled by tritium, using sodium borohydride. Cultured lymphocytes were incubated with labelled FTS for 90 min. Twelve to 15% FTS bound to the cell line and the specificity of the binding was assessed by the strong inhibition of the binding obtained by addition of unlabelled FTS (10^{-8}M). In fact, it was even possible to displace labelled FTS by secondary addition of unlabelled FTS after 90 min incubation. The production of FTS receptors by the T cell line was verified by their disappearance after trypsin treatment and their reappearance after overnight incubation in serum-free medium. It is interesting to note that another T cell line was shown to bind FTS, whereas five B cell and one null cell line were negative. The fact that some T cell lines did not bind FTS indicates that T cells do not express FTS receptors at all stages of T cell differentiation. Preliminary data have shown that normal human peripheral blood lymphocytes express FTS receptors when they are preincubated in serum-free medium, probably to let them shed already bound FTS. Finally, receptors with a high binding affinity for FTS (KD = 10^{-9})

appear to exist on T cells. That these receptors are associated with the biological effects of FTS is likely but remains to be demonstrated.

The biological significance of the receptors is underlined by the high
dissociation constant and the fine specificity (FTS analogues differing only
by one amino acid from FTS, lose most of their capacity to combine with the
receptors). The fact that not all T cell lines show FTS receptors indicates
that a minority of T cells binds FTS, and consequently that FTS acts only on
a T cell subpopulation. It is too early to determine the cell population(s)
in question. However, preliminary analysis of the membrane markers present on
the FTS receptor bearing T cell lines indicates that FTS target cell is a
relatively mature T cell (receptors for $Fc\mu$, low rate of peanut agglutinin
binding). This interpretation would fit well with the presence of FTS receptors
on some peripheral T cells and with the preferential action of thymic factors
in partly T cell-deprived mice (adult Tx or NZB mice).

CONCLUSIONS

The data presented above lead to the assumption that FTS and probably other
thymic factors do not act identically on T cell subsets since 1/ only a portion
of T cells show FTS receptors ; 2/ neonatally or adult Tx mice are significantly
more sensitive to thymic factors than nude mice.

It will be important to determine whether FTS-receptor-bearing cells are
physiologically stimulated by thymic factors within the thymus and/or in the
periphery (especially at their pharmacological doses). It will also be important
to know whether the humoral function of the thymus involves one or several
peptides acting at different stages of T cell differentiation, and lastly what
is the nature of the differentiating signals.

It is likely that the very first stages involving the most immature cells
(lymphoid stem cells) depend upon direct contact with the thymic epithelial
microenvironment (whether or not short range thymic facotrs intervene in this
action). Later on, thymic hormones play an essential role. Their mode of action
is still imperfectly determined. Stimulation of cAMP synthesis probably takes
place, although direct demonstration of such an effect has not yet been clearly
established, perhaps due to the dilution of the thymic hormone target cells
among other cells. Whether or not marker induction involves protein neosynthesis
or membrane rearrangement is also unclear. One should note that T cell markers
are induced within 60 min, whereas function induction takes several days. It is
possible, however, that it is the same signal that operates for marker and

and function induction, the cell being triggered by contact with the thymic hormone and progressing then spontaneously to a new state of differentiation. Before this stage is reached, one is faced with the paradoxical concept of non-functional differentiation where the cell has acquired the markers but not the functions of a T cell, a situation also found in vivo in cortical thymocytes.

REFERENCES

1. Bach,J.F. and Carnaud,C. (1976) Progr.Allergy, 21, 342.

2. Bach,J.F. (1979) Int.J.Immunopharmacol. (in press)

3. Bach,J.F., Dardenne,M., Goldstein,A., Guha,A. and White,A. (1971) Proc.Nat.Acad.Sci. U.S.A. 68,2734.

4. Dardenne, M., Pléau, J.M., Man,N.K. and Bach,J.F. (1977) J.Biol.Chem.,252,8040.

5. Pléau,J.M., Dardenne, M., Blouquit,Y. and Bach,J.F. (1977) J.Biol.Chem., 252,8045.

6. Bricas,E., Martinez,J., Blanot, D., Auger,G., Dardenne,M., Pléau,J.M. and Bach,J.F. (1977) in :"Peptides Proc. 5th American Peptide Symposium (M.Goodman and J. Meinhoger,eds.) J. Wiley, New York, p. 564.

7. Bach,J.F., Bach,M.A., Blanot,D., Bricas,E., Charreire,J., Dardenne, M., Fournier,C. and Pléau,J.M. (1978) Bull.Inst.Pasteur, 76, 325.

8. Stutman,O. (1978) Immunol.Rev. 42, 138.

9. Incefy,G.S., Mertelsmann,R., Dardenne,M., Bach.J.F. and Good,R.A.(1979) Fed.Proc., 38, 1212.

10. Pazmino,N.H., Ihle,J.M. and Goldstein.A.L.(1978) J.exp.Med., 147, 708.

11. Bach,M.A. (1977) J.Immunol. 119, 641.

12. Erard,D., Charreire,J., GAlanaud,P. and Bach,J.F. (1978) J.Immunol. (in press)

13. Bach,M.A., Dardenne,M. and Droz,D. (1978) in : "The Pharmacology of Immunoregulation" (G.H.Werner and F.Floc'h, eds.) Academic Press, p. 201.

14. Pléau,J.M., Morgat,J.L. and Bach,J.F. (1979) C.R.Acad.Sci. (in press).

Cell Lineage, Stem Cells and Cell Determination
INSERM Symposium No. 10
Editor: N. Le Douarin
© *1979 Elsevier/North-Holland Biomedical Press*

THE HEMOPOIETIC SYSTEM AS A MODEL FOR STUDIES ON DETERMINATION AND REGULATION OF DIFFERENTIATION

R.A. PHILLIPS
Ontario Cancer Institute
500 Sherbourne Street,
Toronto M4X 1K9 (Canada)

INTRODUCTION

The study of determination of differentiated function requires model systems in which detailed observations can be made on cells with multiple differentiative potentials. In mammals, there are many systems suitable for studying determination. During embryogenesis there are obviously many cell lineages with multiple differentiative potentials. However, until recently it has been difficult[1] to manipulate embryos in ways that allow study of the determination and the regulation of these complex pathways of differentiation. In adult animals, cell renewal systems such as those of the epithelial layers of skin and gastrointestinal tract and the hemopoietic system offer unique opportunities for the investigation of determination. Of these various systems, the hemopoietic system offers the most advantages. The hemopoietic system produces daily large numbers of lymphoid cells (B and T lymphocytes) and myeloid cells (erythrocytes, granulocytes, megakarocytes, and macrophages). From an experimental point view, the most important advantage of the hemopoietic system is the possibility of studying it as a single cell suspension. Probably because hemopoietic tissue exists essentially as a single cell suspension in vivo, it has been easy to prepare single cell suspensions and to grow hemopoietic cells in vitro. In addition, it is easy to graft hemopoietic tissue; simple intravenous infusion of hemopoietic cells leads to their migration to appropriate sites for differentiation.

The loose structure of hemopoietic tissue and the marked ability of hemopoietic cells to migrate implies that much of the communication between cells is likely to be mediated by factors rather than by cell to cell contact.

Because factors are generally easier to investigate than signals transmitted by cell contact, it is not surprising that a large number of studies have been done to characterize factors involved in the differentiation of the hemopoietic system. The properties of these factors have been reviewed recently by Metcalf[2] and by Burgess et al[3].

In the following sections, I will describe two approaches that we have used to study the differentiation of the hemopoietic system. The first section will summarize experiments designed to study the differentiated cell types within individual clones of hemopoietic stem cells. The second section will describe our attempts to adopt an in vitro system which mimicks as closely as possible the in vivo environment required for hemopoietic differentiation.

IN VIVO STUDIES OF HEMOPOIETIC CLONES

The study of determination requires analysis of clones. Only by analyzing the differentiated progeny of a single cell can one for certain identify cells with multiple differentiative potentials and thereby learn something about the process of determination. Numerous in vivo and in vitro assays have been developed for cells in the hemopoietic system[2]. Although most of these assays detect cells that produce only one type of differentiated progeny, a few assays detect immature precursors that produce colonies containing different types of differentiated progeny. For example, Johnson and Metcalf[4] have described multipotent, in vitro colony-forming cells in the livers of embryonic mice at 12 days of gestation. The most relevant precursors for studies on determination are stem cells. The unique property of stem cells is that they produce both differentiated progency and other stem cells; that is, stem cells have the potential to self-renew[5].

The only clonal assay detecting a cell with extensive self-renewal capacity is the in vivo spleen colony forming assay described by Till and McCulloch[6]. When bone marrow or spleen cells are injected into lethally irradiated syngeneic recipients, some of the injected cells migrate to the spleen and form large macroscopic nodules which can be easily detected and enumerated 10 days after grafting. Till and McCulloch and their colleagues[7,8] demonstrated that each nodule was a colony derived from a single cell, the CFU-S; single colonies contained several types of myeloid cells and other CFU-S[5].

It has been difficult to analyze the lymphoid potential of CFU-S. By both in vivo and in vitro assays, we have been unable to detect functional B or T lymphocytes in spleen colonies (unpublished data). Recently, Lala and Johnson reported the presence of B lymphocyte colony forming cells within spleen colonies[9]. However, since other investigators have not observed such colony forming cells in spleen colonies, more work is required before one can say with certainty that B cell precursors are among the progeny in a spleen colony.

The work of Micklem and his colleagues demonstrated that bone marrow contains stem cells capable of repopulating both the myeloid and lymphoid systems of irradiated mice[10]. Later Wu et al. showed that a common progenitor produced both myeloid cells and thymic lymphocytes but they were unable to determine whether or not the common progenitor was the CFU-S[11]. Several investigators have reported that the injection of individual or pooled spleen colonies into irradiated recipients leads to the regeneration of both myeloid and lymphoid function[12,13]. From the results of these experiments, it has been concluded that CFU-S are the progenitors of both the lymphoid and myeloid systems. However, in none of these experiments could the investigator rule out the possibility that lymphoid regeneration occurred from a contaminant in the spleen colony as opposed to a precursor derived from a colony forming cell.

Because none of the existing colony techniques are suitable for studying the differentiation of lymphocytes from stem cells, we adapted another method of clonal analysis, one originally used to study the differentiative potential of CFU-S[7,8,11]. This technique involves the use of ionizing radiation to induce unique chromosome markers in individual stem cells. Exposure of bone marrow stem cells to ionizing radiation has two effects. First, the majority of this radiation-sensitive population is killed by the radiation[6]. Second, among the surviving stem cells, a high proportion have radiation-induced chromosome translocations[14]. Because the translocations are induced randomly, each is unique and provides an excellent cytogenetic marker for cells derived from such marked stem cells. The presence of identical translocations in two cells identifies them as members of the same clone. In contrast to other clonal assays which require physical proximity to identify members of a clone, the use of chromosome translocation allows the identification of members of the clone even when the differentiative progeny are found in different tissues. Since one property of lymphoid cells is their ability to recirculate through the blood and lymph, this technique is invaluable in determining differentiation pathways of the lymphoid system. This method also makes it possible to study the relationship between myeloid differentiation which occurs primarily in the bone marrow and T lymphocyte differentiation which requires the migration of marrow-derived cells to the thymus where differentiation to functional lymphocytes occurs.

To study more carefully the differentiation pathway of myeloid and lymphoid systems, we modified the method of Wu et al. to allow the study of stem cells with limited or restricted differentiative potential. The details of this modification are described elsewhere[15]. In brief, mice of genotype W/W^v were exposed to a low dose (250-400 rads) of ionizing radiation and then injected with 2 x 10^7 irradiated (700 rads) bone marrow cells from coisogenic normal donors. The use of congenitally anemic W/W^v mice as recipients is essential for these experiments. Because the W mutation results in defective hemopoietic stem cells, the grafted stem cells have a selective advantage over the host stem cells of the W/W^v recipient. However, the presence of defective W/W^v stem cells contributes to the survival of the mice and allows the injection of small numbers of normal stem cells. Under these conditions, the myeloid system, in approximately one-third of the recipients is predominantly repopulated from a single, chromosomally marked stem cell.

The irradiated cells were allowed to grow and to differentiate in the recipients for at least 8 months. This long interval of time was chosen to select for long-lived stem cells with significant self-renewal potential. To study the differentiative potential of marked stem cells in these recipients, karyotypic analysis was done on dividing cells in different tissues. Myeloid cells were studied by examining spontaneously dividing cells in bone marrow which are predominantly myeloid. In addition, spleen colonies were produced by injecting bone marrow cells into irradiated animals; after 12 days individual colonies were dissected from the spleen and dividing cells were examined for the presence of a unique chromosome translocation. As shown by Becker et al.[7] and Wu et al.[8], when a marker is present in a spleen colony, it is present in all of the cells in that colony. To analyze lymphoid cells, splenic lymphocytes were isolated and cultured with LPS, a B cell mitogen, or PHA, a T cell mitogen. After 3 days of incubation, the mitotic cells were analyzed for the presence of a chromosome translocation.

TABLE 1

CLASSES OF STEM CELLS DETECTABLE WITH RADIATION-
INDUCED CHROMOSOME TRANSLOCATIONS

	Potential for Differentiation		
Type of Stem Cell	Myeloid Cells	LPS Blasts (B cells)	PHA Blasts (T cells)
Pluripotent	+	+	+
Myeloid-restricted	+	-	-
T cell-restricted	-	-	+

A total of 50 recipients were examined in this series of experiments. Chromosome translocations occurred in high frequency in 15 mice. Analysis of the 15 relevent animals showed that chromosomally marked, long-lived stem cells followed one of three patterns of differentiation. These patterns are summarized in Table 1. The most common occurrence was the presence of the same translocation in the myeloid system, i.e. in the spontaneously dividing cells in bone marrow and in spleen colonies and in both LPS and PHA blasts. In these recipients the translocation must have occurred in a pluripotent stem cell capable of producing both myeloid and lymlphoid progeny. Another frequently occurring tissue distribution was one in which the chromosome translocation was found only in the myeloid system. In such recipients, the myeloid tissue contained a large proportion of cells with the marker but none of the lymphoid blasts contained the unique chromosome translocation. Presumably such recipients were repopulated by a stem cell already committed to myeloid differentiation. While the lymphoid system in these recipients was normal, it was not possible to determine whether the lymphoid cells were derived from the W/W^V recipient or from unmarked stem cells derived from the normal donor. When bone marrow from a W/W^V recipient showing the myeloid-restricted distribution of an abnormal chromosome was transplanted into a heavily irradiated syngeneic recipient, the irradiated recipient again showed the same abnormal karyotype restricted to the myeloid system. This observation indicates that the translocation occurred in a myeloid-restricted stem cell with significant self-renewed potential. The rarest type of tissue distribution of chromosome markers, observed only in two recipients, was limited to the PHA blasts; neither the myeloid system nor the LPS blasts contained significant numbers of the chromosome translocation which was present in high frequency in the PHA blasts. We interpret this finding to mean that the bone marrow of adult mice contains stem cells already restricted to T cell differentiation. On the basis of other experiments, Kadish and Basch have also postulated the existence of a prethymic stem cell in adult bone marrow[16].

In summary, the experiments using radiation-induced chromosome translocations to mark individual stem cells shows that determination is an early event in the differentiation of the hemopoietic system. Pluripotent stem cells can become committed to differentiate along a specific pathway, e.g., either myeloid or T lymphocyte, without losing their potential for self-renewal. It is perhaps surprising that we did not observe a stem cell committed to B lymphocyte differentiation or a stem cell committed to B and T lymphocyte differentiation. The nature of our experiments makes it impossible for us to make conclusions about pathways where we failed to detect a marker. It is possible that such stem cells do not exist. However, it is also possible that such restricted stem cells do occur but that their frequency is lower than the three types of stem cells detected in this series. Infrequent stem cells or stem cells with limited self-renewal potential are difficult to detect with this method.

IN VITRO GROWTH OF MYELOID AND LYMPHOID PROGENITORS

The technique of radiation-induced chromosome markers is useful for analyzing the progeny of long-lived stem cells. However, it is not suitable for studies on short-lived stem cells which do not have the potential to repopulate a significant proportion of the myeloid or lymphoid systems of a deficient host. This method is also not useful for studies on the regulation of early events in the differentiation of the hemopoietic system. A cell culture system would overcome many of these difficulties. While many investigators have established in vitro clonal assays for late stages in the differentiation of the myeloid system[2], only the procedure described by Dexter generates an in vitro environment that promotes long-term proliferation and differentiation of hemopoietic stem cells. Dexter has recently reviewed the various ways in which the in vitro system mimics the growth and differentiation of stem cells in vivo[17].

There are several unique features of the Dexter culture system. The system as initially described required a high concentration (20-25%) of horse serum; only selected batches of horse serum supported the growth of hemopoietic cells. In addition, the cultures had to be inoculated twice with bone marrow cells. Following the first inoculation of bone marrow cells into the flask, a few cells adhered to the bottom and developed large fat vacuoles. Stem cells, as measured by the spleen colony assay, rapidly died following the first inoculation of bone marrow. When a second sample of bone marrow cells was added to the flask, the stem cells tended to remain in suspension but clustered around the fat cells established from the first inoculation. At this stage one-half to three-quarters of the non-adherent cells could be removed at weekly intervals without depleting the cultures of stem cell activity or of nucleated cells. Following this procedure stem cells could be maintained in vitro for between 6 and 10 weeks.

A recent advance was described by Greenberger who found that the addition of 10^{-7} M hydrocortisone allows the use of almost any batch of horse serum and perhaps even of other sera as well[18]. In addition, it prolongs the survival of stem cells in vitro; we have obtained CFU-S from cultures up to 20 weeks after initiation.

Since T lymphocytes require the thymus epithelium for their differentiation, it is not surprising that Dexter cultures lack functional T lymphocytes; possible T cell precursors are detectable (see below). Functional B lymphocytes are also undetectable in Dexter cultures. B cells are normally produced in bone marrow and since the culture maintains all of the myeloid elements including erythroid precursors, one would expect B lymphocytes or their immediate precursors, pre-B cells, to be present in the cultures. Dexter did not observe any cells with surface Ig in long-term cultures; using a sensitive limiting dilution assay[19,20], we could not detect functional B lymphocytes or pre-B cells and concluded that they must exist at frequencies less than 1 in 10^5. The absence of mature lymphoid cells in the cultures suggested that the in vitro environment selected for myeloid restricted stem cells and that the multipotent and lymphoid-restricted stem cells did not survive in vitro. To test the potential of cultured stem cells to produce lymphoid progeny, we harvested cells from the culture and injected them into irradiated recipients. The cultured stem cells carried a stable chromosome marker, T6, to distinguish them from cells of the irradiated recipient. Two months after injection, karyotype analyses were done on dividing myeloid and lymphoid cells to determine whether or not any of the cultured cells differentiated into LPS-responsive B cells or Con A-responsive T cells. The results of this experiment, published in detail elsewhere[21], showed clearly that cultured stem cells had the potential to produce both myeloid and lymphoid progeny in irradiated recipients; the T6 chromosomes which marked the cultured cells were found in myeloid cells in bone marrow and in both LPS and Con A blasts from splenic lymphocytes. Thus, the long-term cultured cells retain the potential for lymphoid differentiation, and the absence of lymphoid cells in vitro must reflect a defect in the in vitro environment rather than a defect in the cultured stem cells.

Two other interesting observations were made in this series of experiments. First, in some recipients, T6 marked cells were observed only in the lymphoid system; the cultured cells did not make a significant contribution to the regeneration of myeloid cells which must have come from the irradiated host. This observation is consistent with the idea that the separation of the myeloid and lymphoid pathways of differentiation is an early event in the differentiation of the hemopoietic system. The in vitro conditions which are obviously good for myeloid differentiation could lead to a partial exhaustion of myeloid stem cells so that they do not have sufficient proliferative potential to repopulate the myeloid eystem of an irradiated recipient. In contrast, lymphoid differentiation is not detectable in vitro so any lymphoid-restricted stem cells are unlikely to have exhausted their differentiative potential in culture.

The second interesting finding was the close correlation between B and T lymphocyte differentiation. In 28 mice with a detectable proportion of marked cells in either LPS or PHA blasts, it was observed that the proportion of marked cells in LPS blasts was always similar to the proportion of marked cells in Con A blasts (Figure 1). These data clearly indicate there is a strong correlation in the penetration of marked cells into each lymphoid pathway. Although several explanations for this correlation are possible, a likely explanation is that the cultures contain a lymphoid-restricted stem cell with the potential to produce both B and T lymphocytes but not myeloid cells. If separate stem cells for B lymphocytes and for T lymphocytes existed in vitro, we should occasionally have observed mice that had a high proportion of their B lymphocytes derived from the cultured cells and their T lymphocytes derived from host stem cells, or vice versa. No such animals were observed, and we suggest that the correlation represents the existence of a common lymphoid stem cell which is maintained in vitro and which can produce large numbers of B and T lymphocyte progeny when placed in the proper environment such as an irradiated recipient. These data represent the only evidence we have obtained for a common lymphoid stem cell. If such stem cells exist, they should be detectable by applying the techniques of radiation-induced chromosome markers to cultured stem cells. Repopulation of suitable recipients with irradiated, cultured stem cells should produce some recipients with the same radiation-induced translocation in both B and T cells, but not in myeloid cells.

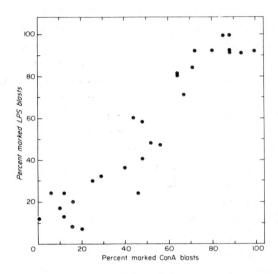

Fig. 1   Correlation between the proportion of nitogen-responsive B and T lymphocytes produced from cultured bone marrow cells. Bone marrow cells obtained from mice with a stable chromosome translocation were cultured for several weeks and then tested for lymphoid potential by injection into irradiated syngenic recipients having a normal karyotype. After two months, splenic lymphocytes were isolated and stimulated with LPS or Con A. Each point in the figure represents the data obtained from one recipient. The ordinate gives the percent of dividing LPS-responsive cells (B cells) with the chromosome marker and the abscissa the percent marked mitoses in cells stimulated with Con A (T cells).

The above experiments show that stem cells from Dexter cultures retain their lymphoid potential. Therefore, it should be possible to modify the tissue culture conditions to permit the differentiation and survival of B lymphocytes and their precursors. Preliminary experiments show that horse serum is especially toxic to B lymphocytes; addition of as little as 1% horse serum markedly inhibits the differentiation of B lymphocytes (unpublished data). Perhaps the addition of hydrocortisone and other hormones, together with the refinements in tissue culture media described by Iscove and his colleagues[22] will eliminate the need for horse serum and allow the use of conditions suitable for B lymphocyte differentiation.

Recent studies in our laboratory indicate that T lymphocyte precursors remain in Dexter cultures for at least 17 weeks. Jacobs and Miller described an *in vitro* colony assay for presumptive T cell progenitors (TL-CFU)[23]. When spleen cells from congenitally athymic mice or bone marrow cells from normal mice are incubated in semi-solid medium containing a conditioned medium prepared from human peripehral blood cells, colonies with 200 cells appear by day 6 of incubation. The cells within individual colonies bear the Thy 1 antigen on their surface, but the original colony-forming cells lack this antigen and are resistant to anti-Thy 1 antibody and complement. The functional properties of this class of cells remains to be elucidated but preliminary experiments indicate that these cells are involved in the regulation of immune responses. Dexter cultures contain large numbers of TL-CFU with properties identical to those TL-CFU obtained from normal bone marrow. If the T cell nature of the colonies can be confirmed, these data will represent the first indications for lymphoid differentiation in long-term cultures of bone marrow.

The *in vitro* culture system offers many advantages over the *in vivo* models used previously. The cell populations can be separated to study the interaction between the monolayer (microenvironment?) and the nonadherent stem cells. Separation could also be used to analyze different subpopulations of stem cells. The ability to sample the same culture repeatedly will make it possible to do detailed kinetic studies on cells at different stages of differentiation of and to study short-lived stem cells that heretofore have been undetectable in *in vivo* assays. Finally, the culture system described by Dexter should make it possible to study *in vitro* some of the factors that influence determination in hemopoietic stem cells.

ACKNOWLEDGEMENTS

Technical assistance was provided by S. Harrison, R. Kuba and W. Holmes. The research was supported by grants from the Medical Research Council and The National Cancer Institute of Canada.

REFERENCES

1. Illmensee, K. and Croce, C.M. (1979) Proc. Natl. Acad. Sci. U.S.A., 76, 879-883.

2. Metcalf, D. (1977) Recent Results in Cancer Research, 61, 1-227.

3. Burgess, A.W., Metcalf, D., Nicola, N.A. and Russell, S.H.M. (1978) Hematopoietic Cell Differentiation, Academic Press, New York, pp. 399-416.

4. Johnson, G.R. and Metcalf, D. (1978) Differentiation of Normal and Neoplastic Hematopoietic Cells, Cold Spring Harbor Laboratory, New York, pp. 49-62.

5. Siminovitch, L., McCulloch, E.A. and Till, J.E. (1963) J. Cell. Comp. Physiol., 62, 327-336.

6. Till, J.E. and McCulloch, E.A. (1961) Radiat. Res., 14, 213-222.

7. Becker, A.J., McCulloch, E.A. and Till, J.E. (1963) Nature, 197, 452-454.

8. Wu, A.M., Till, J.E., Siminovitch, L. and McCulloch, E.A. (1967) J. Cell. Physiol., 69, 177-184.

9. Lala, P.K. and Johnson, G.R. (1978) J. Exp. Med., 148, 1468-1477.

10. Micklem, H.S., Ford, C.E., Evans, E.P. and Gray, J. (1966) Proc. Roy. Soc. London B, 165, 78- 102.

11. Wu, A.M., Till, J.E., Siminovitch, L. and McCulloch, E.A. (1968) J. Exp. Med., 127, 455- 463.

12. Trentin, J., Wolf, N., Cheng, V., Fahlberg, W., Weiss, D. and Bonhag, R. (1967) J. Immunol., 98, 1326-1387.

13. Yung, L.L.L., Wyn-Evans, T.C. and Diener, E. (1973) Eur. J. Immunol., 3, 224-228.

14. Barnes, D.W.H., Evans, E.P., Ford, C.E. and West, B.J. (1968) Nature, 219, 518-520.

15. Abramson, S., Miller, R.G. and Phillips, R.A. (1977) J. Exp. Med., 145, 1567-1579.

16. Kadish, J.L. and Basch, R.S. (1976) J. Exp. Med., 143, 1082-1099.

17. Dexter, T.M., Allan, T.D., Lajtha, L.G., Krizsa, F., Testa, N.G. and Moore, M.A.S. (1978) Differentiation of Normal and Neoplastic Hematopoietic Cells, Cold Spring Harbor Laboratory, New York, pp. 63-80.

18. Greenberger, J.S. (1978) Nature, 275, 752-754.

19. Lau, C., Melchers, F., Miller, R.G. and Phillips, R.A. (1979) J. Immunol., 122, 1273-1277.

20. Andersson, J., Coutinho, A., Lernhardt, W. and Melchers, F. (1977) Cell, 10, 27-34.

21. Jones-Villeneuve, E.V. and Phillips, R.A. (1980) Exp. Hematol., 8, in press.

22. Iscove, N.N. and Melchers, F. (1978) J. Exp. Med., 147, 923-933.

23. Jacobs, S.W. and Miller, R.G. (1979) J. Immunol., 122, 582-584.

Cell Lineage, Stem Cells and Cell Determination
INSERM Symposium No. 10
Editor: N. Le Douarin
© *1979 Elsevier/North-Holland Biomedical Press*

THREE WAVES OF B-LYMPHOCYTE DEVELOPMENT DURING EMBRYONIC
DEVELOPMENT OF THE MOUSE

Fritz Melchers

Basel Institute for Immunology, Grenzacherstrasse 487
CH 4058 BASEL, Switzerland

B-lymphocytes develop from pluripotent stem cells which are
ancestors of erythrocytes, megakaryocytes and platelets, monocytes
and macrophages, granulocytes, and lymphocytes of T-and B-lineage.
Little is known of the hierarchies of cellular developments which
lead to the determinations of these different cell lineages. B-
lymphocytes are characterized by their capacity to synthesize
immunoglobulins(Ig). We expect that for the expression of Ig
heavy (H) and light (L) chains genes the genes for variable (v)
and constant (c) regions of Ig molecules have to be linked on the
DNA level (1). Current estimates of the germ line repertoire of
Ig v-region genes are as high as 50 for each v_H and for v_L,
variable regions linked to H or to L- chains (2). Approximately
15 to 25 genes appear to be carried in the germ line for the c-
region of H- and L-chains. The first cells expressing Ig molecules in the mouse have been found during embryonic development in
fetal liver. These precursor B-cells (pre B-cells) synthesize μ-
H-chains and κ-L-chains as 8S $(L_2\mu_2)$-molecules at a rapid turn-
over (3). The original repertoire of v-region specificities of
50x50 $(v_H x v_L) = 2.5x10^3$ different binding sites carried in the
germ line is expanded during embryonic development and ontogeny
of the lymphoid cell system approximately 100 fold (4) to $5x10^3 v_H$
and $5x10^3 v_L$ or $2.5x10^7$ different v_H/v_L combinations.

The differentiation of pluripotent and multipotent stem cells and precursors to cells of the B-lineage has long been thought to be influenced by the microenvironment in which these cells find themselves or to which they migrate (5). Different microenvironments have been expected to influence the decisions of such stem cells to become committed to the different lineages of the blood cell forming system (6). Recently this concept has obtained impressive support when Zinkernagel et al. (7) demonstrated that precursors of mature T-lymphocytes differentiate in the thymus on epithelial structures encoded for by the K-, I- and D-region genes of the major histocompatibility locus. Similar structures and corresponding genes operating in B-lymphocyte - differentiation have so far not been identified, although the hope remains that knowledge of the sites of differentiation in the organism will lead the way to the identification of structures, and eventually genes, on which B-cells differentiate. The concept of microenvironmental control of precursor differentiation has not been challenged by the findings of Johnsson and Metcalf (8) - although proposed by these authors as a challenge - that single pluripotent precursor cells in culture can give rise to poly-specific colonies containing more than one differentiation form of blood cells. This type of differentiation depends on soluble factors obtained from cells which may well be the normal site of differentiation for such cells. The intriguing possibility exists that such soluble factors from cells, are in fact, surface membrane-derived and thereby abolish the need for cell-cell contact in "in vitro" studies of blood cell differentiation.

Besides the more general biological interest in B-lymphocyte differentiation which centers around the questions of environmentally and genetically controlled steps in the choice of a stem cell to commit its progeny to the B-cell lineage the immune system is concerned with the involvement of the v_H/v_L-binding repertoire determined by germ-line genes in this B-cell development. In particular it has been suggested by Jerne (9) that such germ-line v-regions recognize "self-antigens", maybe in modes

similar to a recognition of "differentiation antigens". Furthermore, this hypothesis predicts that the variability of v-region
genes created during embryonic development and ontogeny is a
result of this original recognition: germ-line specificites of v-
regions are selected against, creating survival values for
mutants which can no longer recognize "self-antigens" and are,
thus, mutated in the binding sites, composed of the hyper-variable
regions of Ig-v-regions. This would, at the same time, explain
acqusition of tolerance against self antigens.

Triggering of committed, mature B-lymphocytes, however, not
only involves v_H/v_L regions on Ig molecules on the surface of B-
cells but also so-called mitogen receptors(10). Mitogens are
best compared to growth hormones and can stimulate, at the appropriate concentrations and with additional activation steps, B-
cells in a polyclonal fashion so that as much as one third of all
B-cells is stimulated to growth and to maturation into IgM- and
IgG-secreting cells (11). Driving forces in B-cell development,
therefore, most likely include mitogens in addition to antigens,
recognized by mitogen receptors in addition to v_H/v_L regions on
Ig molecules. This has recently led to a modification (12) of
the original Jerne-hypothesis, now postulating that mitogen-
receptors and v-regions must share antigenic determinants in
order to account for the negative selection pressure postulated
by Jerne. It is because of this interest in the somatic development of variability in v-region genes in B-cells that immunology
shows interest in B-cell development.

Differentiated B-cells can be identified by their capacity
to make Ig. Early precursors and later antigen-sensitive B-cells
synthesize Ig and insert the synthesized molecule into the surface
membrane (3), do, however, not actively secrete Ig. Final stimulation to Ig-secretion involves the activation of small, resting
B-cells containing Ig and mitogen-receptors in their surface
membrane to growth and the development of secretory cells by
external or internal mitogens. Normally, this stimulation balan-
ces between growth and secretion during the cell cycle (13).

Under the approximate conditions B-cells can, however, either
only grow but not mature to secretion, or mature to secretion but
not grow (14,15). As Ig-secreting cells these final stages of B-
cell development can be identified as plaque-forming cells (16).

Studies of B-cell differentiation "in vitro" from precursor
cells isolated from different organs at different times of development have used the rationale to identify B-cells and any of
their precursors by their capacity to develop "in vitro" and, in
their final stages, driven by the external mitogen lipopolysaccha-
ride (LPS) into Ig-secreting cells. This has, in large parts,
only been possible since a plaque assay was developed for all
cells secreting Ig irrespective of their antigen-binding specificities (17), and since mouse lymphocyte culture conditions have
undergone significant improvements (13,18,19,20).

Murine B-cell development between day 9 and 13 of gestation

The first phase of B-lymphocyte development into LPS-
reactive B-cells, stimulated by LPS to IgM- and IgG- secreting,
plaque forming cells (PFC) can be observed practically simultaneously with the establishment of blood circulation in the embryo.
After day 9 of gestation the main sites, where pre B-cells can be
found, are placenta (21) and embryonal blood (F. Melchers and J.
Abramczuk, in preparation) but not liver (Table I). The frequencies of pre B-cells developing "in vitro" into LPS-reactive
B-cells increase until day 12, thereafter decline rapidly and
simultaneously in placenta and embryonal blood. From the kinetics
of PFC-development it is estimated that LPS-reactivity in these
cells is reached between day 14 and 15 of gestation. The repertoire of v-regions is largely unknown for these cells, must,
however, be heterogeneous since $\sim$ 1 in 100 cells produce IgM
molecules which can lyse TNP-sheep red cells (TNP-SRC) and 1 in
1000 which can lyse SRC. The molecular form of the secreted IgM-
molecules secreted after LPS-stimulation is indistinguishable
from 19S IgM molecules secreted from adult, stimulated B-cells.
On the other hand, precursors of B-cells at day 11 and 12 of

gestation in embryonal blood appear to produce unusual forms of Ig-molecues, namely H-chains only (in preparation). This points to the interesting possibility that the first pre B-cells expressing Ig-molecules may use the recognition of separate v-regions (here of V_H only) and thereby, may reduce the recognition repertoire carried in the germ-line for v_H and v_L from 50x50 = 2.5x10^3 to 50x50 =10^2 (see before).

B-cell development between day 12/13 of gestation and birth
(day 19)

Fetal liver is the second site recognized in embryonic development of the mouse where pre B-cells as well as other blood cell precursors and stem cells can be found. The frequencies of pre B-cells acquiring LPS-reactivity "in vitro" rise from approximately one in 10^6 fetal liver cells at day 13 of gestation to one in 30 at birth (20). At birth, however, the liver cells have actually acquired LPS-reactivity and may no longer be seen as pre B-cells. Acquisition of LPS-reactivity is at that time (day 19 of gestation, equivalent to birth) and occurs for all liver cells at this same time, regardless of when during gestation they have been removed from the embryo and put in culture (22). As for pre B-cells from placenta this shows a very time-accurate preprogramming of the differentiating events which will take place in the pre B-cells. It argues either that the micro-environment of the liver is no longer necessary once the cells have been committed to run through the program pre B - B, or that fetal liver cell suspensions retain "in vitro" the microenvironmental properties which they normally exert "in vivo". In view of the soluble factors derived from such and similar cells which enable pluripotent stem cells to differentiate to the different cell lineages "in vitro" (8, see above) the latter possibility appears equally likely.

The secreted molecules of LPS-stimulated descendents of pre B-cells in fetal liver are mostly 19S IgM, also 7S IgG, and mono- and polymeric IgA. Pre B-cells in fetal liver at day 14 and 15 of gestation synthesize predominantly 8S IgM molecules. It is not clear at present whether H-chains or L-chains alone may be synthesized earlier. The repertoire of antigen-binding IgM-molecules secreted by LPS stimulated B-cells stemming from fetal liver pre B-cells is heterogenous. The extent of its hetero-geneity and its original specificities are currently under inve-stigation (W. Gerhard and F. Melchers, in preparation).

B-cell development for day 16/17 of gestation and during adult life.

The third, and apparently final site of B-cell development is bone marrow. From day 16/17 of gestation and through adult life B-cells are generated from stem cells and pre B-cells in continous waves, so that $3\times10^7-10^8$ B-cells emerge per day into the circulation and into the secondary lymphoid organs (23). Pre B-cells and B-cells very similar to those found in fetal liver (the second site of development) can be identified (24,25). The repertoire of antigen-binding specificities is at the moment indistinguishable from that in fetal liver. It remains obscure why liver does not retain beyond birth the capacity to generate B-cells but exhibits only one wave of development, while bone marrow is a B-cell generating organ for practically the whole life.

Conclusions.

Three sites for B-lymphocyte development during embryonic development of the mouse can be defined. They closely resemble the sites of development of erythrocytes. In this context it will be interesting to see whether the first site of B-cell development, placenta and embryonic blood, is actually seeded by stem cells of extraembryonic origin, i.e. from yolk sac, and whether the unusual H-chain-only expression in these pre B-cells is, in fact, analogous to the expression of a separate fetal hemoglobin (C. Cudennec and J.-P. Thiery, this volume). This may then point to a separate gene for H-chain, which is separate from adult, normal H-chain, but forms a product crossreactive with adult H-chain. It is also tempting to speculate that such an "embryonal H-chain" may be the product of a common precursor for T- and B-cells. Clonal identification with "in vitro" methods of earlier precursors of the B-lineage towards the pluripotent stem cells is needed to probe these speculations.

Very little is known of the genes and their products which regulate B-lymphocyte development. It may be the preoccupied mind of an immunologist which expects molecules operative in growth regulation of mature, immunocompetent cells also to be involved in B-cell differentiation from stem cells. These growth-regulating molecules on B-cells, Ig variable and constant regions, Ia-molecules and mitogen receptors and their genes, as well as the molecules and genes which fit them, are the prime candidates for such a preoccupied mind.

References

1. Brack, C., Hirama, M., Lenhard-Schuller, R. and Tonegawa, S. (1978) Cell 15, 1.

2. Tonegawa, S. Brack, C., Hozumi, N., Matthyssens, G. and Schuller, R. (1977) Immunol. Rev. 36, 73.

3. Melchers, F., von Boehmer, H., and Phillips, R.A. (1976) Transplant. Rev. 25, 26.

4. Weigert, M., and Riblet, R. (1976) Cold Spring Harbor Symp. Quant. Biol. 41, 837.

5. Trentin, J.J., McGarry, M.P.; Jenkins, V.K.; Gallagher,M.Y. Speirs, R.S.; and Wolf, M.N. (1971) in: Morphological and functional aspects of immunity, ed. K. Lindahl-Kiessling, G.A. Alm and M.G. Hanna, Plenum Press, New York, p.289.

6. Moore, M.A.S.;and Owen, J.J.T. (1965) Nature 208, 956.

7. Zinkernagel, R.M., Callahan, G.N., Klein, J. and Dennert, G. (1978) Nature 271, 251.

8. Johnson, G.F.; and Metcalf, D. (1977). Proc. Natl. Acad. Sci. U.S. 74, 3879.

9. Jerne, N.K. (1971) Eur. J. Immunol. 1, 1.

References (continued)

10. Möller, G., ed. (1972) Transpl. Rev. ii, 1.

11. Andersson, J., Coutinho, A., and Melchers F. (1979) J. Exp. Med. 149, 553.

12. Coutinho, A.; Forni, L.; and Blomberg, B. (1978) J. exp. Med. 148, 862.

13. Andersson, J.; Coutinho, A.; Lernhardt, W.; and Melchers, F. (1977) Cell 10, 27.

14. Andersson, J.; and Melchers, F. (1978), Eur. J. Immunol. 4, 533.

15. Andersson, J.; Bullock,W.W.; and Melchers, F. (1974) Eur. J. Immunol. 4, 715.

16. Jerne, N.K.; and Nordin, A.A. (1963) Science 140, 405.

17. Gronowicz, E.; Coutinho, A.; and Melchers, F. (1976) Eur. J. Immunol. 6, 588.

18. Iscove, N.N. and Melchers, F. (1978) J. exp. Med. 147, 923.

19. Melchers, F. (1977) Eur. J. Immunol. 7, 476.

20. Melchers, F. (1977) Eur. J. Immunol. 7, 482.

21. Melchers, F. (1979) Nature 277, 219.

22. Melchers, F.; Andersson, J. and Phillips, R.A. (1977) Cold Spring Harbor Symp. Quant. Biol. 41, 147.

23. Brahim, F.; and Osmond, D.G. (1973) Anat. Rev. 175, 737.

24. Lau,C.A.; Melchers, F.; Miller, R.G.; and Phillips, R.A. (1979) J. Immunol. 122, 1273.

25. Phillips, R.A.; and Melchers, F. (1979) J. Immunol. 122, 1473.

STABILITY OF THE DETERMINED STATE

Cell Lineage, Stem Cells and Cell Determination
INSERM Symposium No. 10
Editor: N. Le Douarin
© 1979 Elsevier/North-Holland Biomedical Press

fs(1)K10, A FEMALE STERILE MUTATION ALTERING THE PATTERN OF BOTH
THE EGG COVERINGS AND THE RESULTANT EMBRYOS IN *DROSOPHILA*

ERIC WIESCHAUS

European Molecular Biology Laboratory, Postfach 10.2209,
6900 Heidelberg, Federal Republic of Germany

In *Drosophila* both the coverings of the unfertilized egg and
the embryo destined to develop in them have clearly defined spacial
patterns and sufficient landmarks to identify their dorsal-ventral
and anterior-posterior axes. In normal development, the anterior
end of the embryo develops at the anterior end of the egg as defined by the coverings, and the dorsal side of the embryo at the
egg's dorsal side. Since it is unlikely that the pattern of the
coverings actively influences the embryonic development in *Drosophila*, the normal correspondence probably indicates that the pattern of the embryo and the pattern of the egg coverings both reflect the same organizing mechanism, i.e. the polarity of the developing oocyte. For a genetic analysis of the process whereby this
primary polarity is established, the useful mutations will be maternal effect mutations which alter both the pattern of the egg
shells and that of the resultant embryo.

In the following pages I will describe such a mutation and some
experiments involving chimeras and genetic mosaics designed to determine the ovarian cell type in which the mutation has its effect.

The mutation is called *fs(1)K10* and is a recessive female sterile located on the tip of the X-chromosome[1]. Its most striking
effect is on the pattern of the outermost egg covering, the chorion.
The most obvious landmark for the dorsal side of the chorion in
normal eggs are two respiratory appendages secreted at the anterior
end (Figure 1). In eggs from *K10* females, the appendages have been
extended onto a ring of appendage material circling the egg as
though its entire circumference has become dorsalized. The chorion
is secreted in the last stages of oogenesis by the follicle cells

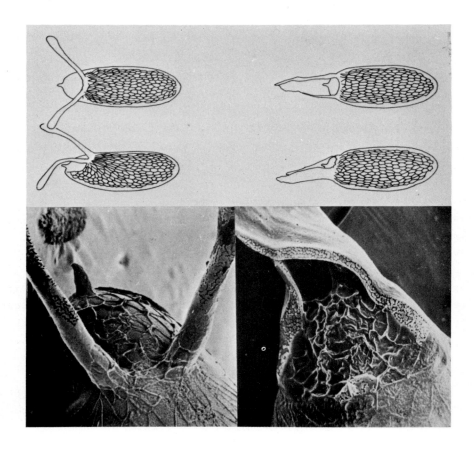

Fig. 1.   Chorion patterns in normal *(left)* and *K10 (right)* eggs.
The upper *camera lucida* drawings show the follicle cell imprints
viewed from the dorsal and lateral side, the lower SEM photographs
show details of the dorsal appendages.

which surround each oocyte[2].   These cells leave imprints on the
chorion which can be seen in the egg after it is laid.   Since the
imprints in the dorsal regions of the chorion are normally much
more elongated than those found ventrally, it is possible to use
their shape in *K10* eggs as an additional criterion for dorsaliz-

ation. The patterns of imprints in the lateral and ventral regions
of *K10* eggs are more elongated than normal, especially in anterior
and middle regions of the egg. No effect of *K10* is detected in
posterior regions, although here the differences between dorsal
and ventral patterns of normal eggs are so small that it would be
difficult to rule out some effect.

The *K10* mutation does not result in a total elimination of dorsal-ventral polarity. The dorsal-most region of a *K10* egg can
always be identified in that the ring of dorsal appendage material
is not continuous but, as in wild type eggs, begins only somewhat
to the right and left of the apparent dorsal midline. Instead,
the chorions of *K10* eggs seem to lack ventral positions and ventral
pattern elements. If one were to describe a cross-section of the
pattern in a normal egg with circumferential values from 0 to 9 in
mirror image symmetry along the right and left sides, with the "0"

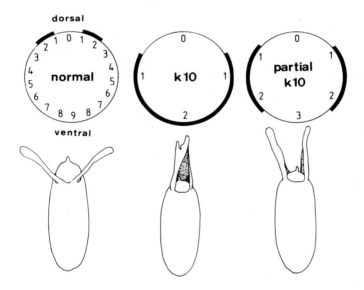

Fig. 2. Schematic diagram describing the modified circumferential
pattern in complete and partial *K10* eggs (see text).

position marking dorsal and the "9" position marking ventral, then
the dorsal appendages would normally be secreted between positions
1 to 2 (Figure 2). The altered phenotype of *K10* eggs can be described in a circumference where the values extend only from 0 to 2
such that now dorsal appendage material is secreted around the
entire egg.

Although the penetrance of the *K10* mutation is one hundred percent, the phenotype of the eggs varies somewhat from one egg to
the next and in about 5% of the eggs the dorsal appendage material
does not extend totally around the circumference but is interrupted
at the ventral side. These eggs can be described using the same
simplified model used for complete *K10* eggs, with the exception
that in such "partial" *K10* eggs, the ventral-most positional value
might reach 3 or 4 (Figure 2). Thus, dorsal appendages would be
secreted only on the two sides, leaving a ventral area which in
fact has only values characteristic of the lateral side of the egg.

Although the model in Figure 2 is intended to be more descriptive than causal, it may tell us about what is happening in the
K10 oocyte because it also adequately describes the pattern of dorsalization observed in embryos which develop in *K10* eggs. Most of
the eggs from *K10* females are not fertilized, probably due to the
altered egg covering interfering with the access of the sperm to
the micropyle. The fraction which reaches the blastoderm stage,
however, develops to form highly abnormal larvae with a pattern of
dorsalization consistent with that observed in the chorion. The
first abnormalities become apparent at the onset of gastrulation
when the ventral region of normal embryos invaginate to form mesoderm[3]. *K10* embryos do not make this invagination. Instead, in the
ventral region, one observes a continuation of the folds which are
normally found only on the dorsal side of the embryo (Figure 3).
This dorsalization is more extreme in the anterior region of the
embryo. Posteriorly, an invagination apparently corresponding to
the posterior midgut or the proctodeum is formed, moves dorsally
and envelops the pole cells. The dorsalization observed in *K10*
gastrula and its anterior posterior extent can also be seen in the
final pattern of the larvae which develop from such embryos. The

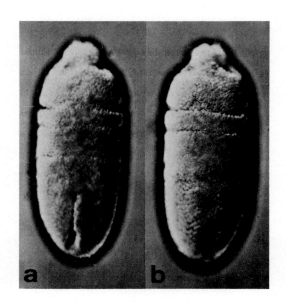

Fig. 3. Dorsal (a) and ventral (b) views of *K10* gastrula showing the absence of the invagination for the mesodermal precursors which normally occur at the ventral side.

anterior ends of such animals consist of a tube of dorsal skin with the characteristic hair pattern of the anterior dorsal region of the larvae (Figure 4). Posteriorly the pattern becomes progress-ively less dorsal and the posterior regions often show spiracles and anal organs, as well as the setae and ventral hypoderm of the last two segments. This anterior-posterior gradient in the extent of dorsalization has also been confirmed by the results of *in vivo* cultures of *K10* embryos to determine the types of imaginal struc-tures they form. It is known from gynandromorph mapping that the anlage for the different imaginal discs occupy defined positions in the blastoderm[4,5]: the labial and humeral discs are situated most dorsally, the eye, the anternal, wing and leg lie in the lateral region and the genital disc lies most ventrally, although in the

extreme posterior of the animal. With the exception of some dorsally derived discs (labial and perhaps humeral), about 90% of the
identifiable discs obtained from cultured *K10* are genital, that is,
discs derived from the posterior ventral region of the embryo
(Wieschaus, unpublished). No eye-antenal, wing or leg structures
are formed in spite of the fact that these midlateral discs represent about 80% of the yield from the control cultures of wild
type embryos.

At present we cannot explain why the dorsalization is much more
extreme in the anterior end of the embryo and why posterior differ-

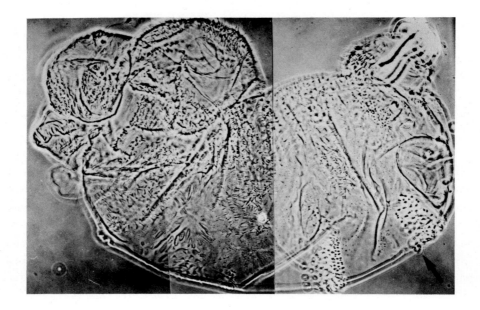

Fig. 4. Abnormal larva developing from a *K10* egg with the dorsalized anterior end to the left. Arrow indicates the normal ventral
hypoderm in the posterior region.

entiation often approaches normal. The phenotype is in any case
reminiscent of the pattern observed in the chorion where the most
obvious dorsalization was the ring of dorsal appendage material at
the anterior end of the egg. The correlation between the patterns
of the chorion and the embryo can be made more precise by using
the partial *K10* eggs to provide an intermediate point. The embryonic pattern observed in these eggs is similar to that found in
complete *K10* eggs but is somewhat more ventralized in the anterior
region. Partial *K10* eggs are twice as likely as complete *K10* eggs
to form ventral hypoderm of segments 7 and 8 and ten times as
likely to form ventral hypoderm in segments 1, 2 or 3 (Wieschaus,
unpublished).

Given the dramatic effect on egg morphology, it is not surprising that the *K10* expression depends on the genotype of the mother.
We have begun morphological studies of oogenesis in mutant and wild
type females to determine the earliest indications of a change in
dorsal-ventral polarity in the mutant oocyte. One of the advantages of a mutation which alters the visible structures of the egg
is that the synthesis of these structures can be followed back into
oogenesis and serve as landmarks or starting points for such an
analysis. The preliminary studies completed so far indicate that
at least after stage 10 of King[2], the most visible effect of the
K10 mutation concerns the migration and secretion of the follicle
cells which surround the developing oocyte. In a normal oocyte,
the follicle cells in the future dorsal region of the egg become
very thick and columnar, especially at the points where the dorsal
appendages will be secreted. In *K10* oocytes, the entire circumference of the oocyte has this thickened appearance and one cannot
distinguish any region with the thinner follicle cells characteristic of the ventral side.

Abnormalities observed in morphological studies do not always
indicate the cell type in which a mutation has its primary effect
and indeed, for *K10*, it is possible to show that the follicle cell
behaviour is actually a *response* to a genetic alteration in the
underlying germ cell itself. This was found using genetic mosaics
in which mutant follicle cells surrounded wild type germ cells or

wild type follicle cells surrounded mutant germ cells. Such
mosaics can be constructed relatively easily in *Drosophila* by
transplanting the precursors for the germ cells between mutant and
wild type embryos[6]. When such transfers are made using *K10* homozygous embryos, the morphology of the egg laid by the mosaic females always corresponds to the genotype of the germ cells and is
independent of the genotype of the follicle cells which actually
secrete the egg shells[1]. These results indicate that the *K10* mutation blocks a function which normally must occur in germ cells
for the egg to have normal shape and polarity and for the follicle
cells to secrete a chorion with proper pattern.

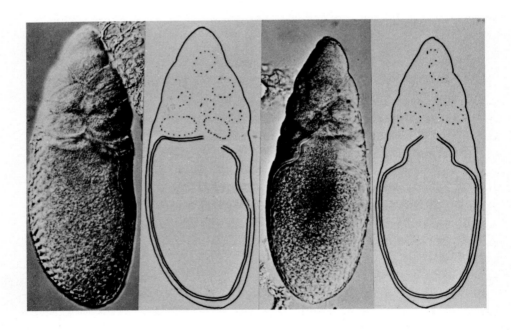

Fig. 5. Oocytes from normal females *(left)* and from females homozygous for *K10 (right)*.

Because the transplantations were made early, at the blastoderm
stage, they do not tell us very much about when the $K10^+$ function
is necessary, that is when the significant transcription at the
K10 locus occurs. For this purpose, there is an alternate technique in *Drosophila* for making mosaics, namely X-ray induced mitotic recombination. As the name implies, mitotic recombination is
a process whereby X-ray induced chromosome exchange alters the normal course of mitosis. Normally when a heterozygous cell divides,
one copy of each of the two homologous chromosomes ends up in each
daughter cell. Following mitotic recombination, the pattern is
changed such that one daughter cell now receives both copies of
the "+" chromosome and the other daughter, both copies of the K10
mutation. We have irradiated females heterozygous for K10 at different times during development and found that production of K10
eggs can be induced even when the irradiations were made with
mature females which had already begun oogenesis. A detailed analysis of these females indicates that most of the clones arise in
the germinal stem cell division prior to the differentiation of
each egg. If a mitosis occurs in the manner traditionally attributed to stem cells, the homozygous K10 daughter has two alternative
pathways open to it, depending on whether it remains in the stemline or begins to form an oocyte. If the cell remains in the stemline, a mosaic female will produce a series of K10 eggs. If on the
other hand, it begins immediate differentiation, then the female
will produce only a single egg of K10 morphology. This means that
we expect the clone sizes to be bimodally distributed if the clones
are induced during stem cell divisions. This is precisely the
distribution one obtains when adult females are irradiated (Figure
5). The fact that the single K10 eggs have a characteristic K10
morphology even though the $K10^+$ allele was present in the cell up
to completion of the final stem cell division indicates that any
transcription at the locus prior to this division is irrelevant for
the K10 phenotype.

If we assume that the females which produce series of K10 eggs
possess single K10 stem cells in their ovaries, then we can calcul-
ate the number of such stem cells by expressing the size of the

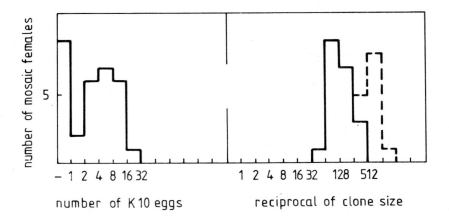

Fig. 6. The number of *K10* eggs laid by mosaic females possessing germline clones produced by X-ray induced mitotic recombination in 5-day old adults. The bimodal distribution indicates that most of the clones probably arise during the germerial stem cell divisions. Females which laid more than 3 *K10* eggs are assumed to have homozygous *K10* clones which have remained in the stemline. The clone size in such females can be estimated by the fraction of the total egg production the *K10* eggs represent. The reciprocal of these clone sizes indicates that the average number of stem cells in each female is about 100.

clones as a fraction of a female's total egg production. Since on an average about 1/100 of such female's eggs are *K10* (Figure 5), we can conclude that the average female possesses about 100 stem cells. The variety of techniques for producing mosaics in *Drosophila* as well as the availability of histochemical markers provide us with additional tools for analysing the division cycles of these stem cells. It is possible to show, for example, that they do not divide in alternating fashion but that instead, that each stem cell undergoes periods of activity followed by periods of relative quiescence[8].

The cell ineage techniques presently available are however inadequate to determine at what stage after the stem cell division

the transcription at $K10^+$ locus occurs. The daughter cell destined
to form an egg does not differentiate immediately but undergoes an
additional series of four incomplete cell divisions to produce a
cluster of 16 interconnected cells only one of which will become
the future oocyte. The other 15 become "nurse" cells and it is
here where most RNA synthesis occurs. The 15 nurse cells are interconnected with the oocyte or with each other by cytoplasmic bridges
left by the incomplete cleavage and, at the end of oogenesis, the
content of the nurse cells are sequentially emptied back into the
oocyte[2]. Thus, in a certain sense one can regard the entire germ
cell complex as a single cell with an extreme degree of intercellular specialization. However it is clear that the temporary division into 16 spacially separate units offers ample opportunity for
different synthesis and rates of deposition, all of which might be
prerequisites for creating the inhomogeneity in the egg which is
later reflected in the pattern of the egg coverings and the embryo.
Since such differences in activity of individual nurse cells might
be detected and studied using genetic mosaics, it is particularly
unfortunate that the attempts to induce mitotic recombination
during these divisions has met with no success. Either these divisions are refractory to the X-ray dosages used in inducing the
mitotic recombination or clones are actually produced but cannot
be recognized due to non-autonomy between the interconnected nurse
cells. If the latter is the case, it can be hoped that discovery
of new cell markers will make such studies possible in the future.

REFERENCES

1. Wieschaus, E., Marsh, J.L. and Gehring, W.J. (1978) Wilhelm
   Roux Arch., 184, 75-82.

2. King, R.C. (1970) Ovarian Development in *Drosophila melanogaster*,
   Academic Press.

3. Poulson, D.F. (1950) Histogenesis, organogenesis and diffraction
   in the embryo of *Drosophila melanogaster* Miegen. In "Biology of
   Drosophila" Wiley, New York, pp. 168-274.

4. Garcia Bellido, A. and Merriam, J. (1969) J. Exp. Zool. 170,
   61-76.

5. Hotta, Y. and Benzer, S. (1972) Nature, London, 240, 527-535.

6. Illmensee, K., Mahowald, A.P. and Loomis, M.P. (1976) Develop. Biol. 49, 40-69.

7. Wieschaus, E. and Szabad, J. (1979) Develop. Biol. 68, 29-46.

8. Schüpbach, T., Wieschaus, E. and Nöthiger, R. (1978) Wilhelm Roux Arch., 184, 41-56.

Cell Lineage, Stem Cells and Cell Determination
INSERM Symposium No. 10
Editor: N. Le Douarin
© *1979 Elsevier/North-Holland Biomedical Press*

THE DEVELOPMENT OF THE THORACIC SEGMENTS OF DROSOPHILA

GINES MORATA and PETER A. LAWRENCE

Centro de Biología Molecular, Universidad Autónoma de Madrid, Canto Blanco. Madrid- 34 and MRC Laboratory of Molecular Biology, Hills Rd Cambridge, England.

INTRODUCTION

The early embryo of <u>Drosophila</u> and the insects in general is composed of a number of segments. These appear to be of approximately the same size with the exception of the cephalic part that is thought to result from the fusion of several segments[1].The segmental organization is preserved in the adult flies.

The epidermal part of each segment is generated from a primordium that may develop into a imaginal disc as in the case of the cephalic, thoracic or genital segments or may remain as a nest of quiescent cells during larval life proliferating rapidly only at the beginning of pupariation. This is the case of the abdominal histoblasts.

In this report we deal mainly with the early development of the cuticular structures of two thoracic segments, the mesothorax and the metathorax. The mesothoracic cuticle derives from two imaginal discs, the wing disc giving rise to the wing, mesonotum and mesopleura and the second leg disc which generates the ventral pleurae and second leg. The metathoracic cuticle also derives from two discs, the haltere disc differentiating the haltere and the metanotum, and the third leg disc. The development of these discs during the larval period has been studied by clonal analysis by different authors[2,3,4]. Here we describe and compare their development with the aim of gaining some general conclusions about the way in which the imaginal primordia are organized.

METHODS. We have used the following techniques:

   Gynandromorph analysis is based on the loss of one X-chromosome
in the first cleavage division of XX female zygotes. This loss produces XO tissue that is phenotypically male and uncovers any recessive marker mutant in the remaining X-chromosome. These marker
mutants change the adult integument making for example yellow (y)
cuticle and bristles instead of the usual dark brown colour, or
forked (f) bristles instead of the straight wildtype. Thus male
cells can be recognised almost everywhere in the adult cuticle.
The most common method of generating gynandromorphs is to use a
ring-shaped X-chromosome which is unstable and become lost early
in development[5]. Gynandromorphs not only give information about
the position of the different primordia in the blastoderm[5,6] but
allow estimation of the number of progenitor cells in different
organs; the more cells contribute to a given structure, the
higher the probability that the structure will include both male
and female cells. This value (the frequency of mosaicism) is taken as a measure of the original number of cells at blatoderm[5,6].

   Clonal analysis consists of marking single cells at different
moments during development; the cell's descendants forming a clone that is recognised in the adult cuticle by the marker mutant
phenotype. The most common method of generating clones takes advantage of X-rays which produce chromatid interchange between homologous chromosomes (mitotic recombination). By this method a
cell heterozygous for a recessive marker mutant (and therefore
phenotypically wildtype) produces, in the division following irradiation, two daughter cells, one homozygous for the marker mutant
and the other for the wildtype allele. The use of X-rays to produce marked clones has the advantage that the event of clone initiation can be precisely timed. Analysing the frequency and size

of clones provides a picture of growth and development of the imaginal discsc[2,3,4].

The Minute technique[7] is a variant of clonal analysis. It makes use of dominant mutants called Minutes of which there are
about 50 different loci in Drosophila. They are recessive lethals
but in the heterozygous condition have a phenotype of fine short
bristles and delayed development. Most if not all, of the delay
occurs in the larval period which increases from 20% to 80% and
which is different in each Minute[8]. The division rate of Minute
cells is reduced in proportion. It was found[7] that the normal
division rate can be restored in wildtype clones (M^+) when they
grow in Minute individuals. These M^+ clones compete out the
surrounding Minute cells and reach a very large size. The M^+ clones are thus given the maximum opportunity to grow, so that the
method tests the developmental potential of individual cells at
specific period of development.

THE DEVELOPMENT OF THE THORACIC DISCS

It has been shown[9] that at blastoderm the different segmental
primordia are already separated, so that clones do not cross from
one segment to another. It should be emphasized that at blastoderm the embryo is merely a single layer of cells that are morphologically identical (with the exception of the pole cells).
The gastrulation and the segregation of the three germ layers takes place some few hours later.

The early development of the mesothoracic cuticle has been studied by clonal and gynandromorph analysis[9,10,11]. It was shown
that at blastoderm or soon after, the imaginal primordium is already subidvided into anterior and posterior groups of precursor
cells[10,11]. The cuticular regions which develop from a specific
group of precursor cells are called compartments[12]. Each of these
compartments begins existence as a group of founder cells that

generate a polyclone[13] . Thus at blastoderm the mesothoracic segment is already subdivided into two different (anterior and posterior) polyclones. At that time however there is no separation between precursor cells of wing and leg discs as between five to 10% of the clones[9,10,11] (depending on the experiment) include structures of wing and second leg. This separation takes place after 7 hours of development. At larval hatching the second leg and wing discs are physically separated and they are also distinguishable from the larval epidermis. Direct counts by Madlhavan and Schneiderman[14] indicate that second leg and wing discs originate from very similar number of cells (42 and 37 respectively).

During the larval period both the second leg and wing disc undergo further segregations. In the wing disc[12] the anterior and posterior polyclones are each subdivided into two polyclones one generating the dorsal part of the compartment and the other the ventral. Both groups of cells also become subdivided into thoracic (proximal) and appendicular (distal) polyclones. Thus after three segregations the wing disc becomes subdivided into eight groups of cells, each differentiating a specific region in the adult cuticle.

In the second leg disc Steiner[10] has found evidence that the anterior polyclone is subdivided into dorsal and ventral polyclones. He did not find evidence that proximo-distal segregation takes place in the leg.

The development of the metathoracic segment appears to be similar to that of the mesothorax. At blastoderm clones can extend from haltere to third leg but they do not cross the antero-posterior compartment boundary[10,15]. At larval hatching the third leg disc contains 45 cells and the haltere 20[14]. There is some evidence[4] that during larval development the haltere disc undergoes a similar pattern of segregations to that of the wing disc although for technical reasons the compartment boundaries cannot be defined as precisely as in the wing disc.

Thus if one compares the number of cells in mesothoracic and metathoracic discs in the first instar, the only difference is that the haltere disc contains about half the number of cells found in the wing disc. This is in good agreement with previous estimates based on mitotic recombination experiments[4].

The relative sizes of the mesothoracic and metathoracic primordia can be estimated by the frequency of mosaicism (FM) in gynandromorphs or by clone frequency after X-irradiation at the blastoderm stage (in this latter case assuming equal cell sensitivity to X-rays). However, while these types of experiments can be easily carried out for the leg discs, the comparison between haltere and wing is difficult because the haltere tissue contains no bristles and the trichomes are very short and densely packed. In such trichomes the markers normally used in gynandromorph or mitotic recombination experiments cannot be scored reliably. Recently we have been able to measure the FM of the haltere disc by using flies mutant for **Tufted** (**Tft**) that differentiate extra bristles on the anterior metanotum, and **hairy** (**h**) that have a number of small evenly distributed bristles on the capitelum[15]. Apart from these extrabristles, the haltere structures appear to be of normal size and there is no reason to believe that these mutants affect the number of haltere cells. However it could be that the FM of the anterior **Tft:h** haltere may be an underestimate since it is possible that some regions of the disc may not be affected by **Tft** or **h**. We found that the FM of the anterior haltere compartment is very similar to that of the anterior wing compartment (16% and 17% respectively). Assuming that the posterior compartment behave in the same way, this result suggests that the number of blastoderm cells contributing to the haltere or the wing cuticle is the same.

The preceding conclusion is reinforced by a series of experiments using mitotic recombination[15] where we compared the number of clones induced at the blastoderm in the haltere and in the wing. The clones in the haltere could be detected because they were mutant for the genes _bithorax_ and _postbithorax_ that transform the haltere tissue into wing[4]. In these experiments 17 clones were found in the wing and 19 in the haltere. For the second and third legs both the FM (20% and 17%) and clone frequency (26 and 30 clones) after mitotic recombination, indicate that they originate from the same number of blastoderm cells.

The number of primordial cells thus appears to be the same, despite the fact that the amount of cuticle produced by the two segments is very different. They also have the same proportion of cells contribution to the anterior compared to the posterior compartment.

Recently we have observed that the FM of the eye-antennal disc, which can be considered to be equivalent to the cuticular part of one cephalic segment, is equal to that of the mesothoracic segment[16]. This indicates that the eye-antennal structures derive from the same number of cells as do the mesothoracic or metathoracic segments. Moreover, the eye-antenna structures are subdivided into anterior and posterior compartments[16] as are all the thoracic segments. Another cephalic disc, the labial disc, is also subdivided into anterior and posterior compartments at blastoderm[17]. In this case despite the small size of the labial disc, the FM (17%, Struhl, personal communication) indicates that it derives from a similar number of cells to that forming the wing or leg discs.

From the preceding discussion it appears that all of the cephalic and thoracic discs so far analysed, share some common features; they all derive from the same or a similar number of cells and are subdivided into anterior and posterior polyclones with

the same proportion of cells in each. One is tempted to speculate
that all the thoracic and cephalic segments may be identical at
blastoderm. The differences between segments would appear later
presumably through the function of such genes as the homoeotic[18]
genes that direct specific segments or polyclones to certain developmental programs.

REFERENCES

1 Anderson, D.T. (1963). J.Embryol.Exp.Morph. 11, 339-351

2 García-Bellido, A. and Merriam, J.R. (1971). Develop.Biol. 24,
   61-87.

3 Bryant, P.J. and Schneiderman, H.A. (1969). Develop.Biol.20,
   263-290.

4 Morata, G. and García-Bellido, A. (1976). Wilhelm Roux'Arch.
   179, 125-143.

5 García-Bellido, A. and Merriam, J.R. (1969). J.Exp.Zool. 170,
   61-75.

6 Hotta, Y. and Benzer, S. (1972). Nature.240, 527-535.

7 Morata, G. and Ripoll, P. (1975). Develop.Biol. 42, 211-221.

8 Ferrus, A. (1975). Genetics. 74, 589-599.

9 Wieschaus, E. and Gehring, W. (1976). Develop.Biol. 50, 249-263.

10 Steiner, E. (1976). Wilhelm Roux'Arch. 180, 9-30.

11 Lawrence, P.A. and Morata, G. (1977). Develop.Biol. 56, 40-51.

12 García-Bellido, A. Ripoll, P. and Morata, G. (1976). Develop.
   Biol. 48, 132-147.

13 Crick, F.H.C. and Lawrence, P.A. (1975). Science. 189, 340-347.

14 Madhavan, M. and Schneiderman, H.A. (1977). Wilhelm Roux'Arch.
   183, 269-305.

15 Lawrence, P.A. and Morata, G. (1979). Submitted.

16 Morata, G. and Lawrence, P.A. (1979). Develop.Biol. In press.

17 Struhl, G. (1977). Nature. 270, 723-725.

18 Morata, G. and Lawrence, P.A. (1977). Nature. 265, 211-216.

Cell Lineage, Stem Cells and Cell Determination
INSERM Symposium No. 10
Editor: N. Le Douarin
© 1979 Elsevier/North-Holland Biomedical Press

HETEROMORPHIC REGENERATION IN THE DEVELOPING IMAGINAL PRIMORDIA OF *DROSOPHILA*

SIEGWARD STRUB

Department of Biology, State University of New York at Stony Brook, Stony Brook, Long Island, New York 11794 (U.S.A.)

ABSTRACT

A new concept on the nature and causes of transdetermination and of homoeotic transformations *in situ* caused by transdetermination events ('indirect homoeosis') is presented. The available data on transdetermination in *Drosophila* imaginal discs, especially foreleg discs, indicate i) that only cells in confined disc regions are endowed with the capacity to undergo transdetermination (homoeosis-competent cells); ii) that transdetermination is initiated when homoeosis-competent cells confront cells possessing widely discordant, possibly opposite, circumferential positional information; and iii) that transdetermined cells undergo terminal regeneration within the allotypic discs. It is therefore postulated that transdetermination represents homoeotic terminal regeneration and is identical to the phenomenon of heteromorphic regeneration observed in several species of lower arthropods. The concept appears also to apply to the class of indirect homoeotic transformations *in situ*, indicating that mutants and phenocopies of the indirect type (which may include *proboscipedia, Antennapedia, ophthalmoptera*, and others) are the result of homoeotic terminal regeneration occurring during development. It is proposed that in developing body appendage primordia of larvae bearing indirect homoeotic mutations, cell death-mediated "*in situ* amputations" expose clusters of homoeosis-competent cells at terminal wounds. Wound healing then creates the conditions necessary for the initiation of homoeotic terminal regeneration. It is speculated that the normal alleles of homoeotic genes of the indirect type might be involved in controlling the proximo-distal outgrowth of the various body appendages in insects.

INTRODUCTION

The term 'homoeosis' describes the replacement of one part of the body by another part[1]. In *Drosophila* three kinds of experimentally occurring homoeotic phenomena are known, namely homoeotic mutations, resulting from the mutant condition of so-called homoeotic genes, homoeotic phenocopies, caused by the treatment of embryos or larvae with certain physical or chemical agents, and transdetermination, arising during culture of imaginal disc tissue *in vivo*. In several species of lower arthropods, a fourth type of experimental homoeosis, heteromorphic regeneration, has been observed following amputation of certain body appendages. (For review see ref. 1).

Current theories about causes and nature of homoeosis fall into two distinct categories.

Certain homoeotic genes, such as those of the *bithorax* complex[2,3] or *engrailed*[4], have been proposed to exert direct control over the establishment and maintenance of developmental pathways. If the presence of mutant alleles or of physico-chemical factors prevent the normal functioning of such genes, cells embark on incorrect pathways, thus producing homoeotic mutants or phenocopies. The strongest criterion to place a homoeotic mutant into this category is the autonomous expression of mutant clones on non-mutant background in X-ray-induced morphogenetic mosaics (see refs. 2,3,4). This type of homoeosis will in the following discussion be called 'direct homoeosis'.

However, as recently pointed out by Denell[5], the phenotypes of a large number of homoeotic mutants are not readily compatible with the notion of their normal alleles controlling basic determinative steps analogous to the manner proposed for direct homoeotic genes. Several mutants are known to produce similar homoeotic transformations, and some even exhibit a pleiotropic homoeotic phenotype[5]. For example, antenna→leg transformations have been reported in *Antp* (*Antennapedia*), *Ns* (*Nasobemia*), ss^a (*aristapedia*),*1(4)29*, *Pc* (*Polycomb*), and others, mid/hind leg→foreleg transformations in *Pc*, *Scx* (*Extra sex comb*), *Msc* (*Multiple sex comb*), *1(4)29*, ss^a, and others, wing→eye transformations in *opht* (*ophthalmoptera*), *eyr* (*eyes-reduced*), and others[1,5,6]. Many of these mutants yield in addition a variety of non-homoeotic pattern abnormalities affecting especially eye, wing, and leg morphology[5,6]. It was therefore postulated[1,5,7-9] that the major effect of this type of homoeotic mutants might be some developmental distortions in the growing imaginal discs, presumably resulting in cell death[5,7], homoeosis being but an indirect consequence thereof (indirect homoeosis; see ref. 5). In this scheme, phenocopy-inducing agents, which as a rule are metabolically harmful[1], simply mimic the conditions produced by a given indirect homoeotic mutant, homoeosis resulting again secondarily. Several authors (refs. 1,5,7-9; Deak, personal communication) proposed that indirectly caused homoeotic phenomena *in situ* result from transdetermination events occurring in the developing imaginal discs.

In contrast to direct homoeosis, however, the exact nature and causes of indirect homoeosis remained basically unknown, as did the function of the wild-type alleles of indirect homoeotic genes. I propose in this article that indirect homoeotic transformations are the result of homoeotic terminal (that is, heteromorphic) regeneration, occurring *in situ* or during culture *in vivo*. It is speculated that the wild-type alleles of indirect homoeotic genes are involved in controlling the proximo-distal outgrowth of the different body appendages.

NATURE AND CAUSES OF TRANSDETERMINATION

Studies on transdetermination in cultured *Drosophila* imaginal disc, especially foreleg disc, blastemas have provided the following basic insights, to be discussed individually below.

• Only cells in confined regions of imaginal discs are endowed with the capacity to undergo homoeosis (homoeosis-competent cells or HC cells).

• Transdetermination is initiated when homoeosis-competent cells are confronted with cells possessing widely discordant, possibly opposite, circumferential positional information.

• The transdetermined cells undergo heteromorphic regeneration, that is, terminal regeneration ("distal transformation"[10]) within an allotypic[11] imaginal disc type.

Locally confined homoeosis-competence. Although indications for a locally confined homoeosis-competence exist for the foreleg[12-15], male[16] and female[16,17] genital, labial[18], and wing[19] discs, the location of the HC cells has only been mapped in the foreleg disc.

Studies by several authors have shown that the foreleg imaginal disc contains a distinct region with a high transdeterminative potential (homoeosis-competent area of HC area) (Fig. 1). The HC area is within the anterior disc half[12], extends into medial and lateral parts[13-15], and appears to be restricted to the

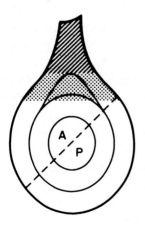

Fig. 1: Approximate location of the HC area in the foreleg disc. The cross-hatched area showed extensive, the stippled area rare (Strub, unpublished data) or no (Karlsson, personal communication) transdetermination in dissociation experiments. Dashed line, approximate location of the anterior-posterior (A/P) compartment boundary (after Steiner, ref. 21).

proximal—most disc region (Karlsson, personal communication). Cells from
other disc parts failed to transdetermine even after extensive proliferation
was stimulated by dissociation[13,15] (see Fig. 1).

    The foreleg disc HC area is mainly, perhaps exclusively, within the anterior
disc 'compartment'[20,21] (Fig. 1). Interestingly, the wing disc structures
formed by transdetermination, too, were almost exclusively typical of the
anterior compartment[20] (Strub, unpublished data), indicating that circumferential and compartmental specificities may be retained during transdetermination.
Transdetermination from antenna to wing[22] and homoeosis *in situ* from eye to
wing[7] also yielded only anterior wing structures. Thus, homoeosis-competence
might be a property residing exclusively in certain cells carrying anterior
circumferential specificities.

    <u>Specific cellular interactions initiate homoeosis.</u> In cultured imaginal
disc blastemas, interactions between non-adjacent cells occur during wound
healing[10,23] or as result of intermingling of undissociated fragments[24] or
of dissociated cells[15,19].

    Exposure of HC cells at a wound and the resulting contacts with non-adjacent
cells is a necessary prerequisite for transdetermination[14]. Intact foreleg disc
blastemas with an unexposed HC area (whole discs; anterior, *An*, halves) did not
transdetermine[12,25]. (For explanation of fragments and nomenclature employed,
see Fig. 2). However, not all contacts of exposed HC cells with normally non-
adjacent cells resulted in transdetermination, as is seen by the failure of
intact[26], gently intermingled (Strub, unpublished data), or dissociated and reaggregated[15] anterior-lateral (*AL*) quadrants, as well as of intact lateral (*La*)
halves[12], to show transdetermination. It appeared that HC cells, in order to
undergo transdetermination, might have to contact cells from opposite circumferential positions in the disc. This was suggested by experiments in which *AL*
quadrants were either gently intermingled, or dissociated and reaggregated, with
cells from the posterior-medial (*PM*) quadrant. In both situations, *AL* cells now
underwent frequent transdetermination (Strub and Nöthiger, unpublished data).

    Several data from intact fragments seem to be incompatible with this notion,
however. In the non-transdetermining *La* halves, wound healing presumably
brought about the juxtaposition of cells from opposite (mid-anterior and mid-
posterior) disc regions (see refs. 10,23). Anterior-medial (*AM*) quadrants and
their complementary *3/4La* fragments, on the other hand, transdetermined
frequently[12], although the healing radial cuts were only 90° apart.

    However, certain peculiarities in the regenerative behavior of fragments
cultured *in vivo* (especially the facts that *AM* quadrants regenerate the whole

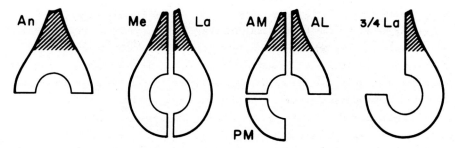

Fig. 2: Foreleg disc fragments mentioned in text. *An*, *Me*, *La*, anterior ("upper"), medial, lateral halves. *AM*, *AL*, *PM*, anterior-medial, anterior-lateral, posterior ("lower") -medial quadrants. *3/4La*, fragment complementary to *AM*. Cross-hatching denotes approximate location of HC area. Central circle indicates approximate borderline of the tarsal material, excised in most experiments.

disc while *3/4La* fragments duplicate[12]) have led to the proposal that in the foreleg disc the circumferential positional information is not evenly spaced, but that the majority of the 'positional values'[27] are clustered in the *AM* quadrant[10] (Fig. 3). In terms of this scheme, HC cells in *AM* quadrants and *3/4La* fragments contacted cells, during wound healing, carrying roughly opposite circumferential values. In *La* halves, however, the HC cells met cells that, although from a physically opposite disc region, did not possess opposite circumferential positional values.

All data mentioned so far, (and others discussed elsewhere[14,15]) are thus compatible with the proposal that transdetermination is triggered whenever HC cells interacted with cells bearing widely disparate, possibly opposite, circumferential positional information. A result not explained however is the dissimilar behavior of medial (*Me*; frequent transdetermination) and *La* (no transdetermination) halves[12]. This difference is not understood[14].

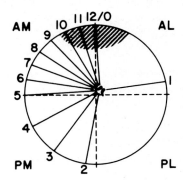

Fig. 3: Proposed spacing of the circumferential positional values (1-12/0) in the *Drosophila* foreleg disc. After French et al. (ref. 10) and Strub (ref. 26). Dashed lines represent borderlines between quadrants (Fig. 2; *PL*, posterior-lateral quadrant). Cross-hatching denotes approximate location of HC area (see Fig. 1).

Do appropriate cellular interactions trigger homoeosis directly, or do they first (as suggested by the traditional concept of the causes of transdetermination[11]) stimulate extra proliferation, as a result of which homoeosis then secondarily occurs? Although no definitive answer can presently be given, it is important to stress that no compelling evidence links proliferation to the *initiation* of transdetermination. The evidence most often quoted in favor of the traditional notion is the positive correlation observed between size of cultured implants and transdetermination frequency[18,25]. However, since transdetermination occurred from smaller to larger discs (labium to leg or antenna[18], leg to wing[25]), the larger size of transdetermined implants may simply reflect the faster growth of the allotypic cells *following* the homoeotic events. Likewise, the finding that in duplicating labial discs only the new halves contained transdetermined areas[18], only proves that transdetermination is an epimorphic process requiring the generation of new tissue material[10,27]. Neither of the above observations, however, provides any evidence as to whether prior growth was needed to stimulate homoeosis. Finally, Hadorn's finding that genital disc fragments in long-term cultures transdetermined only after several transfer generations[11], was most probably due to the fact that the mid-sagittal cuts applied during the first few transfers[11] did not run through an HC area. Only prospective anal and vaginal plate cells, mapping to the central parts of the lateral disc halves, appear to be homoeosis-competent[17]. Indeed, certain transversely cut genital disc fragments transdetermine during their initial stay in an adult host[16,17].

The evidence listed thus appears at least as compatible with the concept that the initiation of transdetermination could be the direct consequence of appropriate cellular interactions, altered proliferation dynamics being but the consequence of the homoeotic events.

<u>Transdetermination appears to be heteromorphic regeneration</u>. In insect legs two different types of non-homoeotic regeneration can occur, intercalary and terminal regeneration, respectively[10,28]. The former process replaces structures normally lying in-between juxtaposed wound edges, but leg segmental borders are not transgressed[28]. During the latter process, initiated e.g. by amputation, all structures and leg segments missing more distally in the appendage are regenerated.

I have recently proposed[28] that the criterion used by cells to embark in intercalary *vs.* terminal regeneration is the disparity in circumferential positional information between the cells confronted at wounds. Less than maximal circumferential disparities, or any proximo-distal disparities, cause the cells involved to engage in intercalary regeneration. However, if cells with maximally discordant circumferential information (regardless of proximo-distal disparities) meet, terminal regeneration is initiated.

It is evident that the proposed trigger mechanisms for terminal regeneration and for transdetermination are identical. Contacts between cells with roughly opposite circumferential positional information are in both cases supposed to activate specific developmental pathways. The responses to the identical signal differ, depending on the type of cells involved: homoeosis-incompetent cells react with terminal regeneration, homoeosis-competent cells transdetermine.

The close relationship between terminal regeneration and transdetermination is further evidenced by the following findings. i) In all types of HC cells-containing foreleg disc blastemas tested (with the exception of *La* halves where some terminal regeneration but no transdetermination was reported[12]) the two processes either co-occurred or were co-absent[12,13,15,28]. ii) Transdetermination, like terminal regeneration within the autotypic[11] disc, preferentially produced the distal structures of the allotypic discs. In transdetermination to leg, whether from antenna[22], wing[29], genital[17], or labial[18] discs, distal, especially tarsal, structures were observed most frequently. Likewise, trans-determinations to wing, both from antenna[22] and foreleg (Karlsson, personal communication; Strub, unpublished data) discs, yielded almost exclusively distal wing material.

Transdetermination thus appears to be homoeotic terminal regeneration. Homoeosis-competent cells, when stimulated to regenerate terminally, do so in an allotypic disc type.

In species other than *Drosophila*, homoeotic terminal regeneration has been studied extensively only in a few phasmids[30-32]. Interestingly, these studies revealed that in the larval antennae of walking sticks, too, HC cells are confined to a narrow portion of the appendage. Only amputations through the two basal antennal segments yielded heteromorphic regeneration, while amputation through any more distal level was followed by terminal regeneration of the excised antennal parts.

NATURE AND CAUSES OF INDIRECT HOMOEOSIS *IN SITU*

If, as suggested, homoeotic transformations of the indirect type *in situ* result from transdetermination events, then the elements of the outlined hypothesis should also apply to indirect homoeotic mutants and the corresponding phenocopies. This indeed appears to be the case.

Indications for localized homoeosis-competence. Strong indications for a local confinement of homoeosis-competence in the developing imaginal primordia exist for the eye and the antenna disc, while no exact information is as yet available for the other discs. The eye→wing transformations seen in *opht* originate exclusively in a narrow section of the anterior eye and the adjacent fronto-orbital head region[7,9]. In antenna→leg transformations produced by *Antp*[73b] and *Ns*, specific and recognizable parts of the first and second, as well as large parts of the third antennal segments always remain present, even in the strongest forms of transformation (Strub, unpublished observations; ref. 33).

Necessity of interactions between non-adjacent cells. *In situ*, normally non-adjacent cells are confronted when cell death eliminates the intervening disc regions.

Three lines of evidence indicate that cell death-mediated interactions between non-adjacent cells are crucial for the initiation of indirect homoeosis[5]. i) Phenocopy-inducing agents, as mentioned earlier, are as a rule metabolically harmful, and some have been directly shown to cause cell death in tissues[1,41,42]. ii) Several of the temperature-sensitive (ts) cell lethal mutants recently isolated produce (with low frequencies) homoeotic transformations after larval heat pulses[9,34]. iii) Many homoeotic mutants considered to be of the indirect type yield a variety of non-homoeotic pattern distortions (see above), indicating that widespread cell death occurs at some stage(s) of development[5,6].

Of course, no direct proof is available that interactions between cells with (close to) maximal circumferential disparities are required to trigger homoeosis *in situ*. An indirect argument presented below suggests however that this might indeed be the case.

Homoeotic outgrowths resemble terminal regenerates. The phenotypes of putative indirect homoeotic mutants and corresponding phenocopies, especially the strong expression classes, represent the most convincing evidence for the notion that indirect homoeosis is the result of homoeotic terminal regeneration. In *pb (proboscipedia)*, distal antenna or leg parts grow out from the labial palps[35,36]. In *Antp-Ns-ss*[a] type transformations, distal leg parts replace certain homologous antennal parts[33,37]. In *opht*, distal wing parts grow out from specific eye regions[7,9]. In *Hx (Hexaptera)*, distal wing, leg, or haltere parts protrude from the humeral region[38]. Even the mid/hind leg→foreleg transformations of the *Pc-Msx-Scx* type could be interpreted as resulting from homoeotic terminal regeneration if it is assumed that a homoeotic switch to foreleg occurred in a nest of HC cells in the mid and hind legs (see Fig. 5).

In the weak expression classes, many homoeotic appendages tend to be distally incomplete. In hemimetabolous insects, distally incomplete appendages were often observed under conditions where terminal regenerates had to start from circumferentially grossly deficient bases[39] that could not be completed by circumferential intercalation[10,28]. The formation of distally incomplete homoeotic appendages in *Drosophila* might be the result of a similar starting situation. If the HC areas in the growing appendage primordia occupied only a limited circumferential sector (which is the case in the foreleg disc, Fig. 1, and seems likely in the eye and the antenna discs; see above), homoeotic appendages would always have to start with a large circumferential deficiency (Fig. 4). In order to reach distal completeness, the homoeotic cells might have to regenerate a large circumferential sector first[10,28], and in attempting to do so they might be in competition with the autotypic material that still occupies a large part of the circumference. The variable success of homoeotically transformed cells in regenerating full circumferences might be one of the main reasons for the large phenotypic variability observed in all putative indirect homoeotic mutants.

THE PUTATIVE DEVELOPMENTAL LESIONS: *IN SITU* AMPUTATIONS

Cell death, as discussed above, appears to play a crucial role in initiating indirect homoeosis *in situ*, but random cell death can be eliminated as a significant factor. Most putative indirect homoeotic mutants exhibit a very high homoeosis penetrance (fraction of animals exhibiting homoeotic features), often approaching 100%. However, two treatments known to induce rather randomly scattered cell death, namely heat pulsing of larvae carrying ts cell-lethal mutations[40], or X-irradiation of larvae[41], induced homoeotic transformations only very rarely if at all[8,34,42-46]. Both treatments instead rather yielded duplicated appendages (which can be interpreted as supernumerary terminal regenerates[34]), a feature not observed in indirect homoeotic mutants.

By inference then, cell death, if it is indeed the trigger of indirect homoeosis, must be very localized, not only insuring that HC cells become exposed at a wound and juxtaposed to cells carrying appropriate positional disparities, but also at the same time not leading to the initiation of supernumerary regenerates.

The simplest way to meet these criteria would be if cell death amputated the developing appendage primordia through proximo-distal levels where clusters of HC cells are located (Fig. 4,A), exposing both homoeosis-competent and homoeosis-incompetent (HIC) cells at the wound. Wound contraction would then appose cells from all[10] (therefore also from opposite) circumferential positions, simulta-

neously initiating homoeotic (in HC cells) and autotypic (in HIC cells)
terminal regeneration. The ensuing competition between allotypic and autotypic
cells for the completeness of the circumference would then decide on the
strength of the homoeotic transformation.

The simplicity of the principle involved and the excellent fit between
predicted and observed phenotypes strongly suggest that the primary developmental lesions of indirect homoeotic mutants might indeed be but cell death-

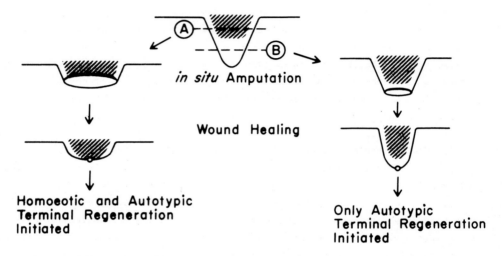

Fig. 4: Schematic representation of the way how cell death-mediated "*in situ-
amputations*" in developing imaginal primordia might trigger (A) or fail to
trigger (B) homoeosis, depending upon whether or not an HC area (cross-hatched)
is being exposed at the wound. It is important to bear in mind that the growing
imaginal discs in *Drosophila* larvae do not have the shapes of body outgrowths
yet, but are basically flat structures. Cell death, in order to amputate prospective distal disc material, thus in actuality would have to eliminate
circular regions located in the center of the discs (compare with Fig. 2).

mediated amputations at appendage levels where HC areas are located.

If this is the case, then one would predict that a class of amputation-
producing mutants should exist whose amputation levels would not expose HC
areas (Fig. 4,B). They would therefore stimulate autotypic terminal
regeneration only, and hence would not be classified as homoeotic mutants.
Prime candidates for this putative class of mutants might be mutations causing
pattern abnormalities (missing, crippled, swollen, fused, etc., segments) in
distal appendage parts.

SPECULATIONS ON THE NORMAL FUNCTION OF INDIRECT HOMOEOTIC GENES

The foregoing considerations indicate that, unlike direct homoeotic genes[2-4], homoeotic genes of the indirect type play no role whatsoever in the establishment or the stability of the developmental pathways affected by the homoeotic transformations that their mutant alleles produce. The fact that the mutant phenotypes include homoeotic features at all seems purely accidental, caused by the coincidence of the levels of cell death-mediated amputations with the location of HC areas.

The proposed action of the mutant genes does however allow us to speculate on the function of the wild-type alleles during undisturbed development. The evidence presently at hand appears to justify the following speculative statements.

Firstly, since mutant alleles of indirect homoeotic genes appear to act by amputating growing appendage primordia at specific proximo-distal levels, their normal alleles might be involved in, and even control, the specification and morphogenesis of the same proximo-distal appendage levels during normal development. Unfortunately, there is still basically a total lack of knowledge of the events and their sequence by which the proximo-distal organization of imaginal primordia is laid down and elaborated during larval development. Further progress in our understanding of the action of indirect homoeotic mutants might be largely dependent on progress to be made with respect to this question.

Secondly, the pleiotropic homoeotic phenotypes observed in some of the putative indirect homoeotic mutants, as well as the frequent occurrence of pattern distortions in non-transformed appendages (resulting from amputations at levels where no HC areas are located?), might suggest that indirect homoeotic genes control the morphogenesis of corresponding proximo-distal levels in different imaginal primordia. Fig. 5 attempts to illustrate this point.

A large number of the presently known homoeotic mutants that could be of the indirect type are located in a narrow portion of the proximal part of chromosome arm 3R, (meiotic map positions around 3-47 to 3-49; *Scx, pb, Antp, Ns, Pc, Msc, l(3)c43^hs1*; ref. 1,6,47), henceforth referred to as the *Antp-Pc* gene complex. Clustering of genes with similar function indicates that they might be under coordinated control[3]. It is therefore conceivable that the *Antp-Pc* gene complex could be the key control element governing the proximo-distal outgrowth of the various body appendages. Since most appendages are segmentally organized, the control of the appendage segmentation pattern might be a major element of this task. Should this speculation be correct, it would mean that the two main

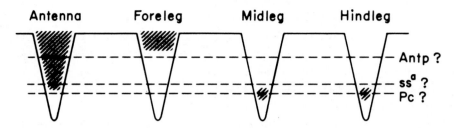

Fig. 5: Speculative diagram of putative amputation levels in different appendage primordia of three homoeotic mutants that might be of the indirect type.
Amputation levels have been chosen according to the extent of the homoeotic
transformation they produce (*Antp* vs *ss^a*) and from the fact that *ss^a* and *Pc* may
show similar pleiotropic homoeotic phenotypes. The locations of HC areas in
the different imaginal discs (except the foreleg disc; Fig. 1) is not known,
and the locations chosen here are completely arbitrary.

clusters of homoeotic genes in the *Drosophila* genome might control the specification of the two types of segmentation that exist in insects, the *bithorax*
gene complex determining body segmentation[2,3], the *Antp-Pc* gene complex on the
other hand controlling the establishment of the appendage segmentation.

FINAL REMARKS

    The overall yet still very preliminary picture emerging from the above
discussion is that in the developing body appendages of *Drosophila*, and probably
of arthropods generally, cells in specific confined areas remain highly labile
with respect to their body segment determination. When a developmental
distortion stimulates such cells to regenerate terminally, they switch their
body segment determination and undergo heteromorphic regeneration, starting
presumably from a homologous proximo-distal level in the allotypic appendage[33].
The direction of the potential homoeotic switch is highly specified for each of
the HC cell clusters, the overall sequence showing a distinct tendency to shift
towards wing[1,11]. On the other hand, it becomes obvious that in the majority
of the cells the state of body segment determination is rigidly fixed and is not
reversed by any of the experimental interferences applied so far.

    The retention, in the developing arthropod body appendages, of localized
clusters of cells with a labile state of body segmentation amidst rigidly
determined cells is a highly puzzling fact. It appears that the presence of
homoeosis-competent cell clusters is without any advantage for the survival of
the animal but is potentially hazardous since the chances for normal regeneration following injury are diminished. It is therefore surprising that

selective pressure during evolution has not (yet?) led to the complete elimination of these potential "trouble spots".

The answer to this question and the general elucidation of the phenomena related with indirectly caused homoeosis is bound to provide us with crucial insights into some of the most important yet presently unsolved aspects of developmental biology.

ACKNOWLEDGMENTS

I wish to thank Dr. Eugene R. Katz, Nicholas Brown, Susan Erster, and Durgadas Kasbekar for most helpful comments on the manuscript.

REFERENCES

1. Ouweneel, W.J. (1976). Adv. Genet., 18, 179.

2. Garcia-Bellido, A. (1977). Amer. Zoologist, 17, 613.

3. Lewis, E.B. (1978). Nature, 276, 565.

4. Lawrence, P.A., Morata, G. (1976). Develop. Biol., 50, 321.

5. Denell, R.E. (1978). Genetics, 90, 277.

6. Lindsley, D.L., Grell, E.H. (1968). Carnegie Institution of Washington Publ., 627.

7. Ouweneel, W.J. (1969). Wilhelm Roux's Arch., 164, 1.

8. Arking, R. (1978). Genetics, 88, s4.

9. Postlethwait, J.H. (1974). Develop. Biol., 36, 212.

10. French, V., Bryant, P.J., Bryant, S.V. (1976). Science, 193, 969.

11. Hadorn, E. (1966). Develop. Biol., 13, 424.

12. Schubiger, G. (1971). Develop. Biol., 26, 277.

13. Strub, S. (1977). Wilhelm Roux's Arch., 182, 75.

14. Strub, S. (1977). Wilhelm Roux's Arch., 182, 69.

15. Strub, S. (1977). Nature, 269, 688.

16. Littlefield, C.L., Bryant, P.J. (1979). Develop. Biol., in press.

17. Mindek, G. (1968). Wilhelm Roux's Arch., 161, 249.

18. Wildermuth, H. (1968). Wilhelm Roux's Arch., 160, 41.

19. Garcia-Bellido, A., Noethiger, R. (1976). Wilhelm Roux's Arch., 180, 189.

20. Garcia-Bellido, A., Ripoll, P., Morata, G. (1973). Nature New Biol., 245, 251.

21. Steiner, E. (1976). Wilhelm Roux's Arch., 180, 9.

22. Gehring, W. (1966). J. Embryol. Exp. Morph., 15, 77.

23. Reinhardt, C.A., Hodgkin, N.M., Bryant, P.J. (1977). Develop. Biol., 60, 238.

24. Haynie, J.L., Bryant, P.J. (1976). Nature, 259, 659.

25. Tobler, H.   (1966).   J. Embryol. Exp. Morph., 16, 609.

26. Strub, S.   (1977).   Wilhelm Roux's Arch., 181, 309.

27. Wolpert, L.   (1971).   Curr. Top. Develop. Biol., 6, 183.

28. Strub, S.   (1979).   Develop. Biol., 69, 31.

29. Garcia-Bellido, A.   (1966).   Develop. Biol., 14, 278.

30. Cuénot, M.L.   (1921).   C.R. Acad. Sci. Paris, 172, 949.

31. Brecher, L.   (1924).   Arch. Mikr. Anat. Entw. Mech., 102, 549.

32. Urvoy, J.   (1970).   J. Embryol. Exp. Morph., 23, 719.

33. Postlethwait, J.H., Schneiderman, H.A.   (1971).   Develop. Biol., 25, 606.

34. Postlethwait, J.H.   (1978).   Wilhelm Roux's Arch., 185, 37.

35. Villee, C.A.   (1944).   J. Exp. Zool., 96, 85.

36. Kaufman, T.C.   (1978).   Genetics, 90, 579.

37. Villee, C.A.   (1943).   J. Exp. Zool., 93, 75.

38. Herskowitz, I.   (1949).   Genetics, 34, 10.

39. Bohn, H.   (1965).   Wilhelm Roux's Arch., 156, 449.

40. Clark, W.C., Russell, M.A.   (1977).   Develop. Biol., 57, 160.

41. Haynie, J.L., Bryant, P.J.   (1977).   Wilhelm Roux's Arch., 183, 85.

42. Russell, M.A.   (1974).   Develop. Biol., 40, 24.

43. Arking, R.   (1975).   Genetics, 80, 519.

44. Simpson, P., Schneiderman, H.A.   (1975).   Wilhelm Roux's Arch., 178, 247.

45. Villee, C.A.   (1946).   J. Exp. Zool., 101, 261.

46. Postlethwait, J.H., Schneiderman, H.A.   (1973).   Develop. Biol., 32, 345.

47.· Martin, P., Martin, A., Shearn, A.   (1977).   Develop. Biol., 55, 213.

Cell Lineage, Stem Cells and Cell Determination
INSERM Symposium No. 10
Editor: N. Le Douarin
© *1979 Elsevier/North-Holland Biomedical Press -*

RENEWAL OF THE PYLORIC EPITHELIUM

C.P. LEBLOND and E.R. LEE

Department of Anatomy, McGill University, Montreal, Canada

On the basis of mitotic activity, cell populations in the adult organism may be classified into three categories. The first comprises *static populations* in which no mitosis is detected; this is the case for most of the neurons in the nervous system. The second category consists of *expanding populations* in which mitotic activity decreases with age; in the adult, mitoses are infrequent; when they occur, the resulting cells are permanently added to the cell population which then slowly increases in size. This group includes the cells of many organs, for instance those of liver and kidney. The third category comprises *renewing populations*, some of which will be the focus of the present study. They are characterized by a high frequency of dividing cells, but without increase in population size. As cells are being produced, other cells are lost, resulting in a balance between cell production and cell loss. Thus, in the epidermis, cells arise in the basal layer, while others are shed from the surface. This renewal process allows for the continuous replacement of a cell population. Usually a renewing cell population includes three cell types: a) stem cell whose mitoses give rise to new stem cells and to cells fated to differentiate; b) differentiating cells at various stages of development; and c) mature or end cells, which are eventually lost.

The renewal process has been the subject of extensive investigations in epidermis, testes, hemopoietic tissues and intestine; however, only a few studies have addressed themselves to the renewal process in the pyloric portion of the stomach. The lack of interest in this area is surprising since it is the site of benign and cancerous lesions. In view of this, we began examining the mode of renewal of cells in the pyloric epithelium and glands. Using single injections or continuous infusion of ^{3}H-thymidine into adult mice, it was possible to localize the regions of cell production, the pathway of migration and the site of cell loss. More recently, we have focused our interests on the ultrastructural characteristics of the proliferating cells. As a result of this work, we are able to propose a model for the origin of the various mucous cell lines which make up the pyloric epithelium.

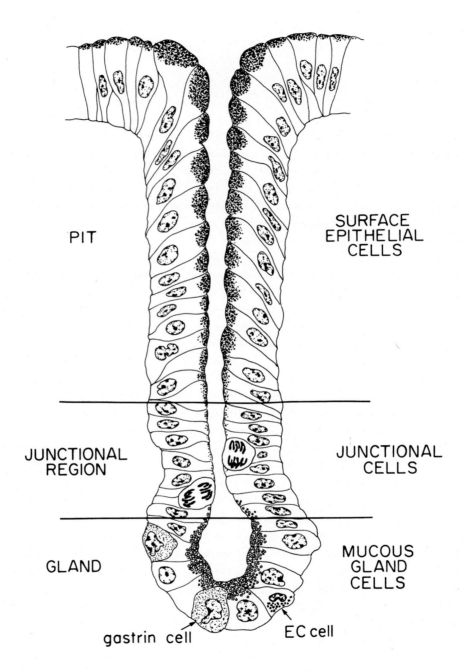

PIT

SURFACE
EPITHELIAL
CELLS

JUNCTIONAL
REGION

JUNCTIONAL
CELLS

GLAND

MUCOUS
GLAND
CELLS

gastrin cell

EC cell

Fig.   1.   A diagram of a gland-pit unit from the mouse pyloric mucosa.

In the adult mouse, the pyloric mucosa may be divided into 3 distinct areas: a) the pyloric pit b) the pyloric gland and lastly c) a region connecting each gland with a pit, the junctional region or isthmus.

The pyloric pits of the mouse stomach are very long, occupying as much as 2/3 of the mucosal thickness (Figure 1). Each tubular shaped pit is lined by a single layer of surface epithelial cells. These cells contain a mucus which produces a deep purple stain when treated by the periodic acid-Schiff technique. At the ultrastructural level, the mucous globules of the surface epithelial cells have a dark mottled appearance, as seen in Figure 2.

The pylorus glands, on the other hand, are small bulbar structures. They are lined by mucous gland cells and scattered entero-endocrine cells. The mucus of the gland cells reacts with the periodic acid-Schiff reagents to produce a pink stain, which is clearly distinguishable from that of the mucus in the surface epithelial cells. When mucous gland cells are examined in the electron microscope their globules contain two distinct components, a small eccentric core and a lighter stained material which is larger and encompasses the core (Figure 3).

The third area or junctional region is particularly striking in that many of its cells are labeled 1 hour following a single injection of ^{3}H-thymidine. Indeed, the presence of numerous mitotic figures in this area confirms the proliferative ability of the cells. As seen in Figure 1, the junctional region is characterized by cells which lack or have only few scattered mucous globules. By using the electron microscope, we have been able to identify several types of junctional cells. Among them, we occasionally find cells which have been termed "undifferentiated cells" (Figure 4). Some of these cells contain no mucous globules in their cytoplasm, but more frequently they have a few scattered small globules. The cytoplasm is rich in free ribosomes and contains only few cisternae of rough endoplasmic reticulum. The Golgi apparatus is smaller than in differentiated cells. In addition, these cells contain small granules which may be lysosomes.

More frequent in the junctional region are cells which have larger and more numerous mucous globules than the undifferentiated cells. The free ribosomes are abundant, the cisternae of rough endoplasmic reticulum are few and the Golgi apparatus is small. Based on the character of the mucous globules however, three types of these cells have been identified: a) immature mucous gland cells which contain characteristic light globules with dense core; b) immature pit cells having a dark irregularly mottled mucous globules like the cells of the pit cell line and c) intermediate cells which produce a mixture of the two

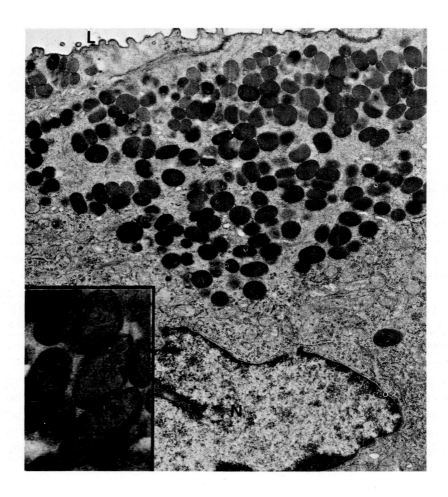

Fig. 2. The surface epithelial cells of the pyloric pits and surface are characterized by dark mottled mucous globules located in the cell apex. L, indicates the pyloric pit lumen and N, the nucleus. x 15,000

The inset shows the mucous globules at a higher magnification. x50,000

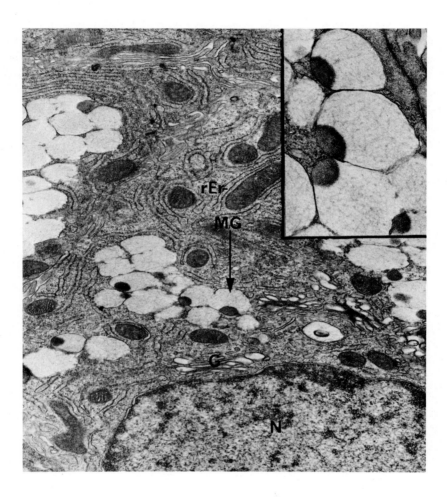

Fig. 3. The mucous gland cells of the pyloric glands contain many characteristic mucous globules (MG). The rough endoplasmic reticulum (rER) is extensive
and numerous Golgi saccules (G) are apparent above the nucleus (N). x15,000
    The inset shows the mucous globules at a higher magnification. After the
fixation used here (glutaraldehyde-paraformaldehyde in cacodylate buffer), the
globules show a light background with a filamentous network, within which a
dense core stands out. x30,000

types of mucus, for they contain globules with a dense core and mottled dark staining globules (Figure 5). These cells are more frequently observed than the undifferentiated ones, but in contrast, are less numerous than either the immature mucous gland cells or immature pit cells. All of the above mentioned junctional cells have the ability to divide as seen by the labeling of their respective nuclei 1 hour following an injection of ^{3}H-thymidine.

These combined observations have enabled us to propose a model for the origin of the various mucous cell lines as seen below. Possibly then, the undifferentiated cell functions as the stem cell of the junctional compartment. When the demand is issued, these rare cells may divide to give rise on the average to another stem cell and to a cell which undergoes differentiation, possibly an entero-endocrine cell, or more frequently an intermediate cell. The intermediate cell would then give rise either to immature gland or pit cells. In sequence these latter two cell types, now being committed, would continue to proliferate and feed into the respective cell lines of either pit or gland.

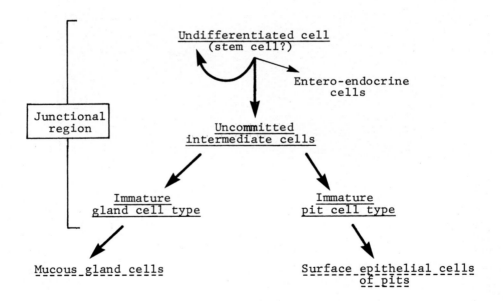

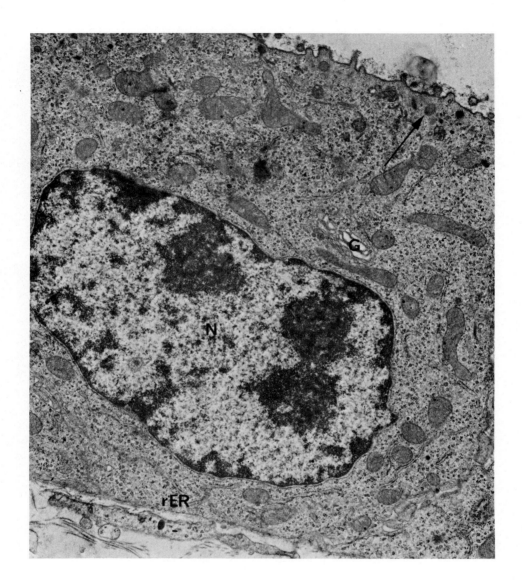

Fig. 4. The undifferentiated cell of the junctional region contains only a few small globules scattered along the apical surface (arrow). Free ribosomes are abundant while rough endoplasmic reticulum (rER) is scant. A small Golgi stack is present above the nucleus (N). x15,000

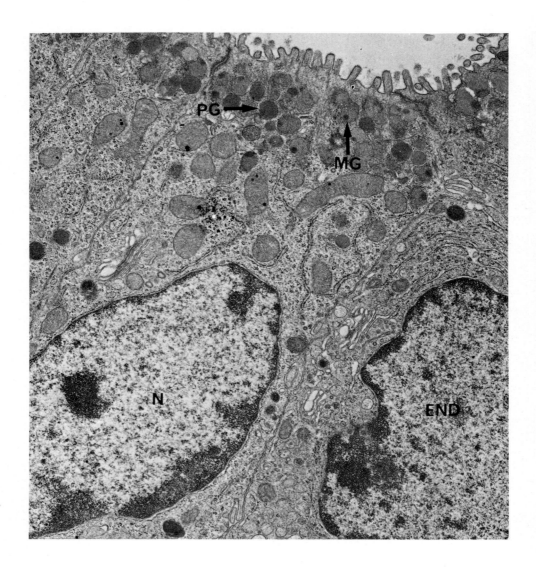

Fig. 5. The nucleus labeled N belongs to an intermediate cell, whose apex contains two types of small mucous globules, dark ones similar to those of the pit cell line (PG) and cored globules similar to those of the mucous gland cell line (MG).

The nucleus labeled END on the right belongs to an entero-endocrine cell of the gastrin type.

As indicated earlier, the cells labeled one hour after a single injection of
[3]H-thymidine are mainly those in the junctional region. In addition, there are
a few labeled surface epithelial cells in the portion of the pits adjacent to
the junctional region. As ^{3}H-thymidine is infused continuously, more surface
epithelial cells become labeled. For example, after two days of continuous
infusion, surface epithelial cells are labeled halfway along the pit or higher,
whereas after three days they are labeled up to and including those on the free
surface. These observations indicate that surface epithelial cells are produced by the division of cells in the junctional region and, to a lesser degree, of cells of the lower pit. With time the new cells migrate along the
walls of the pits to eventually reach the free surface of the mucosa.

As cells approach the upper margins of the pits, the mucous globules of some
but not all cells acquire a dense core. Moreover, most cells show signs of
cytoplasmic deterioration, such as accumulation of vesicles in the cytoplasm
along with lipid droplets, autophagic vacuoles and dense bodies.

Upon reaching the free surface of the mucosa, the surface cells are singly
extruded into the gastric lumen. Some cells, however, die prematurely in the
upper pit region, where they are phagocytosed by neighboring cells; they are
then carried as phagosomes to the free surface where, presumably, they are extruded with the carrier cell. On the average the overall renewal process of
pit cells takes about 3 days.

In the pyloric gland, dividing cells are observed occasionally. Indeed, a
few mucous gland cells are labeled one hour after a single injection of [3]H-
thymidine. These cells are generally located close to the junctional region,
in what is referred to as the upper segment of the glands. As the animals are
exposed to longer durations of ^{3}H-thymidine, cells in the lateral walls and
eventually the basal segment of the gland become labeled. Cell counts reveal
that, by two days of continuous infusion, about 50% of the mucous gland cells
are labeled, but the labeled cells are mainly in the upper segment; after 14
days, only 80% of the gland cells are labeled, and the unlabeled ones predomi-
nate in the basal segment. It thus appears that only few of the cells labeled
early in the upper segment find their way to the basal segment. Only by 24 and
60 days of continuous infusion will nearly all basal cells be labeled. Presumably gland cells are comprised of subpopulations renewing at different rates -
some slowly, others more rapidly; the overall rate decreases with the distance
from the junctional region.

Even though mucous gland cells undergo renewal, it is not clear how the cell
addition is balanced by a cell loss. Preliminary but incomplete evidence indi-

cates that ageing cells may be either phagocytosed or extruded into the gland lumen.

In summary, the various regions of the pyloric epithelium undergo constant renewal. As a result of cell division, primarily in the junctional region, new cells are continually being produced. These junctional cells give rise to the surface epithelial cells which migrate along the pyloric pits to reach the free surface, where they are extruded into the gastric lumen. The junctional cells also give rise to mucous gland cells, but the renewal mechanism is not clear. Only some of the mucous gland cells arising from the junctional region appear to migrate and eventually reach the basal segment of the gland, where they are renewed very slowly. Other mucous gland cells from the upper segment of the gland are fairly rapidly renewed.

ACKNOWLEDGMENTS

This work was done with the support of a grant from the Medical Research Council of Canada.

Cell Lineage, Stem Cells and Cell Determination
INSERM Symposium No. 10
Editor: N. Le Douarin
© *1979 Elsevier/North-Holland Biomedical Press*

THE PRESENCE OF MULTIPOTENTIAL PROGENITOR CELLS IN EMBRYONIC NEURAL RETINA
AS REVEALED BY CLONAL CELL CULTURE

T.S.OKADA, KUNIO YASUDA AND KAZUYA NOMURA
Institute for Biophysics, Faculty of Science, University of Kyoto, Kyoto, 606
(Japan)

INTRODUCTION

In vertebrate animals, the result of cell differentiation is generally very
stable. In spite of the evidence for the maintenance of a complete set of gen-
omes in differentiated somatic cell nuclei by means of nuclear transplantation
experiment, a sudden expression of once repressed genes in the course of cell
differentiation is of very unusual occurrence in vertebrates cells (1). Thus,
an increase or change of the repertoire in the spectrum of differentiative
traits occurs seldomly in once determined or differentiated cells. The situations make us difficult to find any suitable experimental system for the analytical study on the problem of determination in vertebrate cells.

A subject of the problem of determination is to discuss the mechanism of a
programming of multipotentiality of differentiation of a given embryonic cell
into a single pathway as well as of a sudden switch of the differentiation of
once programmed cells. Indeed, the determination in terms of a limitation of
prospective multipotentiality in development in a given embryonic rudiment was
a central problem in the classical era of experimental embryology (2). Most of
the experimental systems established in that period do not seem to meet conditions for modern studies at the molecular and cellular levels of determination.

Studies on cells of eye tissues provide certainly a uniquely potent system
for studying the problem of determination at the cellular and molecular levels.
In these cells, a switch or cell-type conversion of once differentiated cells
into other types occurs rather extensively in the regeneration of lost parts of
eyes in fishes, amphibians and perhaps in early chick embryos (3). A switch
occurs with a definitive pattern, for instance, from pigmented cells of the iris
into lens cells or from those of the tapetum into neural retinal cells. It is
of great advantage of this system that some of differentiative traits involved
can be well identified by molecular markers. For instance, biochemical information on lens and pigment cells has been much accumulated. Particularly, the
specificity of lens cells can be steadily identified by the presence of the

lens-specific molecules, crystallins.

Recent progress in the studies of determination using cells from eye tissues started, when Eguchi and Okada (4) anounced that a complete series of the process of a switch of cell type which is now called *transdifferentiation* can be well followed in conditions of *in vitro* cell culture of dissociated pigmented retinal cells of 8-day-old chick embryos. Soon, a list of examples of transdifferentiation of cells of eye tissues *in vitro* has been extended to cover various eye tissues of both avian and mammalian embryos as well as amphibians, and such instability of cell differentiation revealed in cell culture experiments is not related with the ability of regeneration *in situ* (5, 6, 7, 8, 9).

Methodologically, it becomes possible to obtain the transdifferentiation of lens in the progeny originated from a single retinal cell *in vitro* (4, 10). Thus, the process can be now studied at the clonal level, and this will open a possibility to study a lineage of cells of a clonal origin in terms of changes in the state of determination.

EMBRYONIC NEURAL RETINA IN CELL CULTURE

Neural retina (NR) of avian embryos is an excellent material to observe transdifferentiation *in vitro*. Cells of NR express very extensively the differentiation of cell types which will be never formed in NR *in situ*(11, 12). This material is advantageous for collecting fairly substantial amount of cleanly separated tissue pieces from embryos.

When pieces of NR were dissociated and cultured *in vitro*, both lens and pigment cells were differentiated. The ability of transdifferentiation of these non-neuroretinal cells is retained in chick and quail embryonic NR by about 17 days of incubation, though it becomes less with development (13, 14).

Recently, a number of studies have been carried out as to molecular events leading to the transdifferentiation of lens and pigment cells from embryonic NR *in vitro*. In a typical culture experiment starting from 3.5-day-old chick embryonic NR, the synthesis of delta-crystallin becomes detectable from 9-day cultures and the ratio of synthesis of this specific protein to total soluble proteins is as high as about 40% at 26 days (15). Similar rapid increase is also shown in tyrosinase activity in cultures of 8-day-old embryonic NR (16). As to changes at the transcriptional level, detailed studies have been done recently using 3.5-day-old embryonic NR again (17). It is interesting that this starting material contains already detectable amount of a similar sequence to the most abundant mRNA of crystallins *in situ* (18). By 20 days in culture, the amount of mRNA sequence to hybridize with cDNA prepared to the mRNA sequence of crystallins increases about as much as 500-folds.

Cellular events leading to the transdifferentiation of lens (or pigment) cells from NR *in vitro* must be more complicated than those in lens differentiation in cultures of pigmented retinae. In the latter case, the starting material consists of a homogeneous cell population of pigment cells. Lens differentiation in pure cultures of black cells or in clonal progenies starting from single living black cells is the direct demonstration of the "transdifferentiation" or of a convertion of cell type (4). On the other hand, embryonic NR, though establishing a well-defined tissue layer from early stages, is to differentiate into very diverse pathways *in situ*, such as to develope into photoreceptor visual cells, ganglion cells, supporting cells (Müller cells) and others. In cultures, both lens and pigment cells are differentiated. Thus, there seems to be a great choice of future differentiation of embryonic NR and following questions will immediately arise.

1) Are there any multipotential progenitor (stem) cells, progenies of which will differentiate into most cell types of the *in situ* neural retina plus lens and pigment cells? Or, do cells to differentiate into non-neuroretinal specificities belong to different cell-lines to be separated from other main cell population in embryonic NR to give rise to actual neural retina? In other words, is embryonic NR a mosaic of monopotential cells?

2) Are lens and pigment cells found in cell cultures originated exclusively from, if any, non-committed multipotential stem cells? Or, can such cells that have, at least partially, expressed any neuroretinal traits transdifferentiate into lens and/or pigment cells?

THE PRESENCE OF MULTIPOTENTIAL PROGENITOR CELLS IN EMBRYONIC NEURAL RETINA

Perhaps, one of the most direct method in order to detect the presence of multipotential progenitor cells is clonal cell culture, in which a multipotential progenitor cell, if present, should give rise to "mixed" clones with more than two specificities of differentiation. Extensive studies toward this end has been carried out using cells of 3.5-day-old chick and quail embryonic NR (19). Singly dissociated cells were obtained from cleanly isolated pieces of NR by the treatment with EDTA, without using trypsin, and very small number of cells (500-2,000 cells) were inoculated into separate culture dishes, the substrate of which had been previously coated with collagen. After about 30 days *in vitro*, the overall plating efficiency, (total colonies per plate)/(number of cells inoculated per plate) x 100, was about 0.46%. The following four colony types were obtained: colonies differentiating into lens cells, colonies with pigment cells; colonies with both lens and pigment cells (mixed colonies); and colonies comprised entirely of unidentifiable cells. In early stages of culturing up to about 10 days, neuroblast-like (neuronal) cells appeared in many

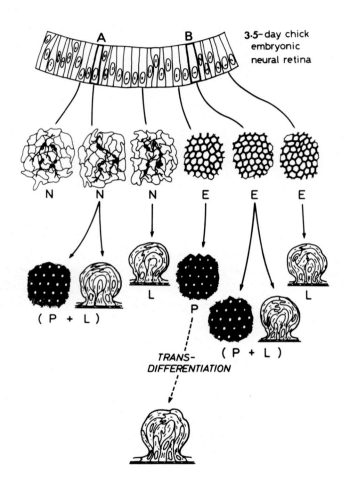

Fig. 1. The multiple pathways in differentiation starting from early embryonic NR as revealed by clonal cell culture. E, Epithelial cells; L, differentiation of lens cells; N, differentiation of neuronal cells; P, differentiation of pigment cells. From Okada et al. (19).

colonies. Unfortunately, there has been yet no irrevocable proof of that all colonies are really *clones* originating from a single cell respectively. However, there are a number of circumstantial evidence which permits us to interpret many, though not all, colonies as clones.

NR of 3.5-day-old avian embryos is a well defined layer of the neuroepithelium, but it is not yet differentiated in terms of that it apparently consists of homogeneous cell population, without showing any divergence into different cell types to be contained in fully developed NR. All cells of NR at this particular stage of embryonic development, however, are not homogeneous in their potentialities in future differentiation. The fact that multiple colony types were formed in clonal cell cultures of this tissue, as schematically summarized in Figure 1, must suggest the heterogeneity in future differentiation potentialities among the constituent cells. But, this does not mean that early embryonic NR is a "mosaic" system of monopotential cells, which have been committed to differentiate into a single pathway.

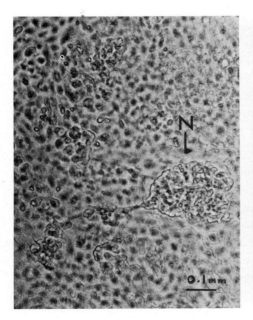 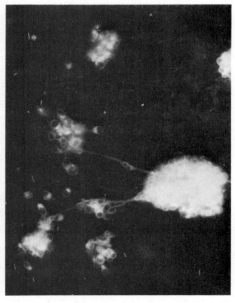

Fig.2. The differentiation of N-cells in a 5-day culture of 3.5-day-old chick embryonic NR. Clusters of N-cells (N) are seen.

Fig.3. A fluorescent microphotograph of the same field as shown in Figure 2 after staining with Merocyanine 540. Note specific fluorescence in N-cells and their axon-like processes.

Reciprocally, the results of clonal cell culture strongly point toward the presence of multipotential progenitor (stem) cells in embryonic NR, since mixed clones with multiple phenotypes appeared often. A clone derived from cell A in Figure 1 is an example expressing very diverse phenotypes. In the early stages of clonal growth by about 10 days, the differentiation of flattened epithelial cells (E-cells) and neuronal cells (N-cells) occurred. After a further culture period of up to about 30 days, both lens cells and pigment cells were differentiated. Cell B is also multipotent to give rise to lens and pigment cells, but no differentiation of N-cells occurred.

In clonal cell cultures of cells of NR of somewhat aged embryos at 8–9–days after incubation, the results are different from those of the similar experiments using 3.5-day-old embryonic NR (10). Of these colonies, either lens or pigment cells were differentiated, whereas no mixed colonies were formed. It seems likely that the determination or the limitation of the multipotentiality in future differentiation of the progenitor cells must occur between 3.5- and 8-9-days of embryonic development of NR *in situ*.

Such a process of the determination may occur in cells growing *in vitro* as well , since recloning of promary clones of 3.5-day-old embryonic NR on Day 9-10 resulted mostly in the monospecific clones with either lens or pigment cells. It was presumed that such a limitation of possible pathways of differentiation occurs during about 8-10 cell generations of clonal cell growth *in vitro* (19). These results indicate that clonal approach by use of cells of embryonic NR suits well for analyzing the problem of determination at the cellular level.

TRANSDIFFERENTIATION FOR LENS FROM NEURONAL CELLS

It has been shown that cells which tentatively designated as neuronal cells, appeared in early stages of in both clonal and mass cultures of NR. In a typical case of mass cultures of 3.5-day-old chick embryonic NR, cells attached to the culture substrate by 24 hours after inoculation are a homogeneous population of epithelial cells. Up to about a week, two cell types can be distinctly distinguished (20). The first type is large flattened cells (E-cells) which establish a monolayer of epithelial sheet directly upon the culture substrate. The second one (N-cell) is much smaller cells which are superimposed on top of the monolayer sheet of E-cells. Since the starting tissue is the neuroepithelium consisting of a single type of cells, such distinction of these two cells types is a first differentiation to occur in culture *in vitro*. Many of N-cells produce long cytoplasmic processes, by which clusters of these cells on the epithelial sheet are interconnected. This was a reason why we tentative designated N-cells as "neuronal". It seems now important to see whether these neuronal cells actually express, even partially, any differentiative traits as neural cells or not. We have taken two approaches toward this end.

The first is by means of the fluorescent microscopic observations of cultured cells stained with a fluorescent dye, merocyanine 540 (MC 540) (21). With appropriate intervals up to 20 days, cultured cells of 3.5-day-old embryonic NR were stained with this dye. Throughout all stages of culture, only N-cells were stained in contrast with the background E-cells which remained completely negative (Figures 2 and 3). In later stages, lens and pigment cells appeared, but they were also negative to the staining.

Although MC 540 is not a specific probe to detect the neural specificity, this dye selectively stains the membrane of electrically excitable cells (21). A clear distinction in the stainability of this dye between two cell types found in early cultures of NR must indicate that the differentiation actually occurs by this stage and N-cells are provided with characteristics more or less common to neural cells.

The second approach is a detection of neurotransmitter molecules and of the activity of enzymes related to their synthesis. In preliminary work using 3-day cultures of 3.5-day-old quail embryonic NR, the presence of several neurotransmitters such as acetylcholine and noradrenaline was detected by the method of Hildebrand et al. (22), using high-voltage paper electrophoresis of the culture homogenates which incorporated radiochemical precursors.

Changes in the specific activity of choline acetyltransferase (CAT) in cultures of chick embryonic NR was studied by Crisanti-Combes et al. (23). They did not use, however, cultures of very early embryonic NR. Above all, it was not shown whether or not lens and/or pigment cells would differentiate in further culturing of their cultures. Thus, we thought it necessary to see the pattern in changes of the activity of this enzyme in transdifferentiating cultures starting from earlier embryonic NR. Using the same culture samples, the amount of delta-crystallin was also measured by Laurll's method of the quantitative immunoelectrophoresis (24).

The activity of CAT in cultures of 3.5-day-old embryonic NR was first detected at 3 days and rapidly increased for the following 2 days to became 2.5 times greater. A decrease in the activity started at 10 days to drop gradually. Nearly concomitant to a drop of the activity of CAT, delta-crystallin became detectable and its amount increased rapidly in further culturing (Figure 4). A rise in the activity of CAT was well paralleled with the increase of N-cells in cultures (Figures 5 and 6). These results show that cells with the activity of

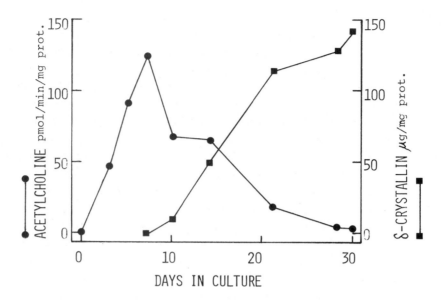

Fig. 4.   Changes in the activity of CAT and in the amount of delta-crystallin in cultures of 3.5-day-old chick embryonic NR.

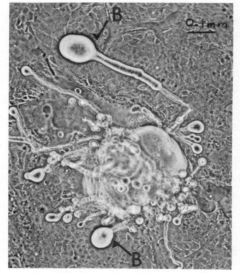

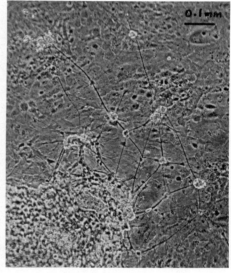

Fig.5.   An appearance of a number of N-cells and of their clusters which are interconnected with axon-like processes in a 8-day culture of 3.5-day-old chick embryonic NR.

Fig.6.   The differentiation of a typical lentoid body with bottle cells (B) in a 20-day culture of 3.5-day-old chick embryonic NR.

CAT which is one of the marker enzymes of neuronal specificity are certainly differentiated in transdifferentiating cultures. The differentiation of those cells occurs *de novo* in cultures, since the activity of CAT is undetectable in NR of 3.5-day-old embryos *in ovo*. Perhaps, small round N-cells, which are stained with merocyanine 504 specifically, may contain this emzyme and they can be assumed to express, at least partially, phenotypes as neural cells.

What is a nature of large flattened E-cells to be observed together with N-cells in cultures of NR ? Unfortunately, no study has yet been done to identify the characteristics of these cells by using any biochemical markers. Crisanti-Combes et al. (25) presumed these cells as Müller cells, based on their ultra-structural similarity with these cells found *in situ* chick embryonic NR.

SEQUENCE OF TRANSDIFFERENTIATION IN CULTURED NR CELLS

The results of clonal culture of 8-day-old chick or quail embryonic NR revealed that E-cells (presumable immature Müller cells) differentiate into either

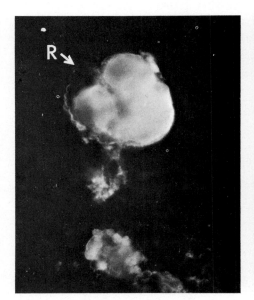

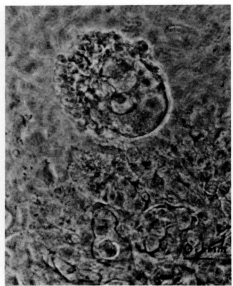

Fig.7. The transdifferentiation of a cluster of N-cells into a lentoid body in a 17-day culture of 3.5-day-old chick embryonic NR. An immunofluo-rescent microphotograph using antibody against delta-crystallin. Note that a part of a cluster (R) still remains to be negative.

Fig.8. A phase-contrast microphotograph of the same field as shown in Figure 7.

lens or pigment cells (10). Can N-cells which are now considered to express the
neural specificity partially, transdifferentiate into lens and/or pigment cells
in the conditions of cell culture ? To answer this question we have conducted
time-lapse cinematographic observations. Cultures were prepared by using 3.5-
day-old chick embryonic NR. After 10-12 days' culturing, when the differentiation of N-cells and E-cells occurred, the locations where N-cells appeared
densely were chosen and photographs were taken every 15 minutes for further culturing of 4-6 days. Not a few N-cells including the cells with short bipolar
processes started to swollen to form bottle cells, the appearance of which is
considered as a stable marker for lens differentiation in cell culture (26).
Often, aggregates of N-cells transdifferentiated directly into lentoid bodies,
which were assemblages of lens cells and stained brightly with fluorescent antibody against chick crystallins (Figures 7 and 8). No indication of the differentiation of pigment cells was observed from N-cells by our cinematographic
observations. On the other hand, the transdifferentiation of pigment cells from
E-cells was seen. Thus, it is now highly probable that cells partially differentiated into neural specificity can transdifferentiate into lens cells. This
posibility has not been taken into consideration in our previous studies (19).

Steps leading to transdifferentiation starting from multipotent progenitor
cells contained in early embryonic NR can be hypothetically summarized in the
following schema.

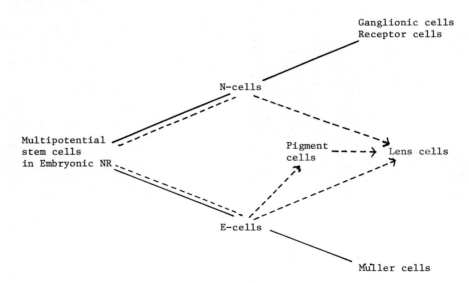

The progenitor cells differentiate into two directions, N-cells and E_1-cells, in the early stage in cultures. In development *in situ*, progenies of N-cells may differentiate into ganglionic and/or receptor cells, while E-cells may differentiate into Müller cells. In cell cultures, progenies of both N- and E-cells massively express foreign differentiations, which are completely inhibited *in situ*. N-cells can transdifferentiate into lens, while E-cells, into pigment cells and lens cells. Pigment cells derived from NR can also transdifferentiate into lens cells. Therefore, we encounter here a sequence in the change of differentiation starting from cells of NR to be terminated with lens cells. Apparent similarity of this sequential change in the expression of cell differentiation from one phenotype to another with the phenomena of transdetermination of *Drosophila* imaginal disks will attract our attention (27).

Further studies on molecular and cellular events on the transdifferentiation of eye tissues *in vitro* will hopefully contribute to our basic understanding of the problem of not only differentiation but also of determination.

SUMMARY

Embryonic neural retina (NR) of a number of vertebrates species is characterized by a unique property to differentiate very extensively into multiple pathways including lens and pigment cells, when the tissue was dissociated and cultured *in vitro*. Clonal cell culture using NR of 3.5-day-old chick embryos revealed the presence of multipotential progenitor (stem) cells in this tissue. These cells differentiate into neuronal cells and epithelial cells in early stages of culturing by about 5 days, and then lens and pigment cells are formed in further culturing by about 20 days. The fact that neuronal cells formed in cultures of embryonic NR partially express the neural specificity has been shown by the stainabily of the cells with merocyanine 504 as well as by the presence of choline acetyltransferase. Time-lapse cinematographical observations suggest that neuronal cells, as well as epithelial cells, in cultures of NR can transdifferentiate into lens cells. A speculative schema is presented for a sequential change in transdifferentiation *in vitro* starting from progenitor cells of NR and terminating with lens cells.

ACKNOWLEDGEMENT

The works reviewed here were supported by a grant for Basic Cancer research from the Japan Ministry of Education, Science and Culture and a research grant from Yamada Foundation. We thank Miss Yohko Katsurayama for help in the preparation of the manuscript. We are grateful to Drs. N.LeDouarin and J.Smith for introducing us the methods for the detection of CAT and neurotransmitters in cultured cells.

REFERENCES

1. Ebert, J.D. and Sussex, I.M. (1970) Interacting Systems in Development, Holt, Rinehart and Winston, New York, pp 1-328

2. Spemann, H. (1938) Embryonic Development and Induction, Yale Univ. Press, New Haven, pp. 1-398.

3. Yamada, T. (1977) Control Mechanisms in Cell-Type Conversion in Newt Regeneration. Karger, Basel, pp. 1-126.

4. Eguchi, G. and Okada, T.S. (1973) Proc. Nat. Acad. Sci., US, 71, 5052-5056.

5. Eguchi, G. (1976) In "Embryogenesis in Mammals". Ciba Foundation Symp., 40, Elsevier, Amsterdam, pp 241-258.

6. Okada, T.S. (1976) In "Tests of Teratogenicity *in vitro*" (J.D.Ebert and M.Marois, eds.), North Holland, Amsterdam, pp. 91-105.

7. Okada, T.S., Yasuda, K., Hayashi, M. and Eguchi, G. (1977) Develop. Biol., 60, 305-309.

8. Yasuda, K., Okada T.S., Eguchi, G. and Hayashi, M. (1978) Exp. Eye Res., 26, 59-595.

9. Yasuda, K. (1979) Develop. Biol., 68, 618-623.

10. Okada, T.S. (1977) Develop. Growth and Differ., 19, 323-335.

11. Okada, T.S., Itoh, Y., Watanabe, K. and Eguchi, G. (1975) Develop. Biol., 45, 318-329.

12. Itoh, Y. (1976) Develop. Biol., 54, 157-162.

13. DePomerai, D.I. and Clayton, R.M. (1978) J. Embryol. exp. Morph., 47, 179-193.

14. Nomura, K. and Okada, T.S. (1979) Develop. Growth and Differ., 21 (in press).

15. Araki, M., Yanagida, M. and Okada, T.S. (1979) Develop. Biol., 68, 170-181.

16. Itoh, Y., Okada, T.S., Ide, H. and Eguchi, G. (1975) Develop. Growth and Differ., 17, 39-50.

17. Yasuda, K., Thomson, I., DePomerai, D.I., Clayton, R.M. and Okada, T.S. (1979) Proc. Ann. Meeting of Jap. Soc. Develop. Biol., Sapporo, Japan.

18. Clayton, R.M. (1977) In "Stem Cells and Tissue Homeostasis" (British Soc. Cell Biol. Symp. 2), Cambridge Univ. Press, Cambridge, pp. 115-138.

19. Okada, T.S., Yasuda, K., Araki, M. and Eguchi, G. (1979) Develop. Biol., 68, 600-617.

20. Araki, M. and Okada, T.S. (1978) Develop. Biol., 60, 278-286.

21. Easton, T.G., Valinsky, J.E. and Reich, E. (1978) Cell, 13, 475-486.

22. Hildebrand, J.G., Barker, D.L., Herbert, E. and Kravitz, E.A. (1971) J. Neurobiol., 2, 231-246.

23. Crisanti-Combes, P., Pessac, B. and Calothy, G. (1978) Develop. Biol., 65, 228-232.

24. Laurell, C. -B. (1966) Anal. Biochem., 15, 45-52.

25. Crisanti-Combes, P., Privat, A., Pessac, B. and Calothy, G. (1977) Cell and Tissue Res., 185, 159-173.

26. Okada, T.S., Eguchi, G. and Takeichi, M. (1971) Develop. Growth and Differ., 13, 323-335.

27. Hadorn, E. (1966) Dynamics of determination. In "Major Problems in Developmental Biology" (M.Locke, ed.), pp. 85-104. Academic Press, New York.

Cell Lineage, Stem Cells and Cell Determination
INSERM Symposium No. 10
Editor: N. Le Douarin
© *1979 Elsevier/North-Holland Biomedical Press*

SELF-ASSEMBLY OF A NERVE: OPTIC FIBERS FOLLOW THEIR NEIGHBORS IN EMBRYOGENESIS.

CYRUS LEVINTHAL AND NEIL BODICK
Department of Biological Sciences, Columbia University, New York, New York.

Although efforts to understand the mechanisms by which ordered connections are established between large arrays of neurons have been underway for many years, there is still no clear picture of the mechanisms involved. One has no hard information as to the way cell-cell interactions or cell interactions with molecules in their environment account for the mapping of one array of neurons onto another. Ever since it was originally suggested by Sperry (1,2,3,), the idea that there is some form of labeling on both ganglion cell axons and tectal cells which accounts for the correct mapping of the optic fibers onto the tectum in lower vertebrates has been widely accepted. In this picture, it is assumed that the labels on the ganglion cells and the labels on the cells in the tectum are such that only when "correct" labels match will the ingrowing fibers come to rest and make synaptic connections. Furthermore, there has, for the most part, been acceptance of the view that the basic mechanisms which account for array matching in the visual system are the same for regenerating fibers as for initial growth during embryogenesis.

Recently, several reports (4,5,6) have presented evidence indicating that the processes involved in the establishment of connections in regeneration are probably different from those used during embryogenesis. Furthermore, Horder and Martin (7) have recently suggested that matching of labels may not be needed to account for any of the experimental results applicable to the establishment of retino-tectal connections. Their interpretation, however, requires that one dismiss a substantial body of experimental evidence (8,9) which seems to point in a different direction. However, regardless of the interpretation given to the experiments concerned with regeneration of a severed optic nerve, it still seems quite likely that the experiments suggesting chemoaffinity or chemical matching of labels do not provide compelling evidence that this mechanism is involved in embryogenesis.

In order to examine the developmental process in detail, we have carried out a morphological study at the electron microscopic level of the first few optic nerve fibers which leave the retina early in embryogenesis. The small tropical fish, the Zebrafish (Brachydanio rerio) was used in these studies, in part because (1) the animals can be bred in the laboratory throughout the year; (2) accurately staged embryos can be obtained with ease; and (3) the dimensions of the structures of interest are sufficiently small that complete serial section electron microscopy is practical. The embryos were studied at a stage when about 1800 optic nerve fibers leave the eye, of which approximately two thirds reach the tectum. In a young adult animal, some 50,000 fibers

connect the retinal ganglion cells to the contralateral optic
tectum. Therefore, the fibers studied in these experiments were
in fact, among the first to leave the eye on the way towards the
tectum. Embryos were obtained and prepared for electron
microscopy with a microperfusion technique described elsewhere
(10).

Individual nerve fibers and their relationship to each other
have been examined by means of computer reconstruction from the
aligned serial section electron micrographs using methods which
have been described previously (10,11).

The essential results of these studies can be described simply.
The fibers which are leaving the eye at this early stage are
found to grow along the retinal surface in small bundles which
arise from groups of adjacent cell bodies in the developing
retina. These small bundles grow from the ganglion cell bodies
to the surface of the retina, then turn and grow towards the
nerve head where they again turn and exit from the eye through
the lumen defined by the choroid fissure. The small bundles
themselves merge into larger and larger groups so that by the
time the nerve fibers reach the optic nerve head, the 1800 or so
nerve fibers are found in approximately 10 bundles distributed
around the circumference of the vitreal surface. In each of
these large bundles, the most recently formed fibers (which arise
from the most peripheral ganglion cells in the retina) are found
to be located in the innermost region, adjacent to the vitreal
surface. Thus, the pattern reflects the fact that the fibers
which arise from the most recently differentiated ganglion cells
grow on top of a layer of the older axons closer to the nerve
head.

As these bundles are followed from the eye towards the brain,
they coalesce, forming first a crescent and then a circular
crossection in which all of the fibers from the most recently
differentiated cell lie along the ventral surface of the structure.
Thus, in this optic nerve, one finds a continuous mapping of
retinal surface position into the optic nerve. Radial positions
of somata are transformed to the dorsal-ventral axis of the
optic nerve while the angular position around the retina is
transformed to the nasal-temporal axis with a discontinuity in
the ventral retina. The two ends of the nasal-temporal axis
represent adjacent ventral ganglion cells.

However, the ventral ganglion cells map to one region of the
tectum. The apparent discontinuity which is introduced
by the choroid fissure is not reflected in the physiological
mapping of the visual field onto the surface of the tectum.
Scholes (13) has recently analyzed this problem in an adult
cichlid fish and found that there are a set of remarkable local
transformations in the positions of the optic nerve fibers
which result in fibers from nasal, rather than ventral, ganglion
cells lying at the end of one axis of the nerve.

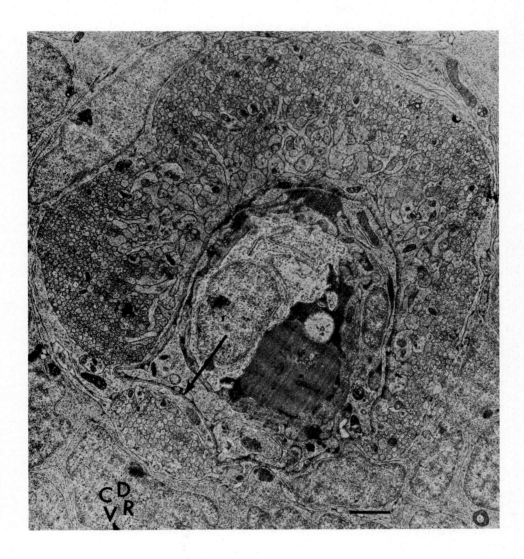

Figure 1. The optic nerve head is crescent in crossection. The youngest fibers are those with irregular profiles shown by reconstruction to have growth cones at their tips. These fibers emanate from cells at the periphery of the eye and occupy the ventral perimeter of the crescent. One large bundle (arrow) has not yet merged into the crescent. D=dorsal, V=ventral, C=caudal, R=rostral, bar=1 micron.

Our studies of the early embryo suggest a plausible mechanism by which the first transformation from retinal position to position in the nerve takes place during embryogenesis. However, we have not as yet examined the developing optic nerve to determine how it might undergo the transformation described by Scholes. The major conclusion indicated by our results is that the first transformation from retinal position to position in the optic nerve is based on the capacity of newly differentiated nerve fibers to follow the axons of neighbors which have differentiated at a slightly earlier time. Since many of these young fibers terminate either before leaving the retina or shortly thereafter, we have been able to examine growing tips. In each case the growth cones at these tips were found to send out processes which follow along and frequently wrap around older adjacent fibers. One can observe, in the reconstruction of these fibers, a pattern which can account for the overall organization of the optic nerve (Figure 3).

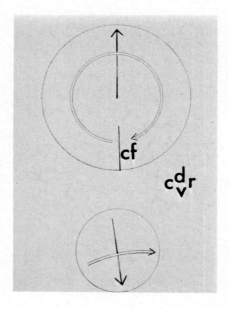

Figure 2. Schematic of positional mapping from the retina to the optic nerve near the place where the nerve leaves the eye. Angular position transforms into the rostro-caudal axis while radial position transforms into the dorso-ventral axis. Note discontinuity at the choroid fissure. cf=choroid fissure, d=dorsal, v=ventral, c=caudal, r=rostral.

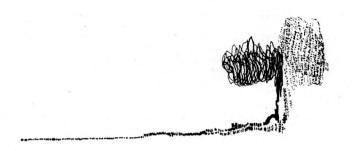

Figure 3. Somata cluster as they spin out fascicles of axons.
Fibers within a fascicle remain adjacent and adjacent fascicles
maintain their relative positions as the fibers course back
toward the tectum. Shown are two cells which have been reconstructed from a cluster containing seven cells.

Thus, a very small number of simple rules can account for
the initial ordering in the optic nerve even when it contains
a very large number of individual nerve fibers. These rules
would be something like the following:

(1) The first ganglion cells to differentiate are those
which are closest to the nerve head. From then on all further
ganglion cells differentiate at a time which is slightly delayed
with respect to their neighbors which have already differentiated.
This rule, if followed by all cells, will produce a wave of
cellular differentiation traveling radially outward from the
fibers which differentiate first (14). In the case of the
Zebrafish those fibers which differentiate first are in the
region just posterior to the choroid fissure. Propogation of
fiber initiation then proceeds both radially and clockwise as the
eye is viewed from outside of the animal.

(2) Each fiber from a differentiating ganglion cell grows
in such a way as to follow the axons of its neighbors. In each
case, a neighbor is defined as a cell which is either in physical
contact or very close to the one under consideration.

(3) The signals which are transmitted between adjacent
fibers and cell bodies are not transmitted across the choroid
fissure.

Even if this picture is correct we still need to consider
two additional problems. First, what provides the guidance for
the very first fibers which leave the eye? Second, how is this
guidance regulated as the fibers get closer to and then reach
the optic tectum?

Further experimental work will be needed to identify those presumptive guiding structures external to the nerve itself. At the moment one can only say that if the type of model we are suggesting is correct then the guidance of the very first fibers must be external to the nerve itself.

ACKNOWLEDGEMENTS

These studies were supported by NSF Grant PCM 78-06636, NIH Grant 5 RO1 NS 09821-08, and the Computer Graphics Facility NIH Grant 5 P 41 RR 00442-10.

REFERENCES

1.   Sperry, R.W., J. Comp. Neurol. Vol. 79, p. 33 (1943).

2.   _____, Anat. Rec. Vol. 84, p. 470 (1942).

3.   _____, Proc. Natl. Acad. Sci. USA Vol. 50, p. 713 (1963).

4.   Chung, S.H. and Cooke, J. Nature, London Vol. 258, p. 126 (1975)

5.   _____, Proc. R. Soc. London B. Vol. 201, p. 279 (1978).

6.   Schmidt, J.T.,J. Comp. Neurol. Vol. 177, p. 279 (1978).

7.   Horder, T.J., and Martin, K.A.C. from Soc. for Exp. Biol. Symp. No. XXXII, Cell-Cell Recognition, Ed., A.S.G. Curtis, Cambridge University Press, (1978)

8.   Yoon, M.G., J. Physiol. Vol. 252, p. 137 (1975).

9.   Levine, R., and Jacobson, M. Exp. Neurol. Vol. 43, p. 527 (1976).

10. Levinthal, C. and Bodick, N. Proc. Natl. Acad. Sci. USA (In Press).

11. Levinthal, C., Macagno, E.R. and Tountas, C. Federation Proceedings, Vol. 33, No. 12 (1974).

12. Macagno, E.R., Levinthal, C. and Sobel, I., Ann. Rev. Biophys. Bioeng. Vol. 8, p. 323 (1979).

13. Scholes, J.H. Nature, London Vol. 278, p. 620 (1979).

14. Hollyfield, J.G., Devel. Biol. Vol. 18, p. 163 (1968).

Cell Lineage, Stem Cells and Cell Determination
INSERM Symposium No. 10
Editor: N. Le Douarin
© *1979 Elsevier/North-Holland Biomedical Press*

AN ANALYSIS OF CELL LINE SEGREGATION IN THE NEURAL CREST

NICOLE M. LE DOUARIN, CHRISTIANE S. LE LIEVRE, GHISLAINE SCHWEIZER and
CATHERINE M. ZILLER.
Institut d'Embryologie du CNRS et du Collège de France, 49bis, Avenue de la
Belle-Gabrielle, 94130 Nogent-sur-Marne (France)

INTRODUCTION

The neural crest, a transient structure of the vertebrate embryo, generates
a variety of cell types that can be classified in 5 categories : nerve cells,
supportive cells of the nervous system, pigment cells, endocrine and para-
endocrine cells and the so-called "mesectoderm", which gives rise to mesenchyme
and its derivatives (connective tissue, bone, cartilage, muscle) (see
Hörstadius[1] ; Weston[2] ; Le Douarin[3],[4] for reviews). Differentiated phenotypes
of neural crest derived cells are expressed after they have accomplished a migration throughout the embryo in an apparently undifferentiated state ; hence
the question arises of when the different cell lines are segregated and under
what kind of stimulus.

During ontogeny, the acquisition by a pluripotent cell of a definite
programme of differentiation is generally not followed by any detectable modification of the cell from either a structural or a chemical point of view. For
this reason, the determined state is usually defined in an operational way ;
this is the ability of a cell population to express a given phenotype even if
it is subtracted from its normal microenvironment, and eventually subjected to
epigenetic influences different from those it would have normally received
during ontogeny. In other words, if a group of embryonic cells is determined,
its evolution proceeds normally without or in spite of additional information
arising from its surroundings. Such an imprecise definition reflects our
ignorance of the molecular changes that are responsible for the restriction of
the developmental capabilities of the cells during ontogeny.

The experiments reported in this article have been devised to investigate
the developmental relationships that exist between the sensory and the autonomic
ganglia, which both arise from the neural crest.

A number of experimental data have accumulated showing that the chemical
differentiation of autonomic neurons remains labile, as far as neurotransmitter
synthesis is concerned, until late in development and appears to be directed
by microenvironmental cues[5],[6],[7],[8]. In the present work we investigated whether
the sensory and autonomic cell lines become segregated early in embryogenesis,

or whether it were possible to evoke changes from sensory to autonomic - or inversely - by experimental disturbances imposed on the differentiating cells.

The principle of the method is based on an observation already described in part previously[8] : if a differentiating autonomic ganglion (the ciliary or the Remak ganglia) is back-transplanted into a younger host at the precise stage where the neural crest cells start migrating, the implanted ganglion cells reacquire migratory capacities and become distributed among the autonomic structures of the host. A possible interpretation of this result is that the grafted autonomic cells display, besides their ability to migrate, a kind of cell-cell recognition mechanism responsible for their localization in the host embryo. This hypothesis implies that the back transplantation of a differentia-ting ganglion can be considered as an *in vivo* "sorting out" experiment, in which the preferential ability of the different cell types to aggregate with each other can be tested. Such a cell-cell recognition process may be interpre-ted as the expression of a determination towards a definite cell line. For this reason, we have transplanted into 2-day chick embryos various types of autonomic and sensory ganglia taken from quails at different stages of development. In addition, pieces of quail neural crest were also implanted in the chick host in contact with the neural primordium of the latter. The "adrenomedullary" level (from somites 18 to 24, see Le Douarin and Teillet[9]) of the neural axis was chosen for the implantation into the host because, in this area, the neural crest produces, in addition to sensory and sympathetic ganglia, the adrenome-dullary cells and the adrenal and aortic adrenergic plexuses. The distribution of grafted cells among the neural crest derivatives of the host can be perceived by virtue of the nuclear marker provided by the quail cells[10,11,12].

EXPERIMENTAL PROCEDURES

1. Graft

- Preparation of the host and transplantation (figure 1)

Host chick embryos at stage 18- to 24-somite were prepared in the following way : a slit was cut in the trunk region of the embryos between neural tube and somitic mesoderm, at the adrenomedullary level of the neural axis, corres-ponding to somites 18 to 24.

The rudiment to be grafted was inserted into the slit and the host embryos were incubated for 4 hours to 7 days thereafter (2 1/2 to 9 days total incuba-tion)

- Preparation of the grafted neural tissues (figure 1)

a) Neural crest : the adrenomedullary trunk neural crests were taken from quail donor embryos at 17- to 24-somite stages. A fragment of neural fold

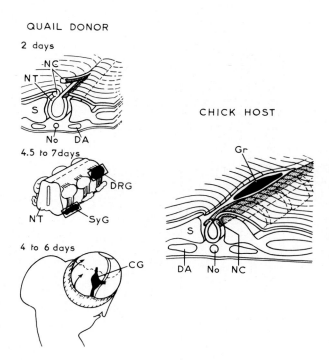

QUAIL DONOR

2 days

4.5 to 7 days

4 to 6 days

CHICK HOST

Fig. 1. Diagram showing the different kinds of grafts of quail tissues into a 2-day chick host embryo. Pieces of trunk neural crest, dorsal root (DRG), sympathetic (SyG) or ciliary (CG) ganglia are inserted into a slit made between the neural primordium and the somites at the "*adrenomedullary*" level of the neural axis (somites 18 to 24). Gr : graft ; DA : dorsal aorta ; NC : neural crest ; NT : neural tube ; No : notochord ; S : somite.

between levels of somites 17 and 24 was unilaterally cut off *in situ* with fine steel needles.

b) Sensory and sympathetic ganglia : they were isolated from 4 1/2- to 7-day old quail embryos. The dorsal trunk region(between the cervical and the sacral level) was incubated for 15 to 20 minutes in a 0.5 % trypsin solution in Ca^{++}, Mg^{++} free Tyrode solution. The neural tissue (sensory and sympathetic ganglion, dorsal and ventral roots and neural tube) were mechanically cleaned from the surrounding mesenchyme and washed in Tyrode solution containing horse serum. Half or one third of a ganglion was grafted.

c) The ciliary ganglia : ciliary ganglia were isolated surgically from 4- to 6-day old quail embryos. The ciliary ganglion was implanted into the trunk region of the host, either whole, or cut into 2 or 3 pieces, depending on the age of the donor.

TABLE I

FINAL LOCALIZATION OF QUAIL CELLS FROM THE GRAFTED NEURAL TISSUES IN THE CHICK HOST DORSAL TRUNK STRUCTURES.

Grafts / Final localization of the grafted cells	DRG	Schwann cells	Sympathetic ganglion	Retroaortic and adrenal plexuses	Adreno Medulla
Trunk neural crest	$\frac{14^{x}}{14^{\#}}$	$\frac{14}{14}$	$\frac{14}{14}$	$\frac{14}{14}$	$\frac{14}{14}$
Ciliary ganglion 4-6 days	$\frac{3^{\bullet}}{32}$	$\frac{32}{32}$	$\frac{20}{32}$	$\frac{14}{32}$	$\frac{18}{32}$
DRG 4.5-7 days	$\frac{14}{21}$	$\frac{21}{21}$	$\frac{19}{21}$	$\frac{16}{19}$	$\frac{15}{19}$

x.Number of cases in which quail cells were found in the host structures.
#.Number of cases observed.
•.In 3 cases a few scattered non-neuronal quail cells were found in the host sensory ganglia.

2. Histology

The trunk region of the host embryo was fixed for histological examination in Zenker's fixative and serial sections were stained according to Feulgen and Rossenbeck's reaction which allows quail and chick cells to be recognized. Falck's method[13] for the detection of monoamine containing cells by formol induced fluorescence (FIF) was applied to some host embryos of 7 to 9 days of incubation. When Feulgen-Rossenbeck's and FIF methods are combined as described previously[8], monoamine-containing cells and quail cells from the graft can be detected on the same section.

RESULTS

1. Graft of a fragment of quail neural crest.

This experiment was carried out as a control to see whether the graft of an additional piece of tissue disturbs the localization of the implanted cells.

A piece of neural crest taken from a quail embryo at the level of somites 17 to 24 was cut off and inserted into a slit made between the somites and the neural primordium at the "adrenomedullary" level of a 20- to 24-somite chick embryo.

Observation of the host at 6 to 9 days of incubation revealed the presence of quail cells in the dorsal root ganglia (DRG) (neurons and satellite cells), the rachidian nerves (Schwann cells), the sympathetic ganglia (neurons and satellite cells), the adrenergic trunk plexuses (aortic and adrenal) and the suprarenal glands (adrenomedullary cells). No quail cells were found in the ganglion of Remak and the myenteric plexuses except for Schwann cells lining sympathetic nerves (Table I). In fact, quail neural crest cell distribution in this case was the same as that observed when isotopic and isochronic grafts of the neural primordium (neural tube + neural folds)are carried out at the same level[9]. In many cases DRG and sympathetic ganglia were found entirely/ mainly made up of grafted cells, while the adrenomedullary cords were also wholly quail in a part of the suprarenal gland. The problem is therefore posed of the behaviour and fate of the host neural crest cells at the graft level. One possibility is that the implanted cells migrate first and occupy all the "sites of arrest" available in their dorso-ventral progression. What is, in such a case, the fate of the host crest cells ? They may either multiply very little and finally disappear or migrate further, penetrate the dorsal mesentery and contribute to the parasympathetic intestinal system (i.e. : ganglion of Remak and enteric plexuses). No answer to this question can be provided by this experiment.

In any case, the distribution and fate of the cells migrating from a supplementary neural crest appears to be the same as in normal development, which means that no detectable modification is imposed on the final localization of the migrating cells by the grafting technique used.

2. Graft of DRG and autonomic ganglia

The grafts of DRG and of ciliary and sympathetic ganglia were observed from 4 hours to 7 days after the graft.

a - Dispersion of the ganglion cells in the host

Migration of the ganglion cells was observed in serial sections of the host for several days following implantation. As early as 6 hours after the graft, quail cells could be seen around the bulk of the implant as if they had peeled off from its periphery. This was mainly apparent on the side of the graft facing the neural tube, and the implanted cells were encountered in many instances migrating in the extracellular material lining the neural tube (figure 2). The

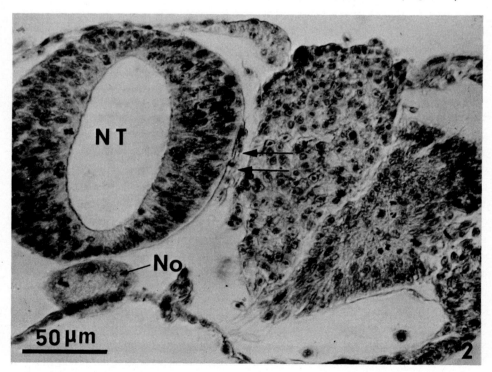

Fig. 2. Graft of a piece of a 4.5-day quail ciliary ganglion at the *adreno-medullary* level (somites 18 to 24) of the neural axis of a 24-somite chick embryo between neural tube and somites. The host is sacrificed 6 hours after grafting. Quail cells (⟹) detached from the ganglion are seen along the lateral aspect of the neural tube (NT), normal migration route of host crest cells. No : notochord. G x 450.

subsequent evolution of the ganglia is somewhat different according to whether they appertain to the autonomic or sensory system. In the case of ciliary and sympathetic grafts, no evident necrosis occurs following implantation. In addition, the grafted ganglion remains whole but its size decreases significantly during the two days following the graft, due to the dispersion of its cells in the somitic mesenchyme. As early as at 5 days of incubation, localization of quail cells in various developing crest derivatives can be recognized ; such is the case, for instance, for some of the cells lining the rachidian nerves, and others located in the primary sympathetic chain ganglia and around the aorta. When the host is 6 day-old the grafted ganglion has usually disappeared and from this stage on the definitive distribution of the grafted cells can be observed.

The evolution of 4.5-7-day quail sensory ganglia differs slightly from that described above in two ways :

1 - necrosis is apparent in most cases during the day following the graft (figure 3).

2 - during the second and third days, the bulk of the ganglion appears fragmented, probably due to resorption of dead cells through host macrophagic activity. As a result, clumps of large neuronal cells associated with smaller satellite elements appear scattered in the host dorsal trunk mesenchyme (figure 4).

From 6-7 days of incubation of the host, definitive localization of grafted cells in host structures is reached.

b - Localization_of_grafted_ganglion_cells_in_host_neural_crest_derivatives.

The results are strikingly different according to the sensory or autonomic nature of the ganglion (see Table I).

Sympathetic and ciliary ganglion cells become located in autonomic ganglia (sympathetic and parasympathetic),   as Schwann cells in rachidian and autonomic nerves,in the suprarenal glands and in the aortic and adrenal plexuses. In no case were quail neurons ever found in host sensory ganglia, whereas these structures contained a few scattered non-neuronal quail cells in 3 out of 32 cases of ciliary ganglion graft. In all the cases observed ciliary ganglion cells had migrated in the dorsal mesentery and had given rise to neural and glial components of the ganglion of Remak and enteric ganglia.

360

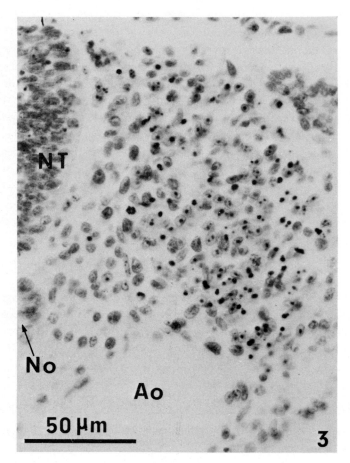

Fig. 3. Graft of a 5-day quail DRG into a chick embryo at the level of somite 20 to 24. The host was fixed 24 hours after the graft. Numerous pycnotic nuclei are observed between the cells of the disrupting quail ganglion. Ao : dorsal aorta ; No : notochord ; NT : neural tube. G x 590.

When sensory ganglia are grafted, numerous quail neurons and satellite cells are associated with the host sensory ganglia (figure 5). In none of the 21 cases observed was the host DRG found to be entirely made up of grafted cells as is the case when a piece of trunk neural crest is implanted. In addition, numerous quail cells participate in the constitution of the sympathetic ganglion, the adrenal and aortic plexuses and the adrenomedulla.

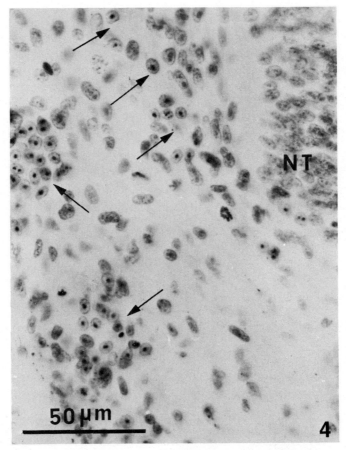

Fig. 4. Graft of a 5-day quail DRG as in figure 3. The host was fixed 30 hours after the   operation. Groups of quail cells (———➤) are scattered in the sclerotome mesenchyme. G x 670.

3. Differentiation of adrenergic cells from the grafted ganglion.

Application of the associated FIF-Feulgen-Rossenbeck techniques to the host embryos showed that CA-containing cells developed from grafted cells in all experimental series : i.e. from trunk neural crest, autonomic and sensory ganglia grafts. These cells were distributed in the adrenergic structures of the host (sympathetic ganglia, adrenergic plexuses of the trunk and adrenomedullary cords).

362

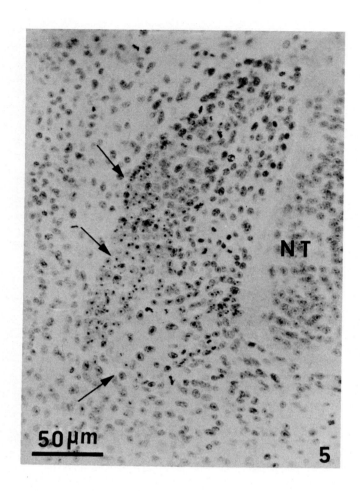

Fig. 5. Graft of a 5-day quail DRG as in figure 3-4. At 4.5 days of incubation of the host, cells from the graft ($\longrightarrow$) are found in the host DGR. G x 370.

CONCLUSION AND DISCUSSION

The experiments described above reveal striking differences in the behaviour of autonomic and sensory ganglia after grafting into a 2-day host. Both types of ganglia can give rise to Schwann cells ; otherwise, the final location of grafted autonomic and sensory ganglion cells in trunk structures of the host is

different. Cells derived from the former aggregate selectively with autonomic ganglia and plexuses and also home to the adrenal medulla. A few non-neuronal

quail cells were found dispersed in a host DRG in only 3 out of 32 cases, but
no quail neurons were ever found in this location.

In contrast, after the graft of sensory ganglia, large neurons of the quail
type were found in the host DRG, while numerous fluorescent quail cells were
also present in the sympathetic structures and in the adrenomedulla.

It therefore appears that the ciliary and sympathetic ganglion cells possess
an "*autonomic*" determination, i.e. compared to the neural crest cell population
they have lost the ability to differentiate into sensory ganglion cells. However, although restricted to the autonomic line, a binary choice still awaits
them : that of becoming either adrenergic or cholinergic. As demonstrated
earlier by several groups (see Patterson[5] and Le Douarin[14]) this choice remains
labile until relatively late in development and is regulated through environmental cues.

In the light of our experiments, the cell population of the 5-7-day old DRG
appears heterogenous. First, they contain differentiating neuroblasts that are
condemned to die following transplantation, whereas no necrosis was evident in
the grafted autonomic ganglia. The neurons and satellite cells which become
localized in the host DRG can be considered as belonging to the already restricted "*sensory*" line. In contrast, the population of DRG cells which migrates
more ventrally, aggregates with the host sympathetic ganglia and plexuses and
homes to the adrenomedullary cords,is not irreversibly committed to the sensory
line. These cells behave as if they were still undetermined and their fate in
normal development is not clear. They may remain in the DRG and finally become
sensory cells, or they may migrate further in a ventral direction and become
components of the autonomic system. In any case, comparison of the results
obtained in the three types of graft carried out indicates that, as expected,
the pluripotentiality to give rise to sensory, autonomic and adrenal cells is
a characteristic of the trunk neural crest, and still exists in the DRG cell
population until at least 7 days of incubation in the quail. In contrast, the
cells of the autonomic ganglia of similar ages are restricted to the autonomic
line and do not have the capacity to give rise to DRG cells. A fact worth empha-
sising is that no satellite cells of the grafted autonomic ganglia were currently
found to home to the host DRG. In contrast, autonomic satellite cells become
localized in the host autonomic derivatives, just as the neurons do. This suggests that sensory and autonomic satellite cells are different in nature and
that some kind of affinity seems to exist between satellite and neuronal cells
of each of the two types of peripheral ganglion. The commitment towards the

TABLE II

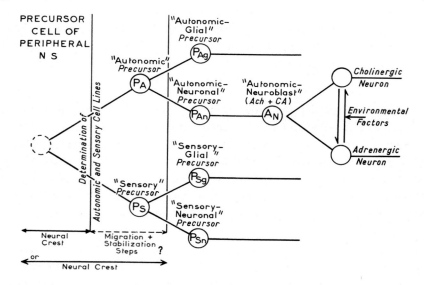

Segregation of the *autonomic* and *sensory* lines in the peripheral nervous system (NS). It is presented as a hypothesis that the sensory and autonomic lines are separated early (either in the neural crest itself or soon after cells have stopped migrating). The determination takes place in a precursor cell from which the satellite and the neuronal lines will respectively derive.

sensory and the autonomic lines very probably takes place in cells that are the precursors of both the neuronal and the satellite cell lines in each type of ganglia (Table II).

However, the problem of when this determinative event occurs -in the neural crest itself or following the onset of migration - cannot yet be decided.

REFERENCES

1. Horstadius, S. (1950) The neural crest : its properties and derivatives in the light of experimental research, Oxford University Press, London, pp. 1-111.

2. Weston, J.A. (1970) In "Advances in Morphogenesis", ed. M. Abercrombie, J. Brachet and T.J. King, Academic Press, New-York, 8, 41-114.

3. Le Douarin, N.M. (1974) Med. Biol., 52, 281-319.

4. Le Douarin, N.M. (1976). In "Embryogenesis in Mammals", Ciba Foundation Symposium, Elsevier, Excerpta Medica, North-Holland, Amsterdam, 71-101.

5. Patterson, P.H. (1978) Ann. Rev. Neurosci., 1, 1-17.

6. Le Douarin, N.M. and Teillet, M.A. (1974). Dev. Biol., 41, 162-184.

7. Le Douarin, N.M., Renaud, D., Teillet, M.A. and Le Douarin, G.H. (1975) Proc. Nat. Acad. Sci., 72, 728-732.

8. Le Douarin, N.M., Teillet, M.A., Ziller, C. and Smith, J. (1978) Proc. Nat. Acad. Sci., 75, 2030-2034.

9. Le Douarin, N.M. and Teillet, M.A. (1973) J. Embryol. exp. Morph., 30, 31-48.

10. Le Douarin, N. (1969) Bull. Biol. Fr. Belg., 103, 435-452.

11. Le Douarin, N. (1973a) Dev. Biol., 30, 217-222.

12. Le Douarin, N. (1973b) Exp. Cell. Res., 77, 459-468.

13. Falck, B. (1962) Acta Physiol. Scand., 56, suppl. 197, 1-25.

14. Le Douarin, N. (1979) In "Current Topics in Developmental Biology", Academic Press, New-York, in press.

Cell Lineage, Stem Cells and Cell Determination
INSERM Symposium No. 10
Editor: N. Le Douarin
© *1979 Elsevier/North-Holland Biomedical Press*

DETERMINATION OF THE NEUROTRANSMITTER PHENOTYPE OF SYMPATHETIC NEURONS IN VITRO

PAUL H. PATTERSON

Department of Neurobiology, Harvard Medical School, 25 Shattuck Street, Boston, Massachusetts 02115, U.S.A.

It is via secretion of their neurotransmitters that neurons exert control over their target cells. The type of transmitter secreted is crucial because target cells often respond in opposite ways to different transmitters. For instance, acetylcholine (ACh) slows the heart beat while catecholamines (CA) accelerate it. Thus it is of interest that it has proven possible to influence experimentally the choice of neurotransmitter and type of synapse formed by developing postmitotic sympathetic neurons in dispersed cell culture. Furthermore, the evidence suggests that there are at least three qualitatively different types of exogenous or epigenetic "factors" which can influence this choice. Discussion of the relative roles of these factors may be of special interest in reference to analogous epigenetic factors operating in other developing systems, such as the blood forming system, covered elsewhere in this Volume. More detailed reviews of much of the material to be presented here are available[1,2].

The neuroblasts of the mammalian superior cervical ganglion begin to produce CA soon after their migration from the neural crest is finished[3,4]. These sympathetic neuroblasts can display noradrenergic (CA-containing) properties even while still dividing[5,6]. At birth, virtually all of these neurons contain CA[7]. When dissociated and placed in culture at this stage, the neurons continue to develop noradrenergically, as judged by morphological[8] and biochemical[9,10] criteria. Under these conditions, the development of cholinergic (ACh-containing) properties is minimal[10,11].

On the other hand, if the culture conditions are appropriately modified, the early noradrenergic development can be reversed and cholinergic differentiation occurs instead. The neurons can synthesize and store ACh[8,10,12] and form functional cholinergic synapses[8,13,15] with the appropriate morphology[8,16]. It is possible to obtain sister cultures in which 100% of the neurons produce CA, or in which more than 90% produce ACh[17] without significantly altering neuronal survival or growth[18]. Thus individual sympathetic neurons have the capacity to become noradrenergic or cholinergic and this decision can be regulated by exogenous cues. In fact the neurons can reverse the initial noradrenergic choice even after beginning to express that phenotype. This has been most dramatically demonstrated in preliminary experiments involving repeated electrophysiological recordings from individual neurons developing over a period of several weeks in microcultures containing heart muscle cells (D. D. Potter and E. J. Furshpan, personal communication). A number of neurons have been observed initially to form noradrenergic synapses on heart myocytes, with no sign of cholinergic function; later, however, the same neurons form cholinergic synapses on the heart cells.

If virtually all of the cultured neurons are noradrenergic at the outset, but can then develop cholinergic functions, it may be possible to identify neurons which express both transmitter properties simultaneously. Such "dual function" neurons have, in fact, been identified in the microcultures with heart cells[16,19]. These neurons can release both CA and ACh at functional synapses with the cardiac myocytes. The frequency of occurrence, and the duration of this dual function stage are under study. The transition from catecholinergic to cholinergic differentiation is largely reciprocal; most of the former CA properties are lost[16,18]. However, the mechanism for high affinity uptake of CA does persist in the cholinergic neurons for some time[16,17,20].

What is the nature of the environmental stimulus that causes the sympathetic neurons to become cholinergic? Such signals can be produced by certain types of nonneuronal cells and are found in a freely diffusable form in the culture medium[18,21] and bound to the membranes of the nonneuronal cells[22]. In both cases the active factors have protein-like properties, and the diffusable factor has an apparent molecular weight of about 50,000 daltons (M. Weber and P. Patterson, unpublished). The particular types of cells that produce the factor(s) are of interest: there is a correlation between the degree of cholinergic innervation a tissue normally receives and its ability to produce this factor in culture[18]. However, since fibroblasts and glioma cells can also produce the factor, the importance of this correlation is not clear[1].

The properties of the diffusable cholinergic factor are clearly distinguishable from those of the well studied protein, nerve growth factor (NGF). The former is not necessary for the survival of sympathetic neurons, does not stimulate growth, but does regulate transmitter choice and synapse type. In contrast, NGF is necessary for the survival of these neurons and does stimulate growth[23,24]. However, NGF does not influence the choice of transmitter; increasing concentrations of NGF in culture promote the differentiation of both catecholaminergic and cholinergic properties. In fact, in cultures producing both CA and ACh, NGF stimulates the production of both transmitters to the same extent[25]. Thus NGF is acting as a permissive influence, whereas the cholinergic factor plays an instructive role.

These findings raised an intriguing question: why is it that nonneuronal cells can cause almost all of the sympathetic neurons to become cholinergic in culture, yet in vivo only a few of them become cholinergic? One possible explanation is that in vivo the cholinergic signal is selectively localized so that only a few neurons receive it. This possibility remains to be definitively tested. An alternative hypothesis is that many or all of the neurons in vivo are exposed to the cholinergic cue, but most are prevented from responding to the signal by an additional factor that is missing from the culture medium. A candidate for such a factor is the normal excitatory input these neurons receive from their spinal cord innervation. In the usual culture experiments this input is missing and furthermore, it had been previously shown in vivo that if the innervation of young sympathetic ganglia is cut, further adrenergic development is reduced[26]. These observations raised the possibility that electrical activity imposed on the sympathetic neurons plays a role in determining the choice of transmitter. Although the spinal cord neurons are not present in culture, their excitatory effect on the membrane potential of sympathetic neurons could be mimicked in several ways: raising the K^+ concentration in the medium, by adding the drug veratridine (which causes an influx of Na^+ ions into the neurons) or by stimulating the cells electrically at a physiological frequency of one/sec.

When mass neuronal cultures were depolarized either in the presence of the cholinergic factor or for 7-10 days before the addition of the factor, the neurons remained primarily noradrenergic. Indeed, depolarization depressed the ratio of ACh production to CA production as much as 300-fold compared with cultures that simply received the cholinergic factor[27]. These changes occurred without a significant alteration in the survival of the neurons, suggesting that the neurons which would have become cholinergic in response to the factor, now remained noradrenergic. It was as if the depolarization, either chronic or accompanying normal electrical activity, stabilized their prenatal instruction to become adrenergic and curtailed their plasticity with respect to transmitter choice. An alternative interpretation is that depolarization is acting as a noradrenergic factor per se. This seems unlikely since all neurons in the nervous system are depolarized occasionally and relatively few are noradrenergic. However, clear evidence for the stabilization idea is lacking until activity can be shown to stabilize another transmitter choice besides the noradrenergic one. Regarding the mechanism of the depolarization effect, Ca^{++} influx appears to be necessary[27,28].

These observations raise the possibility that in intact ganglia the majority of the neurons are preserved in their prenatal noradrenergic condition by electrical input from the spinal cord. A corollary hypothesis is that the small number of ganglionic neurons that are destined to become cholinergic (thost that innervate certain blood vessels and sweat glands) acquire their synaptic input only after they have been influenced by the nonneuronal cells. Inherent in such a mechanism is an interesting possibility. Perhaps the selective formation of synapses between the spinal cord axons and the sympathetic neurons not only establishes the circuitry of the autonomic pathways but also determines the choice of transmitter that is appropriate to the circuitry. This concept emphasizes the potential importance of activity in neuronal differentiation.

In summary, three different types of epigenetic factors have been found to influence the transmitter choice of sympathetic neurons: (i) a permissive factor necessary for any choices to be made, exemplified by NGF, (ii) an instructive cholinergic factor from nonneuronal cells, and (iii) electrical activity is postulated to be a factor that can stabilize choices previously made.

REFERENCES

1. Patterson, P.H. (1978) Environmental determination of autonomic neurotransmitter functions, Annu. Rev. Neurosci. 1:1-18.

2. Bunge, R., Johnson, M. and Ross, C.D. (1978) Nature and nurture in development of the autonomic neuron, Science 199:1409-1416.

3. Cochard, P., Goldstein, M. and Black, I. (1978) Ontogenetic appearance and disappearance of tyrosine hydroxylast and catecholamines in the rat embryo, Proc. Natl. Acad. Sci. USA 75:2986-2990.

4. Coughlin, M.D., Boyer, D.M. and Black, I.B. (1977) Embryonic development of a mouse sympathetic ganglion in vivo and in vitro. Proc. Natl. Acad. Sci. 74:3438-3442.

5. Cohen, A.M. (1974) DNA synthesis and cell division in differentiating avain adrenergic neuroblasts, in Dynamics of Degeneration and Growth in Neurons pp 359-370, Eds. Fuxe, Olson and Zotterman, New York: Pergamon Press.

6. Rothman, T.P., Gershon, M.D. and Holtzer, H. (1978) Cell division and the acquisition of adrenergic characteristics by developing sympathetic ganglion cells, Dev. Biol. 65:322-341.

7. Eränkö, L. (1972) Postnatal development of histochemically demonstrable catecholamines in the superior cervical ganglion of the rat, Histochem. J. 4:225-236.

8. Johnson, M., Ross, D., Meyers, M., Rees, R., Bunge, R., Wakshull, E. and

Burton, H. (1976) Synaptic vesicle cytochemistry changes when cultured sympathetic neurons develop cholinergic interactions, Nature 262:308-310.

9. Mains, R.E. and Patterson, P.H. (1973) Primary cultures of dissociated sympathetic neurons. III. Changes in metabolism with age in culture, J. Cell Biol. 59:361-366.

10. Patterson, P.H. and Chun, L.L.Y. (1977) The induction of acetylcholine synthesis in primary cultures of dissociated rat sympathetic neurons. II. Developmental aspects, Dev. Biol. 60:473-481.

11. Mains, R.E. and Patterson, P.H. (1973) Primary cultures of dissociated sympathetic neurons. I. Establishment of long-term growth in culture and studies of differentiated properties, J. Cell. Biol. 59-329-345.

12. Patterson, P.H. and Chun, L.L.Y. (1974) The influence of nonneuronal cells on catecholamine and acetylcholine synthesis and accumulation in cultures of dissociated sympathetic neurons, Proc. Natl. Acad. Sci. USA 71:3607-3610.

13. O'Lague, P.H., Obata, K., Claude, P., Furshpan, E.J. and Potter, D.D. (1974) Evidence for cholinergic synapses between dissociated rat sympathetic neurons in cell culture, Proc. Natl. Acad. Sci. USA 71:3602-3606.

14. O'Lague, P.H., Potter, D.D. and Furshpan, E.J. (1978) Studies on rat sympathetic neurons developing in cell culture III. Cholinergic transmission. Devel. Biol. 67:424-443.

15. Ko, C.P., Burton, H., Johnson, M.I. and Bunge, R.P. (1976) Synaptic transmission between rat superior cervical ganglion neurons in dissociated cell cultures, Brain Res. 117:461-485.

16. Landis, S.C. (1976) Rat sympathetic neurons and cardiac myocytes developing in microcultures: correlation of the fine structure of endings with neurotransmitter function in single neurons, Proc. Natl. Acad. Sci. USA 73:4220-4224.

17. Reichardt, L.F. and Patterson, P.H. (1977) Neurotransmitter synthesis and uptake by individual rat sympathetic neurons developing in microcultures, Nature, 270:147-151.

18. Patterson, P.H. and Chun, L.L.Y (1977) The induction of acetylcholine synthesis in primary cultures of dissociated rat sympathetic neurons. I. Effects of conditioned medium, Dev. Biol. 56:262-280.

19. Furshpan, E.J., MacLeish, P.R., O'Lague, P.H. and Potter, D.D. (1976) Chemical transmission between rat sympathetic neurons and cardiac myocytes developing in microcultures: evidence for cholinergic, adrenergic, and dual-function neurons, Proc. Natl. Acad. Sci. USA 73:4225-4229.

20. Wakshull, E., Johnson, M.I. and Burton, H. (1978) Persistence of an amine uptake system in cultured rat sympathetic neurons which use acetylcholine as their transmitter, J. Cell Biol. 74:121-131.

21. Patterson, P.H., Reichardt, L.F. and Chun, L.L.Y. (1975) Biochemical studies on the development of primary sympathetic neurons in cell culture, Cold Spring Harbor Symp. Quant. Biol. 40:389-397.

22. Hawrot, E. (1979) Cultured sympathetic neurons: effects of cell-derived and synthetic substrata on survival and development, Devel. Biol., in press.

23. Chun, L.L.Y. and Patterson, P.H. (1977) The role of nerve growth factor in the development of rat sympathetic neurons in vitro. I Survival, growth and differentiation of catecholamine production, J. Cell Biol. 75:694-704.

24. Chun, L.L.Y. and Patterson, P.H. (1977) The role of nerve growth factor in the development of rat sympathetic neurons in vitro. II. Developmental studies, J. Cell Biol. 75:705-711.

25. Chun, L.L.Y. and Patterson, P.H. (1977) The role of nerve growth factor in the development of rat sympathetic neurons in vitro. III. Effect on acetyl-choline production, J. Cell Biol. 75:712-718.

26. Black, I.B., Hendry, J.A. and Iversen, L.L. (1972) Effects of surgical decentralization and nerve growth factor on the maturation of adrenergic neurons in a mouse sympathetic ganglion. J. Neurochem. 19:1367-1377.

27. Walicke, P.A., Campenot, R.B. and Patterson, P.H. (1977) Determination of transmitter function by neuronal activity, Proc. Natl. Acad. Sci. USA 74:5767-5771.

28. Walicke, P.A. and Patterson, P.H. (1979) Consideration of Ca^{++} and cyclic AMP as second messengers in the effects of electrical activity on neuro-transmitter choice by sympathetic neurons, Soc. Neurosci. Abstr. Vol. 5, in press.

Cell Lineage, Stem Cells and Cell Determination
INSERM Symposium No. 10
Editor: N. Le Douarin
© 1979 Elsevier/North-Holland Biomedical Press

MEROCYANINE 540 : A USEFUL STAIN FOR HEMOPOIETIC AND LEUKEMIC CELLS

J. VALINSKY and E. REICH

Laboratory of Chemical Biology, Rockefeller University, New-York, N.Y. 10021
U.S.A.

Merocyanine 540 is a fluorescent dye that was developed as a photosensitizer in the color film industry. Its use as a fluorescent probe of membranes, together with other cyanine dyes, followed the demonstration[1] that small fluorescence changes accompanied the propagation of action potentials in segments of squid giant axons. While exploring the interaction of cyanine dyes with cultured cells we observed that MC540 demonstrated surprising selectivity when used as a vital stain ; and a survey of a wide range of cells and tissues indicated that MC540 stained intact living cells in two different ways[2,3] :

a) The first staining reaction concerned excitable tissues, vertebrate and invertebrate nerve, skeletal, smooth and cardiac muscle, specialized sense and electric organs, and protozoa having large membrane potentials and capable of transmitting action potentials. MC540 staining of these cells was either Ca^{2+} dependent or ionic strength dependent ; staining was inhibited by La^{3+} or by the anti-trypanosomal drug sodium suramin.

b) The second MC540 staining reaction affected immature hemopoietic and leukemic cells, and it is the reaction of interest here. In this case staining required neither Ca^{2+} nor physiological ionic strength, and occurred in isosmotic sucrose solutions. Further, the staining of hemopoietic and circulating leukemic cells was not inhibited either by La^{3+} or by Suramin.

Because MC540 is a sulfonate and carries a negative charge throughout the physiological pH range it is excluded by most normal cells such as fibroblasts, liver, kidney, erythrocytes and granulocytes. The exceptional staining of excitable and immature blood cells therefore occurs because their respective plasma membranes are selectively permeable to MC540 : the selective permeability of excitable cells is dependent in some way on Ca^{2+} or high ionic strength, whereas that of hemopoietic and leukemic cells appears to be an intrinsic property of the membrane at an immature and incompletely differentiated stage of the cellular life cycle. Both staining reactions are accelerated by low level illumination, and in both cases MC540 appears first to enter the lipid phase of the plasma membrane before distributing into other intracellular membrane structures. Staining is essentially irreversible, at least on a time scale of many hours, and it renders cells susceptible to lethal photosensitization by exposure to bright light.

The photosensitizing effects of MC540 are useful for demonstrating some of its staining selectivity. For example, MC540 stains all circulating leukocytes in untreated leukemic patients, but it does not stain any circulating leukocytes of normal individuals. When normal lymphocytes are exposed to mitogenic lectins and illuminated in the presnce of MC540 there is neither a decrease in ^{3}H-thymidine incorporation, nor an increase in trypan blue staining in comparison with control cultures being incubated under identical conditions in the absence of this dye. This result is expected since normal lymphocytes exclude the dye are thereby protected against the destructive effects that follow when it is incorporated into membranes. In contrast, when leukemic lymphocytes are incubated with MC540 in bright light their mitogenic response to lectins is largely abolished, and a parallel increase in trypan blue staining further attests to the loss of viability[3].

A comparable experiment that demonstrates the uptake of MC540 by immature hemopoietic cells is presented in Table I. Here bone marrow cells were assayed

TABLE 1

Effect of Merocyanine 540 on in Vitro and in Vivo Colony Formation by Mouse Bone Marrow Cells.

Treatment	Number of Colonies per 10^5 Cells	
	in Vitro	in Vivo
Untreated	167	20.8 ± 2.6
No colony-stimulating factor	0	-
Merocyanine and light	5.3	0.6 ± 0.9
Merocyanine (dark,wash and light)	30	6.2 ± 2.7
Merocyanine-dark	158	14.4 ± 4.2

Cells from normal mouse bone marrow (C57B1/6J;6×10^6) were incubated with 40 g of merocyanine 540 in 1.0 ml of McCoy's 5A medium for 30 min under the conditions described in the table. The cells were washed once with McCoy's 5A medium containing 15% fetal bovine serum and plated at 5×10^4 cells per 35 mm Falcon tissue culture dish[3]. Colony formation was evaluated microscopically at 50X magnification after 7 days of growth at 37°C in 10 % CO_2/90% air. Colonies containing more than 50 cells were counted.

For in vivo assays, an aliquot (10^5 cells in 0.1 ml of McCoy's 5A medium) of the same cells used in the in vitro assays was injected intravenously into W/W^v acceptor mice which were littermates of the donors. After 10 days of incubation, the animals were sacrificed, and the spleens were removed and fixed in Bouin's fluid. Macroscopic spleen nodules were counted under low magnification.

for colony forming ability in culture (CFU-C)[4], or in mouse spleen (CFU-S)[5].
It is apparent that the precursors of both of these colonies were inactivated
by the combination of MC540 and light. We conclude from this result that MC540
interacts with and penetrates both committed (CFU-C) and pluripotent (CFU-S)
stem cells, just as it does leukemic cells[3]. We have recently extended   studies of MC540 staining to embryonic hemopoiesis in birds and mammals, and have
observed that primitive precursor cells in these systems are also permeable to
this dye. In the early chick embryos essentially all circulating blood cells
are stained up to 4-4 1/2 days of incubation, after which there is a rapid
decrease (to 10% staining) within the subsequent 1-1 1/2 days. In early mouse
embryos a major fraction of the circulating cells is stained during the phase
of hemopoiesis dominated by the yolk sac, and MC540 positive cells disappear
from the circulation following the onset of hepatic hemopoiesis[6].

Several considerations suggest that MC540 staining is determined by membrane
properties that are altered during the maturation that occurs in the course of
normal hemopoiesis. Firstly, a large fraction of normal bone marrow cells, and
a small proportion of cells in normal spleen, lymph nodes and thymus are
stained, whereas few if any circulating leukocytes are stained in normal humans
and mice. Secondly, as seen in Table 1, the proliferative potential of bone
marrow cells is abolished by MC540-mediated photosensitization. These findings
indicate that permeability to MC540 is lost during normal hemopoiesis before
leukocytes enter the circulation, and that this aspect of plasma membrane maturation eith fails to occur in leukemias, or is delayed such that leukemic
leukocytes enter the circulation while remaining MC540 positive.

Because MC540 appears to be   potentially useful for monitoring the
response to drugs both in normal and leukemic individuals, we have recently
adapted the reaction to automated cytodiagnostic equipment, specifically, to
flow microfluorimetry. Typical results obtained with normal and leukemic leukocytes are presented in Fig. 1, and these show that while the scatter-fluorescence
patterns differ in the various leukemic specimens, essentially all circulating
leukocytes stain in each form of leukemia, and the leukemic samples are clearly
distinguished from the normal. Analyses of this kind have been performed on a
significant number of child hood and adult leukemics undergoing drug therapy.

The results obtained so far[7] appear to be of interest both in terms of practical utility, since MC540 gives promise of providing a useful adjunct to therapy and especially prognosis, and because they suggest a view of leukemia and of
stem cell organization and life cycle which is at variance with prevailing concepts. These questions will be considered in detail elsewhere[6].

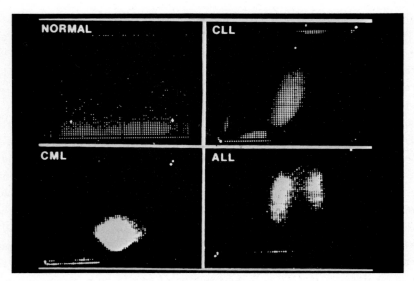

Fig. 1 : Analysis of normal and leukemic leukocytes by flow microfluorimetry after staining with MC 540.
    Washed buffy coat cells were incubated with MC540 and stained under standard conditions as described elsewhere (ref. 3).The stained cells were analyzed by flow microfluorimetry using a B-D FACS-II cell sorting unit. The abscissa represents increasing scatter, the ordinate increasing fluorescence intensity. ALL-acute lymphoblastic leukemia ; CML-chronic myelocytic leukemia ; AML-acute myelocytic leukemia.

ACKNOWLEDGEMENTS :

    This work was supported in part by grant from the Vanneck Foundation and the National Institute of Health, USPHS (CA 08290).

REFERENCES

1. Davila, H.V., Saltzberg, B.M., Cohen, L.B. and Waggoner, A.S. (1973). A large change in axon fluorescence that provides a promising news method for measuring membrane potential. Nature New Biol., 241, 159-160.

2. Easton, T.G., Valinsky, J.E. and Reich, E. (1978). Merocyanine 540 as a fluorescent probe of membranes : staining of electrically excitable cells. Cell 13, 475-486.

3. Valinsky, J.E., Easton, T.G. and Reich, E. (1978). Merocyanine 540 as a fluorescent probe of membranes : selective staining of leukemic and immature hemopoietic cells. Cell 13, 487-499.

4. Mc Culloch, E.A., Mak, T.W. , Price, G.B. and Till, J.E. (1974). Organization and communication in populations of normal and leukemic hemopoietic cells. Biochim. Biophys. Acta, 355, 260-299.

5. Mc Culloch, E.A., Siminovitch, L. and Till, J.E. (1974a). Spleen colony formation in anemic mice of the genotype W/W^V. Science 144, 844-846.

6. Valinsky, J.E. and Reich, E. Manuscript in preparation.

7. Valinsky, J.E., Reich, E., Haghbin, M., Chahinian, M., Ohnuma, T. and Holland, J. (1978). American Society for Hematology Abstracts, Blood.

AUTHOR INDEX